Autoimmunoregulation and Autoimmune Disease

Concepts in Immunopathology

Vol. 4

Series Editors
J. M. Cruse, Jackson, Miss.
R. E. Lewis, Jr., Jackson, Miss.

KARGER

Basel · München · Paris · London · New York · New Delhi · Singapore · Tokyo · Sydney

Autoimmunoregulation and Autoimmune Disease

Volume Editors
J. M. Cruse, Jackson, Miss.
R. E. Lewis, Jr., Jackson, Miss.

31 figures and 26 tables, 1987

KARGER

Basel · München · Paris · London · New York · New Delhi · Singapore · Tokyo · Sydney

Concepts in Immunopathology

Cover illustration

The cells of natural immunity: large granular lymphocytes (smaller cells) attacking K562 erythromyeloid leukemia cells. Stained with giemsa and photographed using a Zeiss photomicroscope equipped with a 63 X plan apochromat lens and phase contrast optics.

The photograph was provided through the courtesy of Dr. George Babcock, Cincinnati, OH, and the costs of color printing provided through the generosity of CARL ZEISS, INC., Thornwood, N.Y., USA.

Drug Dosage

The authors and the publisher have exerted every effort to ensure that drug selection and dosage set forth in this text are in accord with current recommendations and practice at the time of publication. However, in view of ongoing research, changes in government regulations, and the constant flow of information relating to drug therapy and drug reactions, the reader is urged to check the package insert for each drug for any change in indications and dosage and for added warnings and precautions. This is particularly important when the recommended agent is a new and/or infrequently employed drug.

Printed in Switzerland by Meier+Cie AG, Schaffhausen
ISBN 3-8055-4406-5

Jules Bordet

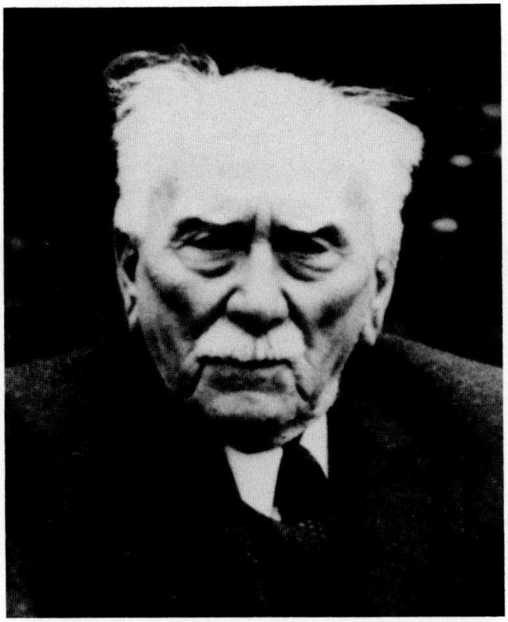

This volume is dedicated to the memory of Jules Bordet (1870–1961), pioneer in immunology and complement research.

Contents

Cruse, J. M.; Lewis, R. E., Jr. (Jackson, Miss.): Regulation of Immune Reactivity to Self 1

Rosenkrantz, K.; Dupont, B.; Flomenberg, N. (New York, N. Y.): Relevance of Autocytotoxic and Autoregulatory Lymphocytes in the Maintenance of Self Tolerance 24

Dighiero, G.; Kaushik, A.; Poncet, P.; Ge, X. R. (Paris): Origin and Significance of Autoantibodies 42

Lattime, E. C. (New York, N. Y.): Natural Cytotoxic (NC) Cell Activity in Murine and Human Systems. Effector Cells from Multiple Lineages with Antitumor Activity 77

Weiler, J. M. (Iowa City, Iowa); Hobbs, M. V. (La Jolla, Calif.): Role of the Third Component of Complement in Immunoregulation 103

Chused, T. M.; McCoy, K. L.; Lal, R. B.; Brown, E. L.; Baker, P. J. (Bethesda, Md.): Multigenic Basis of Autoimmune Disease in New Zealand Mice 129

Eden, W., van (Utrecht); Holoshitz, J.; Cohen, I. (Rehovot): Antigenic Mimicry Between Mycobacteria and Cartilage Proteoglycans: The Model of Adjuvant Arthritis 144

Emery, P.; Williamson, D. J.; Mackay, I. R. (Victoria); Role of Cytokines in Rheumatological Inflammation 171

Charron, D.; Teyton, L. (Paris): Autoimmunity in Rheumatoid Arthritis. A Qualitative and Quantitative Approach to the Role of Ia Antigens 200

Yoo, T. J.; Ishibe, T. (Memphis, Tenn.): Autoimmunity of the Ear 215

Crapper, R. M.; Frazer, I. H.; Mackay, I. R.; Iscaro, A.; Bradford, D. L. (Melbourne): Immunoregulatory Defects Associated with Infection with the AIDS Virus, HTLV-III 243

Gottlieb, A. A.; Gottlieb, M. S.; Scholes, V. E. (New Orleans, La.): Reconstitution of Immune Function in AIDS/ARC 261

Sriram, S.; Ranges, G. E. (Burlington, Vt.): Immunotherapy of Autoimmune Disease with T Cell Subset Specific Antibodies 275

Subject Index 287

Concepts Immunopathol., vol. 4, pp. 1–23 (Karger, Basel 1987)

Regulation of Immune Reactivity to Self

Julius M. Cruse, Robert E. Lewis, Jr.

Department of Pathology, University of Mississippi Medical Center, Jackson, Miss., USA

The finely tuned interaction among lymphoid cell receptors, cytokine molecules and perturbing influences resulting from 'the thousand natural shocks that flesh is heir to'[1] determines whether immune reactivity to self components will remain physiologic or become pathogenic. The present volume represents an assemblage of articles designed to address these phenomena that constitute autoimmunoregulation.

Rosenkrantz, Dupont and Flomenberg discuss the significance of autocytotoxic and autoregulatory lymphocytes in the maintenance of self tolerance, which has been postulated to be based upon clonal deletion/inactivation of cells in the thymus that react against self or the suppression of self-reactive cells by peripherally based regulatory cells. The authors cite evidence in support of each concept, pointing to the role of regulatory cells in preventing autocytotoxic effects.

Although self tolerance is maintained throughout the lifetime of an animal, it can be broken by immunologic intervention resulting in either graft-versus-host (GVH)-like phenomena or autoimmune disease. Irradiation associated with autologous bone marrow transplantation and thymectomy experiments suggest that autoreactive T cell activity is regulated in normal adult animals. Autoimmune diseases offer a natural model for the abrogation of tolerance to self.

Self tolerance occurs first in the thymus where T lymphocytes develop immunocompetence. Thymic lymphocytes demonstrate neonatal tolerance before it is manifested by peripheral lymphoid cells. Dendritic cells are believed to be responsible for the acquisition of self tolerance by

[1] William Shakespeare: Hamlet, Act III, Scene I.

developing T cells. Although thymic epithelial cells have been shown to aid development of H-2 restriction specificities in T cells, future investigations are needed to determine whether they are significant in development of self tolerance.

Whereas the thymus is believed to have a role in the induction of T cell tolerance, maintenance of self tolerance depends partially upon a peripheral mechanism. The elimination of anti-self effector lymphocytes may be attributable to intrathymic inactivation in some cases but due to the presence of peripheral blood regulatory lymphocytes in others.

According to the clonal deletion hypothesis, self-reactive T lymphocytes undergo intrathymic elimination which is supported by the indirect observation that numerous thymocytes die in situ in the thymus. Cytotoxic T lymphocytes reacting with a tolerated alloantigen in actively acquired tolerance experiments are known to be diminished. Thus, it appears that tolerance is accompanied by deletion or inactivation of cytotoxic T lymphocytes. The clonal deletion theory is further supported by mixing experiments in which suppressor cells combined with normal immunocompetent lymphocytes inhibit normal cell activation which is referred to as 'infectious tolerance'.

Autocytotoxic cells, which are apparently under autoregulatory control, are present in the peripheral blood of healthy subjects. Limiting dilution analysis has been employed to demonstrate autoaggressive cells and others that induce down-regulation.

The authors next describe abrogation and reestablishment of self tolerance to demonstrate these autoaggressive and autoregulatory cells. Limiting dilution analysis was used to investigate cytotoxic cells. An autocytotoxic response was observed with relatively low numbers of responder cells where only autocytotoxic cells were present in microcultures. By contrast, autocytotoxicity was suppressed with higher responder cell numbers where regulatory cells were also present in microcultures. Thus, self tolerance was abrogated at the low responder cell dose but was restored with an increased number of responder cells. Limiting dilution procedures have been employed to isolate autocytotoxic and autoregulatory cell lines. Regulatory cells apparently suppress autocytotoxic cell lines by mechanisms other than direct lysis.

It remains to be determined whether autocytotoxic and autoregulatory cells represent physiologic or aberrant immune cellular activity directed against self antigens. Thus, autoreactivity, whether by autoreactive T cells or autoreactive antibodies, is an apparently normal function of the immune response. Therefore, low levels of autoimmune reactivity might represent a normal and beneficial effect whereas increased or uncontrolled autoreactivity might represent an autoaggressive mechanism of injuring the host. Complicated regulatory circuits may be operative in the mechanism whereby regulatory cells act, rather than by causing direct lysis of autoaggressive cells in acquired tolerance. Similar interaction among inducer-transducer-effector cells may be operative in autoregulatory cells. Idiotype-anti-idiotype recognition may also play a significant role in down-regulation of autoreactive T lymphocytes. A 'veto' cell model has been described in which the 'veto' cell is able to down-regulate responses against itself regardless of its remaining cellular functions or specificity. Cloned cytotoxic T cells have been demonstrated to act as 'veto' cells. Thus, self tolerance may be dependent upon both clonal deletion and specifically interacting suppressor cells. Thus, autoaggressive lymphocytes with the capability of participating in disease states have been clearly demonstrated in the blood of healthy subjects.

Dighiero and associates present a lucid discussion of the origin and significance of autoantibodies. Following an introductory review of Burnet's concept of clonal deletion, forbidden clones and pathogenic autoantibodies, the authors emphasize the physiological effects of natural autoantibodies and their relationship to the pathogenic variety. As models, they investigated autoantibodies against mouse erythrocytes as well as those specific for DNA and cytoskeletal proteins under both physiologic and pathologic conditions in murine and human systems. They also considered the significance of autoreactive B cells and their relationship to natural and pathogenic autoantibodies.

Autoantibodies have been described in both normal and autoimmune mouse strains with specificity for X, HB, HOL and I red blood cell antigens. Whereas, anti-X autoantibody is associated with autoimmune hemolytic anemia in the NZB mouse, anti-HB autoantibodies appear in all mouse strains and have physiologic but no known pathologic significance. Normal unimmunized mice produce antibodies against an autoantigen termed HB which is a normally hidden autoantigen exposed only by bromelin treatment. Such antibodies have been demonstrated in both autoimmune NZB and in normal nonautoimmune strains.

The classic autoimmune hemolytic anemia observed in NZB mice involves the interaction of autoantibodies with an exposed labile glycoprotein red cell surface autoantigen. Features of murine hemolytic anemia resemble those in man. The plasma of all mouse strains differing in H-2 haplotypes has been found to contain SEA-X, which is a soluble analogue of red cell bound X antigen, although anti-X autoantibody is found only in the NZB strain even though B cells binding X autoantigen were detected in all mice studied. Anti-X autoantibodies are principally IgG. NZB mice also possess an IgG autoantibody reactive with autoantigen in dried red cell smears and on stromata of erythrocytes but not accessible on intact red cells. Further studies with monoclonal autoantibodies led the authors to propose that various red cell autoantibodies may be implicated in the development of naturally occurring hemolytic anemia in NZB mice.

The blood sera of normal nonimmunized animals and man have been found to contain natural autoantibodies against various autoantigens that include tubulin, actin, thyroglobulin, myoglobin, fetuin, albumin, transferrin, collagen and cytochrome c. Thus, natural autoantibodies against cytoskeletal proteins and DNA have been found in the IgG fractions of healthy humans. Antibodies have also been shown naturally in normal serum against brain antigens, thymus cells, carbohydrate components, denatured collagen, elastin, gelatin, red cells, gamma globulin, thyroid, gastric parietal cells, and lymphocytes. Monoclonal antibodies in humans have often been found to represent the expansion of a clone synthesizing a natural autoantibody under physiologic conditions. The authors examined 612 different monoclonal immunoglobulins to determine whether some manifested antibody activity against actin, tubulin, myosin, thyroglobulin, dsDNA, myoglobin, fetuin, albumin, and transferrin. No relationship was found between antibody activity of the monoclonal immunoglobulins and a patient's clinical status.

The authors next investigated autoreactive B cells responsible for natural autoantibodies by the development of hybridoma cell lines producing natural monoclonal autoantibodies and determining their antigen binding specificity. Murine and human lupus monoclonal autoantibodies were investigated with respect to polyspecificity among lupus and/or DNA autoantibodies, their idiotypic and structural characteristics and the immunogen in lupus that stimulates their production. Results suggest that monoclonal anti-DNA autoantibodies have limited heterogeneity with respect to specificity. Based upon the relatively low immunogenicity of DNA, investigators have examined whether DNA released from natural cell turnover or complexed with foreign proteins or DNA autoantibodies induced by a self or nonself cross-reacting antigen might be a stimulating immunogen in lupus. Heparan sulfate has been suggested as a target for anti-DNA autoantibodies associated with glomerular damage in SLE. Common features of natural autoantibodies against different autoantigens such as DNA, cytoskeletal proteins and isologous red blood cells include cross-reactive idiotypes, secretion by LylB cells, and their presence in significant amounts among normal serum immunoglobulins. The development of autoantibodies against autoantigens that are exposed or not necessarily hidden challenges the clonal deletion theory as an only mechanism for self tolerance. Cross-reactive idiotypes are common among naturally occurring monoclonal antibodies. There is even a sharing of idiotypes among monoclonal anti-DNA autoantibodies from murine and human sources. Investigation of the epitope recognized by autoantibodies reveals multispecific binding by most natural autoantibodies, unlike the more restricted specificity by the induced variety. Available data suggest that multispecific autoantibodies recognize corresponding structures on many different antigens and that B lymphocytes might bear a polyspecific receptor with the ability to interact with antigens from various sources. Thus, antibody induced by one of the binding antigens might still have the capacity for cross-reactivity.

The same germ-line genes may encode for autoantibodies as well as antibodies against foreign antigens. Studies employing CBA/N mice which carry the Xid gene, in contrast to normal mouse strains, fail to produce anti-DNA autoantibodies following mitogenic challenge even though they possess the genetic information. Such results imply that the Xid gene may have a regulatory role. The article concludes with postulates concerning the possible raison d'être for naturally occurring, relatively low concentrations of autoantibodies and their relationship to their pathogenic counterparts in patients or experimental mice with autoimmune disease.

Lattime presents a novel review of autoimmunoregulation with respect to the cells of natural immunity significant in surveillance against tumor development. Lymphoid cells that mediate natural cytotoxicity do not have markers characteristic of T cells, B cells or macrophages. Natural killer (NK) cells with activity against lymphoid tumors were described prior to a description of natural cytotoxic (NC) cells with activity against nonlymphoid tumors. These act in conjunction with cytotoxic T lymphocytes (CTL). In addition to NK cells, which include both NK and NC, activated killer (AK) have also been described. All of these cell types have been defined in murine systems and investigations into human equivalents continue. NC activity requires a longer (12–24 h) assay than the assay for NK which is only 4 h. In a study of murine nonlymphoid tumor lines, some were found susceptible to NC, others to NK and the remainder to both NK and NC acting in combination. The classic NC target is the WEHI-164 cell line which appears to have very low susceptibility to NK activity.

NC cell function, which is a property of null cells, was not eliminated by removal of NK and T cells from effector cell populations. In addition to the null cell population, T and B lymphocyte lineage cells have the capacity to mediate NC activity, as well as cells expressing NK-associated Qa-5 and NK 1.1 antigens. Cells positively selected from various defined lineages are able to mediate NC activity assayed by lysis of WEHI-164 target cells. In studies on lymphokine regulation of cells, NK activity is augmented by interferon (IFN) and interleukin-2 (IL-2), but not interleukin-3 (UL-3). Whereas NC activity is augmented by both IL-2 and IL-3, it is not affected by IFN. Investigation of their mechanism of action suggests that NC effector cells must come into contact with target cells for which they show specificity leading to the production of a soluble cytotoxic factor which causes target cell lysis. Although MHC restriction is not required for NC lysis, NC effector-target cell interaction involves specificity. Lattime presents a discussion of the three phases of NC lysis including target recognition, programming for lysis and target mechanism. There are both similarities and differences in the interaction of NC and NK cells with their targets with respect to target recognition and effector cell binding. Whereas future studies must be aimed at the potential role of NC and/or NK cells in surveillance against spontaneously developing tumors in vivo, there is convincing evidence that NK and NC cells are associated with removal of circulating tumor emboli. Investigations also show that tumor cell lines succeptible to NC and NK cells induce tumors with less efficiency than do NC/NK-resistant cell lines. Nontumor activities have been ascribed to NK cells in their role in regulating normal hematopoiesis and the association of NK activity with rejection of bone marrow grafts. In addition, NK cells have been associated with surveillance against pathogenic microorganisms including herpes, cytomegalovirus, hepatitis, trypanosomes, Shigella, and malaria. Recently, tumor necrosis factor (TNF) has been shown in association with NC cell activity and is produced upon stimulation of NC cells. A common feature of multilineage cells with NC activity might be their ability to produce TNF. A human equivalent of the murine NC effector cell has been initially characterized based on the cell surface phenotype, lymphokine regulation and target cell interaction. The article concludes with a consideration of culture-generated cytotoxic populations, cloned cell lines and their relationship to NC.

In addition to its better known properties, complement is now recognized as a significant regulator of the immune response. Although initial studies employed in vivo systems to depress hemolytic complement, in vitro assays have demonstrated immunoregulatory actions of individual complement proteins and degradation products. C3 has been the subject of many investigations on immune regulation by complement since it is of critical importance in both classic and alternative pathways, is present in serum in a greater concentration than any other complement protein and was the target of in vivo cobra venom factor (CoVF) treatment of animals to reduce C3 levels. C3 receptors on lymphocytes and macrophages participate in immunoregulation. Immunoregulatory macrophages secrete C3 which may in turn regulate lymphokines and participate with antibody to localize antigen in tissues. The authors discuss the role of C3 and its fragments in immune regulation. Following a brief review of C3 structure and activation, Weiler et al. describe early investigations of a role for complement in immunoregulation in vivo. Complement activators such as CoVF were administered to experimental animals to achieve complement depletion with a striking reduction in total hemolytic complement (CH50) which was found associated with suppression of the primary immune response to T-dependent antigens but no suppression of antibody formation to T-independent antigens. Additional observations in CoVF-conditioned animals suggested impaired ability to localize antigen in the spleen, to form germinal centers, etc. Markedly elevated levels of complement activation fragments such as C3a could have produced suppressive effects.

Other early investigations employed antibodies against C3 in an effort to suppress CR^+ B cells but not CR^- B lymphocytes. Three to four separate C3 receptors are now known and whereas one receptor might suppress, another might augment an immune response. Animals with a genetic deficiency of individual complement components constitute the only true models for complement depletion studies. For example, C3-deficient humans have increased susceptibility to infection but have no known impairment of the immune response. This is in contrast to C4-deficient animals and humans who do have impaired immune responsiveness, although the mechanism is unknown. Although C3 is apparently not necessary for an autoimmune response to occur, C3 fragments are known to down-regulate immune responses. The inhibition of NK-mediated lysis of target cells by C3 has been attributed to C3a fragments in C3 preparations. C3a has also been reported to inhibit mitogen- and antigen-induced stimulation of leukocyte inhibitory factor. C3a inhibits polyclonal and antigen-specific antibody responses in vitro. It has been suggested that C3a may act through augmentation of nonantigen-specific suppressor T cells. C3a apparently does not regulate IL-2 production but IL-2 may eliminate suppressive effects of C3a. Macrophages bearing C3a receptors may be requisite for T cell regulation by C3a. Prostaglandin production by macrophages, which is augmented by C3a, results in diminished T helper cell function of elevated T suppressor cell activity. Although C3a is able to regulate immune responses in vitro, this fragment is rapidly degraded in vivo to C3a-des-arg by anaphylatoxin inactivator yielding a product that is without any immunoregulatory function.

Numerous studies suggest that C3b and its fragments exert immunoregulatory actions. Human lymphocyte blastogenesis in response to antigen but not mitogen is inhibited by C3b, C3c, and C3d. C3b is postulated to act directly on B lymphocytes and not on T helper cells.

C3d-K inhibits both mixed lymphocyte and proliferative responses of human spleen T and B cells to antigen and mitogen. It interferes with synthesis of IL-2 leading to inhibition of IL-2-induced T cell mitogenesis. Thus, its action is directly on the lymphocyte. A product of C3 degradation termed fraction 2 inhibits antigen- and mitogen-induced proliferative responses of T and B cells, rat memory B cell responses, mixed lymphocyte responses and cytotoxic T cell but not NK cell generation. Although similar, fraction 2 is distinct from C3a. Fraction 2 is also capable of increasing vascular permeability. A small molecular weight fragment produced by C3 degradation induces immunosuppression. It is a significant down-regulator of immune responsiveness during C3 breakdown. A C3 alpha chain fragment termed 'soluble C3d' can regulate B cell activation. Another immunoregulatory low molecular weight fragment derived by CoVF-convertase-treated C3 has been described. Immunoregulatory fragments derived from degradation of C3b include C3d-K, which has been mapped on the alpha chain of C3, fraction 2, C3d, C3-FP and LMF that inhibit T and B cell responsiveness. All of these fragments inhibit proliferation induced by mitogen.

Clinical observations revealed that C3 deficiency does not lead to abnormal immune responsiveness. C3 fragments including C3a and C3b down-regulate an immune response. Thus, a C3 deficiency would interfere with an individual's ability to attenuate an immune response. Whereas C3a has a short half-life of only seconds in vivo, C3b fragments have a longer half-life permitting them to exert immunoregulatory activity for a longer period of time. The authors suggest that C3 is fixed in areas of increased antibody synthesis and that it down-regulates lymphocyte responses. They propose that C3 degradation products diminish lymphocyte activation in areas of complement consumption in immune complex disease. The article concludes with suggestions for future research into the role of complement proteins in immunoregulation which might herald advances in therapy.

Chused and associates present an up-to-date analysis of the multigenic basis of autoimmune disease in New Zealand mice. Following the demonstration that New Zealand black (NZB) mice developed autoimmune hemolytic anemia, it was shown that crosses with other strains, such as the New Zealand white (NZW), could lead to animal models of other diseases, such as lupus erythematosus in the $(NZB \times NZW)F_1$ hybrid which develops antibodies against DNA and gp70 leading to immune complex glomerulonephritis. As observed in humans, female mice of an appropriate autoimmune strain are more severely affected than are males. Factors that have a role in the development of autoimmune disease of New Zealand mice include: polyclonal activation of B cells which participate in the occurrence of hemolytic anemia; increased IgM synthesis in young mice; altered NZB lymphocyte subset distribution with age; IL-2 receptor expression by B lymphocytes in older animals when disease occurs, which might be related to diminished B cell responsiveness to regulatory T cell signals; loss of T lymphocyte suppressor action in aging NZB mice; increased T amplifier activity and disappearance of T helper function; resistance to the induction of tolerance by B cells of NZB and NZB F_1 mice; and interference with tolerance induction in helper T cells of $(NZB \times NZW)F_1$ hybrids. Studies of NZB × NFS RI lines demonstrate a sequence of genetic 'gates' that govern the occurrence of autoimmune hemolytic anemia. Four interacting genes apparently control development of hemolytic anemia which shows a close correlation with hyperactivity of B lymphocytes and resistance to B cell tolerance induction. When B lymphocyte abnormalities occur, a separate gene may govern the synthesis of autoantibodies against erythrocytes. Yet another gene may induce hemolytic anemia through an isotype switch. Renal disease is not correlated with either hemolytic anemia or B lymphocyte hyperactivity in NZB × NSF RI lines. It has been postulated that the genes governing renal disease only partially intersect those linked to development of hemolytic anemia. The authors postulate that impairment of T cell tolerance induction in $(NZB \times NZW)F_1$ hybrid mice manifested at immunologic maturity in contrast to the defect in T suppressor cells in aged parental NZB mice might help to explain the occurrence of antibodies to DNA and immune complex glomerulonephritis in the hybrid.

More genes appear necessary to develop autoimmune disease in NZB mice than previously believed. At least five or six separate genes and perhaps more are required for hemolytic anemia development. The authors postulate that spontaneous autoimmune disease in man may have a similar but more complex genetic mechanism than that observed in mice. The multiple genes involved in spontaneous autoimmune disease render identification and determination of mechanisms of action of the individual genes difficult. Nevertheless, it is anticipated that isolation of New Zealand mouse genes that might serve as gene probes could be useful in future investigations of human autoimmune disease.

Van Eden, Holoshitz, and Cohen present a lucid discussion of antigenic mimicry between mycobacteria and cartilage proteoglycans. Essentially everyone has the potential for development of autoimmunity, which may occur as a consequence of infection by selected microorganisms. Immune reactivity against microbial antigens may encompass the stimulation of T lymphocytes capable of reacting with self. Likewise, counter autoimmune regulatory T lymphocytes may also occur in response to separate epitopes on the same microbial stimulants.

A well-known example of the association of autoimmune disease with infection is the role of streptococcal infection with development of acute rheumatic fever. The inoculation of rats with streptococcal bacterial cell wall peptidoglycan-polysaccharide fragments has been shown to lead to experimental arthritis. Many cases of rheumatoid arthritis are associated with or may be precipitated by infection with streptococci.

HLA-B27 antigen has been associated with certain autoimmune rheumatological disorders. A cross-reactive epitope shared among HLA-B27, *Yersinia* and *Klebsiella* has been reported. Unlike experimental autoimmune diseases in which animals are immunized with self antigen preparations, such as rats immunized with myelin basic protein to induce experimental autoimmune encephalomyelitis (EAE), adjuvant arthritis (AA) can follow inoculation of susceptible Lewis rats with *Mycobacterium tuberculosis*. T cell lines have been employed to show conclusively that AA is an autoimmune disease. The *M. tuberculosis*-specific T cell line termed A2 is able to passively transfer AA into irradiated syngeneic recipients. A T lymphocyte could simultaneously demonstrate specific immune reactivity against a bacterial antigen and autoimmune reactivity.

It is now well known that immunization with collagen type II can lead to the development of autoimmune arthritis. Collagen type II and complete Freund's adjuvant (CFA) may act synergistically to induce arthritis. Besides collagen, cartilage also consists of proteoglycans. Evidence of structural mimicry between *M. tuberculoisis* and proteoglycans was demonstrated by proliferation of the A2b cell line to proteoglycans as well as to *M. tuberculosis*. Synovial fluids of rheumatoid arthritis (RA) patients containing proteoglycans specifically stimlulated the A2b clone. Passive transfer of the A2b cell line into previously unsensitized recipients renders them capable of responding with delayed-type hypersensitivity (DTH) reactivity to both *M. tuberculosis* and proteoglycans. Experimental evidence suggests that the core protein, or possibly oligosaccharides linked to it, comprising proteoglycan molecules, could be sites for target antigenic determinants in adjuvant arthritis. In addition to the A2b arthritogenic lymphoid cell clone, monoclonal antibodies against mycobacteria may demonstrate reactivity against proteoglycans, indicating shared epitopes between mycobacteria and cartilage. *M. tuberculosis* and joint cartilage mimicry may lead to immunologic injury of joints associated with AA.

Structural mimicry between selected antigens of microorganisms and mammalian tissues revealed as serological cross-reactivities suggest a mechanism for inducing some types of autoimmunity. Examples include common epitopes shared between group A streptococci and host tissue antigens. Human myocardial sarcolemmal membrane proteins have been shown to be cross-reactive with streptococcal M proteins which could account for carditis resulting from autoimmunity in acute rheumatic fever. Poststreptococcal glomerulonephritis patients develop antibodies against heparan sulfate proteoglycans in glomerular basement membranes which share antigenic determinants with streptococcal hyaluronic acid.

The development of rheumatoid factors following bacterial immunization sugget that immunoglobulin constant regions may possess epitopes that cross-react with bacterial peptidoglycans. Likewise, anti-DNA antibodies in SLE patients might be associated with microbial infection. Anti-DNA antibodies have been found reactive not only with nucleic acid antigens but with phospholipid cardiolipin as well, which could account for a biologically false-positive test for syphilis in SLE patients.

In contrast to the unexplained role of autoantibodies in the pathogenesis of both RA and SLE is the pathogenic effect of autoantibodies against acetylcholine receptors in myasthenia gravis. Shared antigenic determinants have been demonstrated among acetylcholine receptors, *Proteus*, and *Klebsiella* microorganisms. *Klebsiella* share antigens with B-27 lymphocytes of ankylosing spondylitis (AS) patients. Whether or not this structural mimicry is involved in the pathogenesis of AS remains to be demonstrated. It has been suggested that the thyroid-stimulating antibodies in Graves' disease might result from a host response to bacterial infection by *Yersinia enterocolitica* which contains an antigen that could stimulate antireceptor antibodies. Such a concept is substantiated by the finding of *Yersinia* infections in many cases of Graves' disease.

Antigenic mimicry between mycobacteria and proteoglycans might have a role not only in adjuvant arthritis but in RA as well. Not only bacteria but some viruses such as those associated with diabetes mellitus and multiple sclerosis have epitopes cross-reactive with normal tissues.

The authors suggest that autoimmunity may be commonplace but its expression down-regulated. They propose that the presence of self-recognizing lymphocytes in healthy subjects and the capacity to raise autoreactive lymphocytes experimentally to induce autoimmune disease refutes Burnet's 'forbidden' clone hypothesis.

T suppressor cells may prevent recognition of self antigens by self-recognizing clones. The A2 cell line used in the adjuvant arthritis model was able to induce either disease or protection depending upon whether the recipients were irradiated or nonirradiated, respectively. A protective, nonarthritogenic subclone of A2 was subsequently discovered and termed A2c. It could not only prevent but could therapeutically assist rats with AA. Based on experimental evidence suggesting that the A2c clone represented a supressor inducer T cell, the authors propose that a single suppressor inducer T cell clone might lead to control of autoimmune disease and restoration of self tolerance. Experimental evidence suggests that immunization with a complex antigen stimulates not only clones specific for various epitopes but also others that suppress or control expansion of clones specific for cross-reactive epitopes that could lead to autoimmune disease. Self tolerance is restored naturally after recovery from adjuvant arthritis.

The MHC-linked Ir genes influence autoimmune disease susceptibility in man and animals. The control mechanism could involve epitope selection or immune regulation or both. The authors suggest that most

MHC alleles may have been selected based on their ability to facilitate recognition of or regulate responses to antigenic determinants critical for defense against microbial infectious agents.

Emery, Williamson and Mackay present an in-depth account of the role of cytokines in synovial inflammation in RA. IL-1, IL-2, IFN-γ, colony-stimulating factor (CSF), osteoclast-activating factor (OAF), and fibrogenic and vascularization factors all constitute cytokines especially significant in the pathogenesis of RA.

Following a discussion of the background, biochemistry, sources, actions, and assay methods, the role of IL-1 in rheumatological diseases is presented. IL-1, which is produced mainly by macrophages, refers to a family of molecules that activate (T and B) lymphocytes. Their actions may be local or systemic. Besides their local effects in activating certain cell types such as T cells, among other actions, they may induce fever, activation of acute phase reactants, serum cation alterations and neutrophil release from bone marrow.

IL-1 detected in synovial effusions of RA patients is produced by synovial cells and rheumatoid synovial dendritic cells. In rheumatic diseases, IL-1 stimulates lymphocytes leading to their intrasynovial proliferation, affects immune system cell interactions and effector mechanisms in joints, promotes bone resorption and mediates both destruction and repair of connective tissue matrix, among other effects. Systemic effects of significance in rheumatological diseases produced by IL-1 include reduction in cations in serum, such as iron, promotion of muscle proteolysis and activation of acute phase protein formation by the liver. IL-1 is postulated by the authors to account for the continuing inflammation in rheumatoid joints through a positive feedback mechanism.

Following a presentation of the background, biochemistry, sources, actions and assay techniques for IL-2, the authors discuss the role of this cytokine in rheumatological diseases. Depressed cellular immune responsiveness is reflected by skin testing as well as the diminished transformation of blood lymphocytes in vitro by antigen or mitogens. The decreased production of IL-2 which was most marked by synovial membrane lymphocytes and also manifested by blood lymphocytes, correlates with disease manifestations. The addition of exogenous IL-2 to lymphocytes from RA patients restores their lymphocyte-transforming activity to normal.

Although there is no doubt that the IL-2 system is abnormal in RA, it is unclear whether the IL-2 level in rheumatoid joints is deficient or excessive, but a deficiency is most probable. It is believed that relative quantities of IL-2 regulators associated with initial presentation of antigens are critical to the level of immune rsponsiveness and disease production.

Following a consideration of the background, biochemistry, sources, actions and assay methods for IFN-γ, the authors discuss its role in rheumatological diseases. IFN-γ has been shown to increase synovial fibroblast proliferation and to suppress hemopoiesis. Most of its other effects are stimulatory with exceptions. During differentiation, IFN-γ may induce new surface markers and cause proliferation of T and perhaps NK cells. It enhances not only expression of class I MHC antigens but of class II MHC antigens in a broad spectrum of cell types. It induces IL-1 production by macrophages which acquire antigen-presenting capability. IFN-γ is believed to have a significant effect in synovial inflammation. It enhances HLA-DR expression on dendritic cells of the synovial membrane in RA as well as of fibroblasts, synovial cells, in addition to activated T and B lymphocytes. The authors postulate that IFN-γ could perpetuate the immune response in the synovium by facilitating HLA-DR antigenic expression which would augment antigen presentation to helper T cells leading ultimately to formation of more cytokines including IFN. The role of IFN-γ in initiating other autoimmune processes including autoimmune thyroid disease through aberrant HLA-DR expression on thyrocytes in well known. IFN-γ could have a similar role in inducing aberrant HLA-DR expression in other diseases such as RA.

CSFs represent a family of glycoproteins capable of controlling proliferation and differentiation of hemopoietic progenitor cells. After reviewing the background, biochemistry, sources, action and assay methods, the authors discuss the possible role of CSFs in rheumatological diseases. These cytokines may be derived from activated T cells, macrophages, fibroblasts and endothelial cells which may all be present in the rheumatoid synovium where they may stimulate mature cells to function. One of these, for example GM-CSF, may act on human peripheral blood neutrophils to cause degranulation and superoxide formation following chemotactic stimuli, increased antibody-dependent cytotoxicity and inhibition of migration. All of these effects could isolate and activate these cell types in areas of inflammation. Although colony-stimulating activity has been demonstrated in synovial fluid, efforts have not yet deciphered which CSFs were present. CSFs are postulated to possibly have a significant role in effector cell activation at areas of inflammation in addition to their better known role in governing hemopoiesis in the bone marrow.

Cytokines may also have nonimmunological effects as evidenced by their association with fibrosis and angiogenesis. IFN-γ from T cells and IL-1 from macrophages may stimulate fibroblasts to produce collagen. Mast cells have also been implicated in fibrosis. Histamine from mast cell granules stimulate growth of fibroblasts. The elevated levels of mast cells in RA synovium have been correlated with inflammation. Mast cells are increased in the skin in scleroderma, which is hypothesized by some investigators to result from increased activity of intimal fibroblasts. Angiogenesis factors have also been shown to stimulate an intensive mast cell reaction which could account for the association of mast cells, fibrosis and angiogenesis in diseases such as scleroderma.

Tumor angiogenesis factor has also been demonstrated in synovial fluid. EM studies of RA synovium have shown a resemblance between new vessels in RA synovium and those found in tumors. It has been postulated that OAF, which is associated with bone destruction, might represent a combined effect of several immune cell products. CSFs could induce bone resorption as they facilitate osteoclast precursor cell differentiation.

The authors conclude the article by emphasizing impaired cytokine regulation in rheumatological disease; the effects of cytokines on inflammation; correlation of the cytokine profile with a particular disease, and the possibility that identification of a cytokine defect could offer new therapeutic approaches.

It is becoming increasingly apparent that the aberrant expression of class II histocompatibility antigens by tissue cells may have a pivitol role in the induction of autoimmunity with pathogenic sequelae.

Charron and Tetyon present a precise qualitative and quantitative analysis of Ia antigen participation in autoimmunity associated with RA. Among the immunologic reactions within the synovial membrane and synovial fluid, both adherent and nonadherent cells in the synovium pannus of RA reveal hyperexpression of Ia antigens. Since the human HLA-D region and the mouse I region control the immune response, it is now recognized that Ia antigens determined by this region serve as effector molecules whose expression is precisely regulated. Aberrant Ia antigen expression by cells on which they are not usually expressed may perpetuate autoimmunity.

The HLA-D region consists of HLA-DR, DQ, and DP subregions each determining class II glycoproteins comprised of an alpha chain and a beta chain. Thus the authors' research has been aimed at quantitative as well as qualitative expression of these Ia antigens in such pathologic conditions as RA. Susceptibility to RA may be associated with certain HLA-D region genes that increase relative risk, possibly by permitting recognition of autoantigen as well as foreign antigen. This could be followed by proliferation or cytotoxicity resulting in local tissue injury. Charron and Tetyon developed an in vitro model to investigate HLA-class II antigen expressed by synovial lining cells in culture to elucidate their role in RA. Serologically defined antigens associated with RA include DR4, and potentially DR1, as well as the recently described MC1, which represents the determinant with greatest disease association in RA. Employing the mixed lymphocyte reaction (MLR) typing, DW4 has shown a close association with RA. Biochemical and molecular biology techniques have demonstrated molecular variants within complex haplotypes such as the DR4 haplotype. Different numbers of DR molecules may be expressed by haplotypes. In seropositive juvenile rheumatoid arthritis (JRA), which is closely associated with DR4, structural studies have revealed that molecular variants are significant in disease susceptibility, whereas DR4 is not an important disease marker. Most of the serologically homozygous (DR4/DR4) JRA patients have been shown to be heterozygous by cellular DW typing and biochemical (2D PAGE) analysis. In both JRA and diabetes mellitus, evidence suggests that combinatorial determinants facilitate increased susceptibility to the respective diseases. Hybrid class II molecules may be formed in heterozygous individuals.

In RA, aberrant expression of Ia antigens has been demonstrated on nonimmune cells that do not usually manifest them; there is accentuated HLA-class II antigen expression on cells normally expressing them, and there is differential expression of DR, DQ and DP HLA-class II subsets. RA patients exhibit more Ia-positive peripheral T lymphocytes than do normal controls. In addition, there is hyperexpression of class II antigens locally in the synovial pannus in RA. The positive signals that control HLA expression in vivo may be lost during in vitro cultures. Since one of the in vivo acting lymphokines may be IFN-γ, the addition of IFN-γ to in vitro cultures led to the induction of all three HLA-D subregion products as well as Ii mRNA. A proteoglycan of the chondroitin-sulfate (CS) class, is associated with Ia antigens. Its coprotein consists of the invariant chain. Chondrocytes, that express Ia antigens in RA, synthesize cartilage CS. This proteoglycan might interfere with processing and function of Ii and perhaps Ia metabolism.

Future studies must be directed not only to class II antigen expression at the cell surface but to quantitative expression and biosynthesis of class II molecules as well as an analysis of posttranslational glycosylation, acylation, and phosphorylation. Investigations must also address the invariant chain, proteoglycan, and membrane receptors in affected tissues. All these factors may play a critical role in disease perpetuation and be significant in assessing possible future anti-Ia therapy.

Yoo and Ishibe present a fascinating and unique account of autoimmunity associated with auditory dysfunction. Diseases considered with hearing loss include Ménière's disease, otosclerosis, autoimmune sensory hearing loss, among others. The authors have developed an animal model of ear disease in which type II collagen immunization of animals led to sensory hearing loss, vestibular dysfunction, degeneration in the spiral ganglion, crista ampullaris, vacuolar degeneration in the utricles, endolymphatic hydrops and otospongiosis-like lesions. Available experimental evidence suggests cellular and humoral immune responsiveness to native type II collagen as a part of the pathogenesis. Immunopathologic changes in the model resemble those in human disease equivalents, and the disease can be passively transferred with either lymphoid cells or serum.

Although immune reactions are associated with a number of diseases of the ear, future investigations must determine whether or not autoimmune phenomena represent an etiology for human ear lesions. Autoimmunity against type II collagen has been proven in relapsing polychondritis. One fifth of patients with autoimmunity sensorineural hearing loss (AISNHL) develop immunity to either type II or type IV collagen. Type II collagen autoimmunity and immune complexes in lesions may occur in selected otosclerosis patients. Autoimmunity to type II collagen has also been implicated in the etiology of Ménière's disease. Type II collagen autoimmunity in the inner ear could lead to immunoglobulin and complement deposition as well as immunologic injury of the endolymphatic duct resulting in impaired resorption of endolymph and consequently endolymphatic hydrops.

The authors describe several animal models of autoimmune ear disease. Rats immunized with native bovine type II collagen developed autoimmune sensorineural hearing loss. This represents the collagen-induced ear disease model for the AISNHL, spiral ganglion degeneration and cochlear vasculitis. In a guinea model of autoimmune hydrops and saccular degeneration, endolymphatic hydrops were induced in guinea pigs that had been immunized with native bovine type II collagen. Anatomical targets of the immune responsiveness include structures containing type II collagen such as membranous labyrinth, subepithelial layer of the endolymphatic duct, spiral ligament and endochondrial layer of the capsule.

In the animal model for degeneration of the crista ampullaris and vestibular dysfunction, the crista ampullaris, which contains type II collagen, manifests vacuolar degeneration and vestibular dysfunction develops. In another animal model, rats immunized with native type II collagen developed otospongiosis-like lesions, which could have significance for a better understanding of human otosclerosis. There is a close resemblance between immunopathologic alterations in human ear disease and those in the collagen-induced autoimmune ear disease model (CIAED). The passive transfer of CIAED with lymphoid cells from type II collagen-immunized guinea pigs to previously unsensitized recipients was successful and lesions were demonstrated to be induced by immunologic injury. To determine whether serum could transfer CIAED, Wistar rats were immunized with native bovine type II collagen, the antisera collected and fractionated, and the γ-globulin fraction administered to previously unsensitized recipient rats. The results demonstrated that CIAED could be transferred by immune serum in the rat.

To investigate the epitope of type II collagen participating in the induction of CIAED, cyanogen bromide was employed to cleave a CB-11 peptide from type II collagen. This CB-11 peptide was significant to the production of arthritis in mice and antibodies against it were detected in the blood sera of mice in which CIAED had been induced. Deafness followed 10 months postimmunization of mice with CB-11 peptide. Hearing loss was accompanied by severe histologic alterations and dense precipitates in the tunnel or Corti. Thus the mechanism of injury to the inner ear is suggested to be an immunologic reaction. The available evidence suggests that CB-11 peptide represents one of the type II collagen molecule epitopes capable of inducing type II collagen-induced ear disease.

The article concludes with a consideration of other factors that influence collagen-induced autoimmune ear disease. Significant variables include the species of animals, the genetically determined immune responsiveness of the species or strain employed in experiments, whether the antigen is incorporated into Freund's adjuvant, the duration of immunization, preexisting infection of animals prior to immunization and the nature of the antigen.

Crapper, Frazer, Mackay, Iscaro and Bradford present an up-to-date account of immunoregulatory defects associated with infection with the AIDS virus, HTLV-III. They describe the spectrum of immune defects in homosexual men and their relationship to infection with HTLV-III virus. Homosexual men exhibit diminished cellular immunity which is accentuated by infection with HTLV-III virus. Precise causes of immune deficiency in males seronegative for HTLV-III are unknown but appear associated with sexual promiscuity, passive anal intercourse, and active infection with CMV. Of course, HTLV-III virus alone is fully capable of depressing immunity and inducing AIDS. T helper cells are decreased either by direct lysis by HTLV-III or autoimmune injury. HTLV-III lysis is not the only mechanism of injury to T helper cells since only activated T cells rather than resting lymphocytes are sites of replication and damage by the virus and only few peripheral blood lymphocytes possess the HTLV-III genome and fewer still contain replicating virus.

HTLV-III viral infection might initiate an autoimmune response, which is well established for several viral agents. Anti-lymphocyte antibodies in blood sera of HTLV-III-infected individuals show specificity for T helper lymphocytes. This could be attributable to immunologic cross-reactivity between viral and host antigens, host cell membrane alterations induced by the virus or immunologic reactivity against HTLV-III envelope proteins attached to the surface of uninfected CD4 lymphocytes. This would render T helper cells bearing surface-anchored antibody susceptible to cytotoxic effects mediated by cells or complement.

Twenty to forty percent of men seropositive for HTLV-III infection exhibit persistent lymphadenopathy, which increases with the length of HTLV-III infection. Such patients reveal diminished T cell responsiveness compared with homosexual men not manifesting lymphadenopathy attributable to decreased T helper and increased T suppressor cells. These alterations in T cell levels are further accentuated in males manifesting constitutional symptoms.

T suppressor cells are increased in many infections including the acute HTLV-III type. The elevation in CD8-positive (Ts) lymphocytes is attributable principally to expansion of the cytotoxic T lymphocyte population recognizing viral encoded antigens in association with class I MHC molecules. There is an increase of CD8, possibly suppressor, cells in seronegative homosexual males and a greater increase in seropositive individuals. The authors suggest that the rise in T suppressor cells in seronegative individuals might be associated with infection by cytomegalovirus (CMV) which is known to affect essentially all homosexual men. There was a marked reduction in T helper cells in seropositive males manifesting systemic symptoms. Immune function was found to improve in both seronegative and seropositive homosexual males who were willing to alter certain homosexual life-style factors including sexual promiscuity and receptive anal intercourse. Thus, immune system function appeared to improve in many with diminished sexual activity.

Gottlieb and Scholes provide an informative account of reconstitution of immune function in AIDS/ARC patients. Following a review of the basic clinical and immunologic features of AIDS, which is known to be caused by the retrovirus, human immunodeficiency virus (HIV), they define the various immune system defects that include a striking decrease in T helper lymphocyte numbers and function, diminished ability of the lymphocytes to produce IL-2 and IFN-γ, variable effects on NK cell function, and nonspecific activation of B lymphocytes manifested as hyperglobulinemia and diminished capacity to mount a specific antibody response to microbial antigens. The principal immune defect is in the T helper cell subset.

HIV infection leads to several levels of immune system dysfunction. While some HIV-infected individuals may manifest relatively mild immunodeficiency, others develop devastating deficiency of the immune system, which may be associated with increased infection and development of malignant tumors.

Investigators are currently seeking a drug that will destroy the virus and a vaccine that may protect those not yet infected. Problems include the need for an effective drug to cross the blood-brain barrier and the difficulty posed by the virus being integrated into the DNA of host cells thereby protecting the virus from easy elimination. Future approaches will include the use of an effective antiviral agent combined with an immunorestorative agent for treatment of AIDS and AIDS-related complex (ARC) patients. Agents tested to restore the immune system of AIDS victims include INFs, IL-2, thymic factors and γ-globulin in addition to pharmacologic immunomodulators such as azimexon, cimetidine and Immuthiol. AZT (3'-azido-3'-deoxythymidine) has antiviral actions and showed some beneficial effects clinically such as weight gain, increased T helper cells and restoration of delayed hypersensitivity to recall antigens in some patients. Isoprinosine treatment of AIDS/ARC patients provided marginal clinical and immunological improvement. Thymopentin

(TP-5) also produced limited effects. Ribavirin, which inhibits reverse transcriptase action of HIV, produced marginal clinical effects.

The authors describe the use of leukocyte-derived immunomodulators such as IMREG-1 to enhance DTH reactions to recall antigens. The production of antigen-induced leukocyte migration inhibition factors (LIF), and macrophage migration inhibition factor (MIF), which are associated with the delayed hypersensitivity response, are accelerated and augmented in vitro by treatment of peripheral blood lymphocytes with IMREG-1. In vitro effects appear closely correlated with delayed hypersensitivity reactions in vivo. IMREG-1 affects human T helper lymphocytes in several respects that include increased production of IL-2 which augments formation of IFN-γ and IL-2 receptor expression. There is an accentuated formation of migration inhibiting lymphokines. The ability of IMREG-1 to augment T helper lymphocyte function in vitro suggested that it might be a candidate for modulation of immunodeficiency in patients with impaired T helper cell activity, such as those with AIDS or ARC. IMREG-1 was able to enhance IL-2 formation by peripheral blood lymphocytes derived from AIDS/ARC patients. IFN-γ was also augmented in association with the increased formation of IL-2. Some AIDS patients treated with IMREG-1 manifested enhanced IL-2 production by peripheral blood lymphocytes and restored delayed hypersensitivity indicating that immune system function in response to antigenic challenge had been reestablished. None of the patients demonstrated toxicity in response to IMREG-1 and no adverse effects on laboratory hematological or biochemical parameters were found.

Twenty-nine AIDS patients treated with IMREG-1 gained weight and demonstrated clearing of oral candida in those presenting with this infection. It reduces the rate of destruction of T4 (helper) lymphocytes but does not lead to their activation which would further promote viral infection and expression. The authors conclude that administration of IMREG-1 reconstitutes the impaired immune system and clinically improves AIDS/ARC patients. They suggest that future AIDS therapy might include an antiviral agent useful for control of viral expression with short-term administration and an immunomodulator to improve T4 helper cell function.

The volume concludes with an assessment by Sriram and Ranges of immunotherapy of autoimmune disease with T cell subset-specific antibodies. The T cell plays a critical role in self-nonself recognition, therefore disordered regulation of T cell function is often associated with autoimmune disease. Anti-T cell antibodies have been used in the past for various purposes including control of allograft rejection in organ transplantation. The most recent include anti-T cell monoclonal antibodies developed through hybridoma technology. As T cell subsets have become better defined, monoclonal antibodies have been raised against them. Monoclonal antibodies specific for the T4 or Leu-3 antigen of human lymphocytes or the corresponding L3T4 antigen of mouse lymphocytes identify helper/inducer cells. Anti-L3T4 antibodies inhibit all class II MHC antigen restricted T cell function including proliferation of T cells, antibody responsiveness, and T lymphocyte killing of class II associated antigen. L3T4 antigen is believed to facilitate binding of the Ia antigen complex with the T cell receptor. The authors investigated the role of anti-L3T4 antibodies in vivo as a potential therapy for autoimmune disease. They studied its effect in experimental allergic encephalomyelitis (EAE) and collagen-induced arthritis (CIA) as well as the lupus-like disease in (NZB × NZW) F_1 mice. Their results appear promising for the use of similar antibodies in immunotherapy of human autoimmune disease.

In the EAE model, administration of 100 μg of anti-L3T4 antibodies injected for 2 days preceding and following immunization with myelin basic protein (MBP) diminished clinical and histologic disease in immunized animals compared with controls. The antibody preparation also proved effective in preventing chronic relapsing EAE which bears a resemblance to multiple sclerosis in man. For any therapy to be clinically useful, it must be effective when begun even following the appearance of clinical signs. Clinically there were fewer relapses in the anti-L3T4 antibody-treated group, compared with saline-injected controls, and histologically there was a corresponding decrease in the inflammatory response in the brain and only limited demyelination in the spinal cord.

Anti-L3T4 antibody prevented development of type II collagen-induced arthritis in mice. The treatment was more effective if administered prior to immunization with the type II collagen rather than if it was delayed until day 28, when the disease incidence was similar in experimental and control groups.

Anti-L3T4 antibodies inhibited the production of anti-DNA antibodies and prolonged survival in (NZB × NZW)F_1 hybrid mice that spontaneously develop a lupus-like syndrome resembling systemic lupus erythematosus in humans. The antibody treatment was effective even when begun after the production of anti-DNA antibodies and following the onset of renal disease.

With respect to the mechanism of action of anti-L3T4, the antibody inhibits all class II MHC antigen-restricted functions in vitro. It may interfere with binding of L3T4 antigen on the T cell with that of the antigen-presenting cell. The antibody apparently eliminates rather than blocks $L3T4^+$ cells.

Potential adverse side effects of treatment with anti-L3T4 antibodies include a reduction of helper T cells in lymphoid organs and in the circulation leading to a blood picture resembling that in AIDS. Therefore, anti-L3T4 antibodies might have greater use in short-term depletion of specific T cell subsets rather than for prolonged use in therapy of autoimmune diseases. $L3T4^+$ cells return to normal once the antibody is discontinued.

Unraveling some of Nature's best kept secrets related to the intricate interactions of cell receptors and cytokines that maintain homeostasis of the immune system reveals many autoimmune reactions to be normal physiologic responses. This is in contrast to earlier concepts that autoimmunity was exclusively pathogenic. It is anticipated that future research will illuminate the autoimmunoregulatory mechanisms participating in this marvelous process.

The editors express genuine gratitude to the investigator/authors who have taken valuable time from their research to prepare these interpretive articles. We express appreciation also to Dr. Robert M. O'Neal, Chairman of the Department of Pathology, University of Mississippi Medical Center, for his generosity in permitting us to assemble this volume. Special recognition is due Dr. Thomas Karger and his staff in Basel and New York for splendid cooperation and assistance in preparing the manuscripts for publication.

Dr. Julius M. Cruse, Department of Pathology, University of Mississippi Medical Center, 2500 North State Street, Jackson, MS 39216 (USA)

Concepts Immunopathol., vol. 4, pp. 24–41 (Karger, Basel 1987)

Relevance of Autocytotoxic and Autoregulatory Lymphocytes in the Maintenance of Self Tolerance

Karen Rosenkrantz[a,b], *Bo Dupont*[a], *Neal Flomenberg*[b]

[a] Human Immunogenetics Laboratory, and [b] Effector Lymphocyte Biology Laboratory, Memorial Sloan-Kettering Cancer Center, New York, N.Y., USA

Immunological tolerance to self is an essential property of healthy organisms [1]. Although protective immune responses are generated against an almost endless array of foreign antigens, aggressive responses toward self antigens do not normally occur. The mechanisms which maintain self tolerance are still largely unknown. Theoretical models have been focused on two concepts: the clonal deletion/inactivation of autoaggressive cells in the thymus [2, 3], or, alternatively, the suppression of such cells by regulatory cells in the periphery [4]. In this review, we will attempt to highlight some of the evidence supporting each of these models – emphasizing current data which suggests that regulatory cells play an important role in preventing autocytotoxic responses. In addition, we will include work from our laboratory which demonstrates that autocytotoxic cells and autosuppressor cells capable of down regulating autoaggressive responses are present in the peripheral blood of healthy human individuals [5, 6].

Immune System's Concept of Self Is Acquired during Development and Actively Maintained thereafter

The immune system's definition of self appears to be shaped during ontogeny. Over 40 years ago, Owen noted that dizygotic twins sharing a common intrauterine blood supply were tolerant of each others tissues. This observation led Burnet and Fenner [7] to propose that any foreign antigens encountered early in the course of development would be regarded as self. This hypothesis was confirmed in 1953. Independently,

Hasek [8] and Billingham et al. [9] demonstrated that tolerance could be artificially induced by exposure to antigen neonatally or in utero.

Once established, self tolerance appears to be actively-maintained throughout an organism's lifetime. In adult animals self tolerance can be broken by a variety of immunological manipulations, leading to graft-vs.-host (GVH)-like syndromes or autoimmune diseases [10–18]. Irradiated animals repopulated with autologous bone marrow and treated with cyclosporin A for several weeks develop a syndrome similar to GVH disease when the cyclosporin A is discontinued [11–13]. In rats, this syndrome can be adoptively transferred with T cell populations to irradiated syngeneic animals, but not to normal syngeneic animals. Thymectomy or deletion of specific lymphocyte subsets similarly promotes the onset of autoimmune reaction [14–18]. These experiments suggest that normal adult animals possess a regulatory mechanism which controls the activity of autoaggressive T cells.

Studies to assess the mechanism by which self tolerance is induced and maintained have been hampered by a paucity of available experimental models. Because of the difficulties in studying tolerance to autologous antigens, investigators have turned to alternate strategies. One approach has been to study tolerance induced toward an antigen normally considered to be non-self – an alloantigen, a hapten, or a virus. However, the mechanisms which establish and maintain neonatal tolerance may be quite different from those that act in tolerant states established later in life. In addition, tolerance induced toward foreign antigens is not necessarily mediated by the same processes which control tolerance toward self. An alternate approach has been to rely on natural or experimental models in which self tolerance has broken down (i.e. autoimmune diseases) hoping that studying the pathology will shed light on the normal physiological processes.

Intrathymic Events in Self Tolerance

The thymus is a site where T cells normally develop immunocompetence [19–23] and has been implicated as the site where self tolerance is first established [24]. Unresponsiveness resulting from neonatal tolerance induction is first demonstrable in thymic lymphocytes, before it becomes apparent in peripheral lymphoid populations [25, 26]. In order to more specifically identify the cell populations within the thymus responsibile for tolerance induction, experiments with bone marrow chimeras and other transplantation studies have been utilized.

One thymic cell population which induces lymphocyte tolerance appears to be of hematopoietic origin. Even when lymphocytes mature in the presence of an allogeneic thymus, they do not mount proliferative responses or cytotoxic responses to syngeneic cells [27–31]. It has been postulated that marrow-derived HLA class II-expressing dendritic cells migrate to the thymus and become resident therein [32]. These dendritic cells are thought to be the cells responsible for inducing self tolerance in developing T lymphocytes [27–29, 31].

The role of thymic-derived cells (i.e. epithelial cells) in establishing self tolerance remains more controversial. Lymphocytes which mature in vitro in an allogeneic thymus, developing from embryonic rudiments, are unable to mount cytotoxic responses against lymphocytes derived from either the stem cell or thymic donor [28]. In this system, tolerance appears to be engendered by both types of cells. In vivo studies of cultured thymus grafts, however, have produced more ambiguous results. Investigators have utilized pretreatment with deoxyguanosine or tissue culture at low temperatures to selectively destroy cells of hematopoietic origin in thymus grafts, and have then studied the capacity of such thymic grafts to induce tolerance [27, 29–31, 33]. When these pretreated grafts are transplanted into normal allogeneic mice, host-derived lymphocytes may be either nonresponsive [27] or strongly responsive [29–31] to stimulator cells from the thymic donor. Similarly, when pretreated grafts were transplanted into *athymic* (nude) mice, host lymphocytes may be either nonresponsive [30] or strongly responsive [27] to cells derived from the thymic donor. Evidence has been presented that thymic epithelial cells can imprint T cells with H-2 restriction specificities [31]. Further work will be necessary to discern whether thymic epithelial cells also play a role in the induction of self tolerance.

Proponents of the clonal deletion theory propose that self-reactive T cells are eliminated in the thymus [2, 3, 24]. Experimentally, the intrathymic deletion process is difficult to directly demonstrate, though a large number of thymocytes die in situ [34, 35]. Therefore, the evidence supporting an intrathymic deletion mechanism is largely indirect. In experimental models of acquired tolerance of alloantigens, there is a reduction of cytotoxic T lymphocytes against the tolerated alloantigen [36, 37]. Similarly, in studies utilizing limiting dilution analyses of induced tolerance toward alloantigens, proteins, or modified syngeneic cells, it has not been possible to demonstrate any cells reacting with the tolerogen [25, 28, 38]. This has lent support to the notion that in tolerant states, potentially reactive CTL are deleted or permanently inactivated.

The failure to demonstrate suppressor cells in 'mixing' experiments has also been used historically as evidence to support the clonal deletion theory [39]. When a lymphocyte population containing suppressor cells is mixed with a normal immunocompetent population of cells, the suppressor cells inhibit the activation of the normal cells, so-called 'infectious tolerance' [40]. When tolerance is established by prior clonal elimination of reactive cells, normal cells are free to respond when cocultured with the tolerant populations. In many experimental systems, the state of tolerance cannot be transferred by cell populations from tolerant to nontolerant animals [39, 41].

Extrathymic Events in Self Tolerance

While strong evidence suggests that the thymus plays a role in T cell tolerance induction, there is evidence that the maintenance of self tolerance is at least in part mediated by a peripheral mechanism. For example, in some experimental models, a clonal reduction of precursor lymphocytes directed against the tolerogen may, in fact, be the consequence of a highly efficient peripheral regulatory cell population rather than an intrathymic process. In murine models of neonatal tolerance to alloantigens, limiting dilution analysis techniques indicate a reduction in the precursor frequency of cytotoxic lymphocytes specific for the tolerogen, consistent with a clonal inactivation of the relevant effector lymphocytes [25, 28, 38]. However, these reductions are, at least in some cases, produced by demonstrable suppressor cells [38]. In a similar model system, tolerant mice were injected with repeated doses of anti-I-J antiserum directed against suppressor cells. This treatment markedly abrogated the reductions in precursor frequency associated with the tolerant state [25]. Thus, the apparent purging of anti-self effector cells may in some cases reflect intrathymic inactivation. In other cases, however, it may reflect a population of regulatory lymphocytes present at a very high frequency in the peripheral blood.

In normal healthy individuals, the clonal 'deletion' of anti-self effector cells appears to be incomplete. Peripheral blood mononuclear leukocytes do not in general develop cytotoxicity against autologous target cells. However, utilizing peripheral blood mononuclear cells from healthy individuals, an autoaggressive response has been demonstrated when T lymphocyte subsets have been isolated and tested [42–44] or when exogenous growth factors are added to the cultures [45]. These studies suggest that autocytotoxic cells are present in the peripheral blood of normal individuals. Since experimental manipulations are necessary in order to demonstrate the presence of such autocytotoxic cells, an autoregulating mechanism must be present within peripheral blood which normally prevents the expression of these autoaggressive responses.

The isolation and identification of peripheral cells capable of regulating such autocytotoxic cells has proven to be a difficult task. Much of the descriptive data on regulatory cells are derived from experimental models in which animals are rendered tolerant to allogeneic tissues, modified syngeneic cells, or to other antigens [46–49]. In murine studies, deletion of lymphocyte subpopulations leads to autoreactive responses (50, 51] and autoimmune diseases [15, 17, 18]. In addition, cell lines have been isolated which can prevent the development of autoimmune syndromes [52]. Such studies suggest that some murine autoregulatory cells may be at least phenotypically similar to the regulatory cells characterized in other experimental systems [46–49].

The inherent limitation of most of these experimental models is the fact that autoaggressive and autoregulatory responses are not being studied within normal, healthy individuals. Ideally, one would like to use an experimental model in which one breaks and then reestablishes self tolerance within the same experiment using cells isolated from a single healthy individual. We have utilized limiting dilution analysis to demonstrate that autoaggressive cells and cells capable of down regulating autoaggressive cells are normally present in the peripheral blood of healthy human donors [5, 6].

Breaking and Reestablishing Self Tolerance – Demonstration of Autoaggressive and Autoregulatory Cells in Normal Peripheral Blood

Limiting dilution analysis has been utilized previously to assess the frequency of precursors of a variety of lymphocyte subpopulations and to demonstrate complex interactions between a variety of synergistic and antagonistic cell populations [53–56]. The technique of limiting dilution

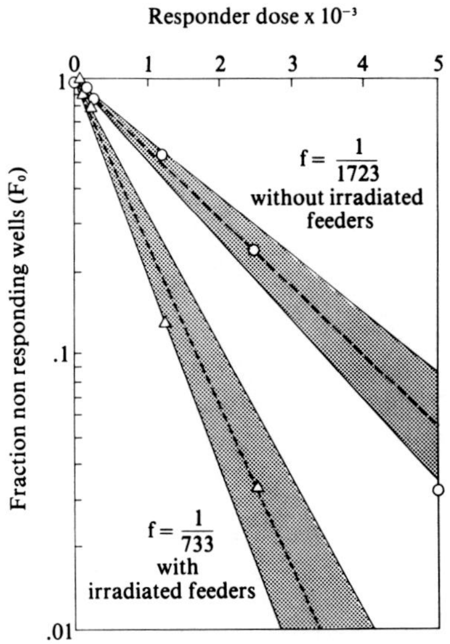

Fig. 1. Limiting dilution analysis of the allocytotoxic response. Increasing numbers of responder RWK PBL (HLA-A2, w33, B7, w35, w6, Cw7, DR2,6) were stimulated by KR PBL (HLA-A1, B8, w6, Cw7, DR3,4) in 10% RWK serum and 15% IL-2 human-conditioned medium with (△) and without (0) 10,000 irradiated RWK PBL per well; 96 wells were plated at each responder dose. Cytotoxicity was measured against KR PHA lymphoblasts. 10×10^3 and 50×10^3 responder dose points are not shown as all wells were positive. In the absence of additional irradiated responder cells, f = 1/1723 ($p > 0.05$). In the presence of additional irradiated responder cells, f = 1/733 ($p > 0.05$).

analysis is well described [57–60]. To utilize limiting dilution analysis in the study of cytotoxic cells, one titrates increasing numbers of the responder cell population into microcultures, together with fixed numbers of stimulator cells and a source of interleukin-2 (IL-2) and other lymphokines. After 10 days of culture, individual microculture wells are assayed for cytotoxicity toward ^{51}Cr-radiolabelled target cells.

To analyze the data, each well is scored as exhibiting positive (+) or no (–) cytolytic activity. A threshold value for cytotoxicity is established based upon the chromium release observed in a control plate, which is seeded with stimulator cells, but no responder cells. The threshold value is equal to the mean chromium release of the control plate plus 3 SDSDs [58–60]. Wells exhibiting chromium release above this value are scored as positive, while wells exhibiting chromium release below this value are scored as negative.

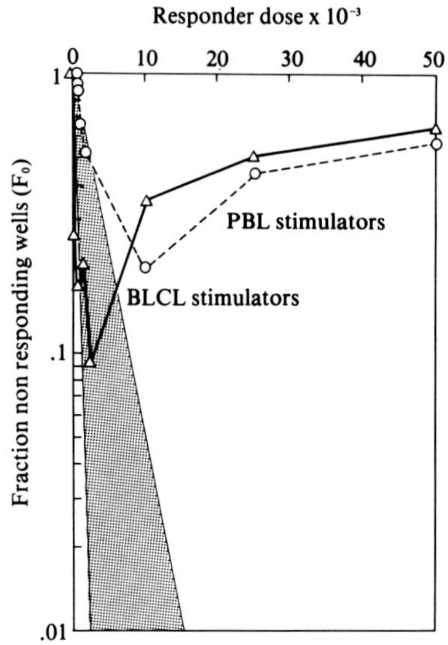

Fig. 2. Limiting dilution analysis of the autocytotoxic response. NF PBL (HLA-A26,28, B14, w41, w6, Cw8, DR1,3) were stimulated by irradiated autologous PBLs (0) or BLCLs (△) in 10 % NF serum and 10 % IL-2 conditioned-medium prepared from a gibbon cell line, MLA-144; 48 wells were plated at each responder dose. Cytotoxicity was measured against NF PHA lymphoblasts. Shaded area represents the experimental range of allospecific cytotoxic T lymphocyte precursor frequencies. When PBLs were used as stimulator cells, positive wells at the point of inflection (responder cell dose = 10,000 cells/well) exhibited a mean percentage cytotoxicity of 12.0 % with a range of 5.9–35.8 %. On the control plate (stimulator cells alone), the mean chromium release + 3 SD corresponded to 5.5 % cytotoxicity. When B-LCL were used as stimulator cells, positive wells at the point of inflection (responder cell dose = 2,000 cells/well) exhibited a mean % cytotoxicity of 15.4 % with a range of 5.3–32.1 %. The mean chromium release + 3 SD for the control plate corresponded to 5.3 %.

The fraction of *nonresponding* wells is plotted as a function of cell dose in semilogarithmic form (Fo plot) (fig. 1). If the relationship between these two parameters is linear (so-called single hit kinetics) ($p > 0.05$), then the precursor frequency for the cytotoxic cell can be calculated from the slope of the regression line. For more details concerning the mathematics, the reader is referred to other reviews [58–61].

Limiting dilution analyses of allocytotoxic responses following specific priming with irradiated allogeneic peripheral blood mononuclear leukocytes (PBL) are consistent with a single hit kinetic model. Figure 1 illustrates data from one such study. All wells at responder cell doses

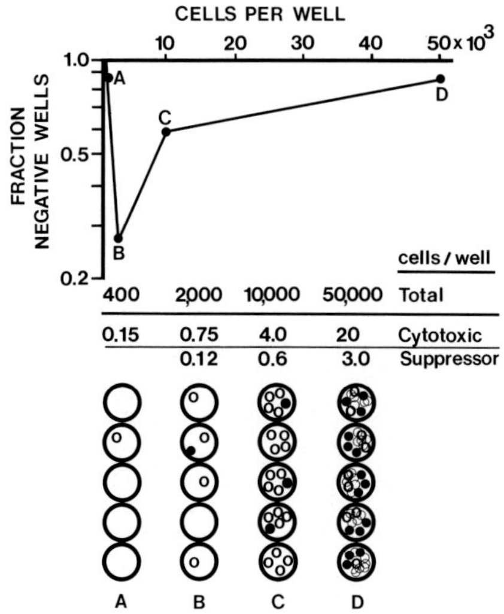

Fig. 3. Biphasic responses in limiting dilution analyses: a two-cell model. A hypothetical experiment is shown as an Fo plot. The composition of microtiter wells from points A, B, C, and D of the graph are illustrated below. The large open circles represent the individual microculture wells. Small open circles represent autocytotoxic cells, while closed circles represent regulatory cells. At low responder cells numbers (points A and B) individual wells receive predominantly autocytotoxic cells and generate autocytotoxic responses. At higher responder cell number (points C and D), microwells receive regulatory cells and the autocytotoxic response disappears.

greater than 10,000 cells per well are positive. In this assay, precursor frequencies for the allocytotoxic cells range from 1/700 to 1/1,700, depending upon the experimental conditions. These values are in agreement with data obtained in several laboratories [62, 63].

In contrast, following sensitization with autologous irradiated PBL, cytotoxic responses toward autologous phytohemaglutinin (PHA)-activated lymphoblasts exhibit a distinctive biphasic response. As depicted in figure 2, strong autocytotoxic responses toward autologous PHA-activated lymphoblasts or Epstein-Barr virus B-transformed lymphoblastoid cell lines (B-LCL) developed at low responder-cell doses. Indeed, in some experiments, one hundred percent of the test wells may exhibit positive respones at the inflection point of the curve (the point of maximum cytotoxicity). In this experiment, the percent cytotoxicity observed in these microtiter wells ranges from 5 to 32%. However, as cell dose is fur-

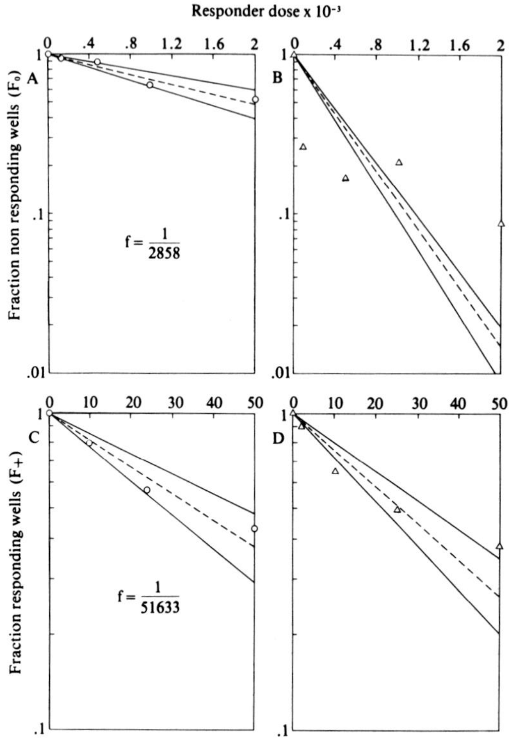

Fig. 4. Kinetic analysis of the autocytotoxic response. *A* Fo plot of autologous PBL stimulation [f = 1/2858(p > 0.05)]. *B* Fo plot of autologous BLCL stimulation (p < 0.01). *C* F+ plot of autologous PBL stimulation [f = 1/51633 (p > 0.05)]. *D* F+ plot of autologous BLCL stimulation (p < 0.05).

ther increased, in contrast to the allocytotoxic response, the autocytotoxic response disappears.

This biphasic response is consistent with the action of two-counterpoised cell populations: an autocytotoxic cell population and a very low frequency regulatory cell, capable of suppressing the autocytotoxic cell (fig. 3). At lower responder cell numbers, individual wells receive only the autocytotoxic cells and an autocytotoxic response is generated. At higher responder cell numbers, microwells begin to receive the regulatory cell and the autocytotoxic response is suppressed. In effect, one sees the breaking of self tolerance at low responder cell dose, and its subsequent reestablishment as the responder cell dose is further increased. At low cell dose, the autocytotoxic cell is dominant. The frequency of this popu-

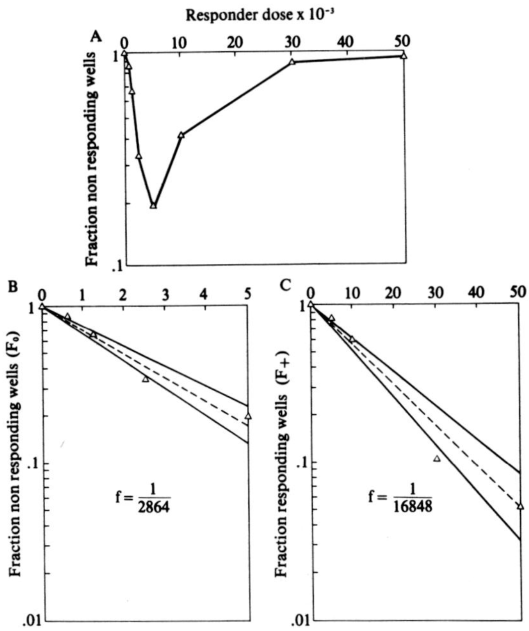

Fig. 5. Autocytotoxicity is generated using autologous human-conditioned medium. *A* NF PBLs (HLA-A26,28, B14, w41, w6, Cw8, DR1,3) were stimulated with irradiated autologous PBL in 10 % NF serum and 15 % autologous IL-2 human-conditioned medium; 96 wells were plated at each responder dose. Cytotoxicity was measured against autologous PHA lymphoblasts. *B* Fo plot of *A* [f = 1/2784 ($p > 0.05$)]. *C* F+ plot of A [f = 1/16848 ($p > 0.05$)].

lation can therefore be calculated from the descending limb of the biphasic curve (from the origin to the inflection point). In this case, when autologous PBL were utilized as stimulator cells, the precursor frequency for the autocytotoxic cell was 1/2,900 (fig. 4). (When autologous B-LCL are utilized as stimulator cells, the response does not conform to the single-hit kinetic model, and, therefore, the precursor frequency cannot be calculated from these equations.) The ascending portion of the curve reflects the cell doses at which the regulatory population is dominant. One can, therefore, calculate the frequency of the regulatory population from the data from this portion of the biphasic curve. Here the fraction of *responding* rather than *nonresponding* wells is plotted as a function of cell dose (F + plot). This reflects the reciprocal biology of an inhibitory cell population [59]. A positive cytotoxic response is, in effect, a negative

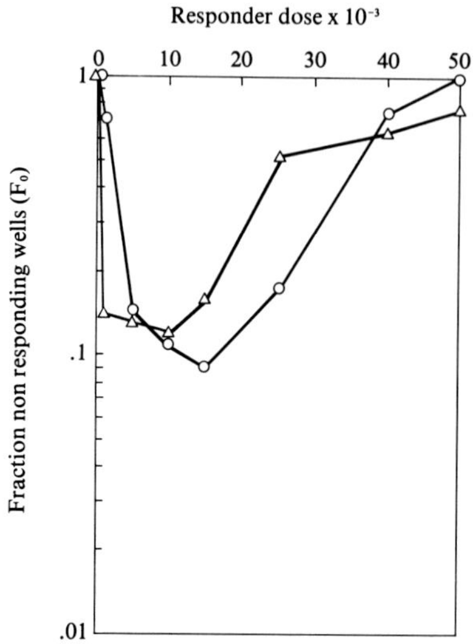

Fig. 6. Comparison of B lymphoblastoid cell lines and PHA lymphoblasts as targets for autocytotoxic cells. KR PBL (HLA-A1, B8, Bw6, Cw7, DR3,4) were stimulated with autologous PBL in 10 % KR serum and 15 % IL-2 human-conditioned medium. Ninety-six wells were plated at each responder dose. Cytotoxicity was measured against autologous PHA lymphoblasts (0) and autologous B-LCL (Δ).

suppressor response. The precursor frequency of autoregulatory cells is 1/51,600 as shown in figure 4.

It seemed possible, though unlikely, that the autocytotoxic responses observed in these experiments were the consequence of foreign serum proteins. Experiments were performed in autologous serum utilizing an autologous IL-2 preparation. Similar biphasic curves were demonstrated (fig. 5). In addition, experiments were carried out to ensure that the cytotoxic response was not due to nonspecific effect of lectin used in activating the target cells. Following stimulation with autologous-irradiated PBL, the autocytotoxic response toward autologous B-LCL was measured. Again, a biphasic response was seen (fig. 6). These cytotoxic responses, therefore, cannot be attributed to foreign proteins or lectin and thus appear to represent bona fide responses to self antigens.

Autocytotoxic and Autoregulatory Cells

Autocytotoxic and autoregulatory cell lines have recently been isolated utilizing these limiting dilution techniques [6]. Microcultures were initially seeded with responder cell doses which usually fall near the inflection point (the point of maximum cytotoxicity). Each microculture was separately expanded into a cell line utilizing standard T cell culture techniques. Three of 37 cell lines lysed autologous PHA-activated lymphoblasts. These cells express phenotypes normally associated with mature T cells (i.e. CD2+, CD3+). Five additional cell lines were isolated which prevented the development of autocytotoxicity against autologous PHA-activated lymphoblasts in fresh microcultures. These regulatory cells were incapable of lysing autocytotoxic cell lines suggesting that suppression was mediated by a mechanism other than direct lysis of the autocytotoxic cell. Whether these cells directly exert this suppressive effect or induce the development of other suppressor effector populations remains unclear. However, like regulatory cells described in experimental systems of acquired tolerance [47–49], the autosuppressor cell lines express classical T cell phenotypes (e.g. CD2+, CD3+). Therefore, utilizing limiting dilution analysis techniques, cells capable of autocytotoxicity and their regulatory cell populations can be isolated from normal peripheral blood, separately characterized, and recombined to study their interactions.

The functional significance of autocytotoxic and autoregulatory cells remains to be established. Autocytotoxic cells may represent the cellular components of Ehrlich's horror autotoxicus [64]: truly aberrant cells with receptors directed at self antigens and without physiologic function. Alternatively, they may represent cells recognizing self antigens, but with physiologic functions such as intercellular communication or regulation. It is also possible that these cells normally recognize self-MHC products together with foreign antigen, but are capable of binding to self antigens with sufficient affinity that they trigger the lysis of autologous target cells under the appropriate conditions.

Autoreactivity appears to be a normal component of the immune response. The existence of autoreactive antibodies and autoreactive T cells isolated from the blood of normal healthy individuals have been extensively documented [65–74]. Autoproliferative T cells have recently been shown to provide helper activity in vivo [74]. Thus, autoreactive responses, when present at low level, may be an integral component of the immune system and may only become truly autoaggressive and harmful to the host when they are not adequately controlled. The balance between autocytotoxicity and health versus autoaggression and diseases may thus be more quantitative than qualitative.

In our own studies, the regulatory cells appear to act by a mechanism other than direct lysis of autoaggressive cells. In studies of acquired tolerance, complex regulatory circuits have been described [47–49]. Studies of autoregulatory cell populations may well reveal a similar cascade of inducer-transducer-effector cell populations and soluble factors.

Complex networks based on idiotype-anti-idiotype interactions are a general feature of many postulated regulatory systems [46–49, 53]. There is evidence that suppressor cells with anti-idiotypic specificity play a role in neonatally-induced tolerance [37, 75, 76], in resistance to GVH-like syndromes [77] and in unresponsiveness to MHC-incompatible tissues [78]. These findings raise the question as to whether cell networks based upon idiotype-anti-idiotype recognition may also be important in the down regulation of autoreactive T cells.

There may be several distinct mechanisms involved in autoregulation. A simple two-cell regulatory system has also been proposed [79–81]. In the 'veto' cell model, a 'veto' cell is capable of downregulating responses directed against itself – irrespective of its other cellular functions or its specificity. It has been demonstrated that cloned cytotoxic T lymphocytes can function as 'veto' cells [82, 83]. A cytotoxic T lymphocyte from individual 'A' with lytic specificity only toward cells from individual 'B' can nonetheless suppress anti-A directed responses from individuals B, C, D, E, etc. Whether such a cell would also prevent the development of anti-A reactivitiy remains to be tested.

Summary and Conclusions

The state of self tolerance may well be an amalgam of many processes including (but not necessarily limited to) clonal deletion and specific suppressor cell networks. Cells with autoaggressive potential are clearly present in the blood of healthy individuals and have been implicated in diseases states. Given the critical importance of maintaining self tolerance, it is not at all surprising that several mechanisms appear to play a role in this process. Attempts to harness and manipulate these various mechanisms in order to prevent allograft rejection or to treat autoimmune diseases should prove to be exciting areas of investigation in the years ahead.

Acknowledgements

This work was supported by grants from the US Public Health Services, National Institutes of Health, NCI-CA-22507, CA-08748, CA-23766, and CA-33050, and a grant from the XOMA corporation. Dr. Rosenkrantz was supported by a Clinical Scholar's Award from NIH grant CA-09512. Dr. Flomenberg was supported by a Clinical Scholar's Award from the Norman and Rosita Winston Foundation.

We would like to express our thanks to Robert Knowles for helpful discussions and to Donna Williams and Carol Bodenheimer for expert technical assistance.

References

1 Jerne, N.K.: The natural-selection theory of antibody formation. Proc. natn. Acad. Sci. USA *41:* 849 (1955).
2 Burnet, F.M: The clonal selection theory of acquired immunity (Cambridge University Press, London 1959).
3 Nossal, G.J.V.; Pike, B.L.: Evidence for the clonal abortion theory of B lymphocyte tolerance. J. exp. Med. *141:* 904 (1975).
4 Gershon, R.K.; Kondo, K: Cell interactions in the induction of tolerance. Immunology *18:* 723 (1970).
5 Rosenkrantz, K.; Dupont, B.; Flomenberg, N.: Generation and regulation of autocytotoxicity in mixed lymphocyte cultures. Evidence for active suppression of autocytotoxic cells. Proc. natn. Acad. Sci. USA *82:* 4508 (1985).
6 Rosenkrantz, K.; Dupont, B.; Williams, D.; Flomenberg, N.: Autocytotoxic and autosuppressor T cell lines generated in autologous lymphocyte cultures (submitted, 1986).
7 Burnet, F.M.; Fenner, F.: The production of antibodies (MacMillan, London 1949).
8 Hasek, M.: Parabiosis of birds during embryonic development. Cesk. Biol. *2:* 265 (1953).
9 Billingham, R.E., Brent, L., Medawar, P.: Actively acquired tolerance of foreign cells. Nature, Lond. *172:* 603 (1953).
10 Van Bekkum, D.W.; De Vries, M.J.: Radiation chimeras (Academic Press, New York 1967).
11 Glazier, A.; Tutschka, P.J.; Farmer, E.R.; Santos, G.W.: Graft-versus-host disease in cyclosporin A treated rats after syngeneic and autologous bone marrow reconstitution. J. exp. Med. *158:* 1–8 (1983).
12 Hess, A.D.; Horwitz, L.; Beschorner, W.E.; Santos, G.W.: Development of graft-vs.-host disease-like syndrome in cyclosporine-treated rats after syngeneic bone marrow transplantation. I. Development of cytotoxic T lymphocytes with appar-

ent polyclonal anti-Ia specificity including autoreactivity. J. exp. Med. *161:* 718 (1985).
13 Cheney, R. T.; Sprent, J.: Capacity of cyclosporine to induce autograft-versus-host-disease and impair intrathymic T cell differentiation. Transplant. Proc. *17:* 528 (1985).
14 Wick, G.; Kite, J. H.; Witebsky, E.: Spontaneous thyroiditis in the obese strain of chickens. IV. The effect thymectomy and thymo-bursectomy on the development of the disease. J. Immun. *104:* 54 (1970).
15 Penhale, W. J.; Irvine, W.J.; Inglis, J. R.; Farmer, A.: Thyroiditis in T-cell depleted rats: suppression of the autoallergic response by reconstitution with normal lymphoid cells. Clin. exp. Immunol. *25:* 6 (1976).
16 Kojima, A.; Prehn, R.T.: Genetic susceptibility to post-thymectomy autoimmune diseases in mice. Immunogenetics *14:* 15 (1981).
17 Sakaguchi, S.; Takahashi, T.; Nishizuka, Y.: Study on cellular events in post-thymectomy autoimmune oophoritis in mice. II. Requirement of Lyt-1 cells in normal female mice for the prevention of oophoritis. J. exp. Med. *156:* 1577 (1982).
18 Sakaguchi, S.; Fukuma, K.; Kuribayashi, K.; Masuda, T.: Organ-specific autoimmune diseases induced in mice by elimination of a T cell subset. I. Evidence for the active participation of T cells in natural self-tolerance; deficit of a T cell subset as a possible cause of autoimmune disease. J. exp. Med. *161:* 72 (1985).
19 Miller, J. F. A. P.: Immunological function of the thymus. Lancet *ii:* 748 (1961).
20 Good, R. A.; Dalmasso, A. P.; Martinez, C.; Archer, O. K.; Pierce, J. C.; Papermaster, B. W.: The role of the thymus in development of immunological capacity in rabbits and mice. J. exp. Med. *116:* 773 (1962).
21 Zinkernagel, R. M.; Callahan, G. N.; Althage, A.; Cooper, S.; Klein, P. A.; Klein, J.: On the thymus in the differentiation of 'H-2 self recognition' by T cells. Evidence for dual recognition? J. exp. Med. *147:* 882 (1978).
22 Fink, P.J.; Bevan, M.J.: H-2 antigens of the thymus determine lymphocyte specificity. J. exp. Med. *148:* 766 (1978).
23 Boehmer, H. von; Haas, W.; Jerne, N. K.: Major histocompatibility complex-linked immune responsiveness is acquired by lymphocytes of low-responder mice differentiating in the thymus of high-responder mice. Proc. natn. Acad. Sci. USA *75:* 2439 (1978).
24 Jerne, N. K.: The somatic generation of immune recognition. Eur. J. Immunol. *1:* 1 (1971).
25 Nossal, G. J. V.; Pike, B. L.: Functional clonal deletion in immunological tolerance to major histocompatibility complex antigens. Proc. natn. Acad. Sci. USA *78:* 3844 (1981).
26 Wood, P.J.; Streilen, J.W.: Ontogeny of acquired immunological tolerance to H-2 alloantigens. Eur. J. Immunol. *12:* 188 (1982).
27 Boehmer, H. von; Schubiger, K.: Thymocytes appear to ignore class I major histocompatibility complex antigens expressed on thymus epithelial cells. Eur. J. Immunol. *14:* 1048 (1983).
28 Good, M.F.; Pyke, K.W.; Nossal, G.J.V.: Functional clonal deletion of cytotoxic T-lymphocyte precursors in chimeric thymus produced in vitro from embryonic antigen. Proc. natn. Acad. Sci. USA *80:* 3045 (1983).
29 Ready, A. R.; Jenkinson, E.J.; Kingston, R.; Owen, J. J. T.: Successful transplan-

tation across major histocompatibility barrier of deoxyguanosine-treated embryonic thymus expressing class II antigens. Nature, Lond. *310:* 231 (1984).

30 Jordan, R. K.; Robinson, J. H.; Hopkinson, N. A.; House, K. C.; Bentley, A. L.: Thymic epithelium and the induction of transplantation tolerance in nude mice. Nature, Lond. *314:* 454 (1985).

31 Lo, D.; Sprent, J.: Identity of cells that imprint H-2-restricted T-cell specificity in thymus. Nature, Lond. *319:* 672 (1986).

32 Barclay, A. N.; Mayrohofer, G. J.: Bone marrow origin of Ia-positive cells in the medulla of rat thymus. J. exp. Med. *153:* 1666 (1981).

33 Jenkinson, E. J.; Franchi, L. L.; Kingston, R.; Owen, J. J. T.: Effect of deoxyguanosine on lymphopoiesis in the developing thymus rudiment in vitro. Application in the production of chimeric thymus rudiments. Eur. J. Immunol *12:* 583 (1982).

34 Bryant, B. J.: Renewal and fate in the mammalian thymus. Mechanisms and inferences of thymocytokinetics. Eur. J. Immunol. *2:* 38 (1972).

35 McPhee, D.; Pye, J.; Shortman, R. D.: The differentiation of T lymphocytes. V. Evidence for intrathymic death of most lymphocytes. Thymus *1:* 151 (1979).

36 Beverly, P. C. L.; Brent, L.; Brooks, G.; Medawar, P. B.; Simpson, E.: In vitro reactivity of lymphoid cells from tolerant mice. Transplant. Proc. *5:* 679 (1973).

37 Brooks, C. G.: Neonatally induced transplantation tolerance. In vitro evidence supporting a clonal inactivation mechanism. Eur. J. Immunol. *5:* 741 (1975).

38 Stockinger, B.: Cytotoxic T-cell precursors revealed in neonatally tolerant mice. Proc. natn. Acad. Sci. USA *81:* 220 (1984).

39 Siskind, G. W.: Immunologic tolerance; in Paul, Fundamental immunology (Raven Press, New York 1984).

40 Gershon, R. K.; Kondo, K.: Infectious immunological tolerance. Immunology 21: 903 (1972).

41 Gammon, G.; Dunn, K.; Shastri, N.; Oki, A.; Wilbur, S.; Sercarz, E.: Neonatal T-cell tolerance to minimal immunogenic peptides is caused by clonal inactivation. Nature, Lond. *319:* 413 (1986).

42 Parkman, R.; Rosen, F. S.: Identification of a subpopulation of lymphocytes in human peripheral blood cytotoxic to autologous fibroblasts. J. exp. Med. *144:* 1520 (1976).

43 Good, M. F.; Nossal, G. J. V.: A method for the accurate determination of antihapten cytotoxic T lymphocyte precursors. Correction for apparent anti-self reactivity. J. immunol. Methods *52:* 149 (1982).

44 Reimann, J.; Miller, R. G.: Generation of autoreactive killer cells under limiting dilution conditions. J. Immun. *131:* 2128 (1983).

45 Altman, A.; Katz, D. H.: Existence of T cells manifesting self reactivity indistinguishable from alloreactivity. J. Immun. *125:* 1536 (1980).

46 Jerne, N. K.: Towards a network theory of the immune system. Annls Inst. Pasteur, Paris *125C:* 373 (1974).

47 Green, D. R.; Flood, P. M.; Gershon, R. K.: Immunoregulatory T-cell pathways. A. Rev. Immunol. *1:* 439 (1983).

48 Dorf, M. E.; Bennacerraf, B.: Suppressor cells and immunoregulation. A. Rev. Immunol. *2:* 127 (1984).

49 Tada, T.: Help, suppression, and specific factors; in Paul, Fundamental immunology (Raven Press, New York 1984).

50 Murphy, D. B.; Herzenberg, L. A.; Okumura, K.; Herzenberg, L. A.: A new I subregion (I-J) marked by a locus (Ia-4) controlling surface determinants on suppressor T lymphocytes. J. exp. Med. *144:* 699 (1976).
51 Gibson, J.; Basten, A.; Walker, K. Z.; Loblay, R. H.: A role for suppressor T cells in induction of self-tolerance. Proc. natn. Acad. Sci. USA *82:* 5150 (1985).
52 Cohen, I. R.; Holoshitz, J.; Eden, W. van; Frenkel, A.: T lymphocyte clones illuminate pathogenesis and effect therapy of experimental arthritis. Arthritis Rhem. *28:* 841 (1985).
53 Eichmann, K.; Fey, K.; Kuppers, R.; Melchers,L.; Simon, M. M.; Weltzien, H. O.: Network regulation among T cells; conclusions for limiting dilution experiments. Springer Semin. Immunopathol. *6:* 7 (1983).
54 MacPhail, S.; Stutman, O.: Suppressor T cells activated in primary in vitro response to non-major histocompatibility alloantigens. J. exp. Med. *156:* 1398 (1982).
55 Bach, S. H.; Leshem, B.; Kuperman, O. J.; Bunzendahl, H.; Alter, B. J.; Zarling, J. M.: Allosensitization to obtain anti-tumor immunity; in Fefer, Goldstein, The potential role of T cells in cancer therapy (Raven Press, New York 1982).
56 Cohen, D. J.; Lee, H. M.; Monanakumar, T.: Mechanisms of CML hyporesponsiveness in long-term renal allograft recipients. Hum. Immunol. *14:* 279 (1985).
57 Skinner, M. A.; Marbrook, J.: An estimation of the frequency of precursor cells which generate cytotoxic lymphocytes. J. exp. Med. *143:* 1562 (1976).
58 Miller, R. G.; Teh, H. -S.; Harley, E.; Phillips, R. A.: Quantitative studies of the activation of cytotoxic lymphocyte precursor cells. Immunol. Rev. *35:* 38 (1977).
59 Lefkovits, I.; Waldman, H.: Limiting dilution analysis of cells in the immune system (Cambridge University Press, London 1979).
60 MacDonald, J. R.; Cerottini, J. C.; Ryser, J. E.; Maryanski, J. L.; Taswell, C.; Widmer, M. B.; Brenner, K. T.: Quantitation and cloning of cytolytic T-lymphocytes and their precursors. Immunol. Rev. *51:* 93 (1980).
61 Taswell, C.: Limiting dilution assays for the determination of immunocompetent cell frequencies. J. Immun. *126:* 1614 (1981).
62 Lindahl, K. F.; Wilson, D. B.: Histocompatibility antigen-activated cytotoxic T lymphocytes. II. Estimates of the frequency and specificity of precursors. J. exp. Med. *145:* 508 (1977).
63 Ryser, J. E.; MacDonald, H. R.: Limiting dilution analysis of alloantigen-reactive T lymphocytes. I. Comparison of precursor frequencies for proliferative and cytolytic responses. J. Immun. *122:* 1691 (1979).
64 Ehrlich, P.; Morgenroth, J.: Über Hamalysine. Berlin klin. Woschr. *38:* 251 (1901).
65 Cairns, E.; Block, J.; Bell, D. A.: Anti-DNA autoantibody-producing hybridomas of normal human lymphoid cell origin. J. clin. Invest. *74:* 880 (1984).
66 Cairns, E.; St. Germain, J.: Bell, D. A.: The in vitro production of anti-DNA antibody by cultured peripheral blood or tonsillar lymphoid cells from normal donors and SLE patients. J. Immun. *135:* 3839 (1985).
67 Schwartz, R.: Autoantibodies and normal antibodies. Two sides of the same coin. Harvey Soc. Lect. *3* (November, 1985).
68 Howe, M. L.: Isogenic lymphocyte interaction. Responsiveness of murine thymocytes to self antigens. J. Immun. *100:* 1090 (1973).
69 Weksler, M. E.; Moody, C. E.; Kozak, R. W.: The autologous mixed lymphocyte reaction. Adv. Immunol. *31:* 271 (1981).

70 Glimcher, L. H.; Longo, D. L.; Green, I.; Schwartz, R. H.: Murine syngeneic mixed lymphocyte response. I. Target antigens are self Ia molecules. J. exp. Med. *154:* 1652 (1981).

71 Dos Reis, G. A.; Shevach, E. M.: The syngeneic mixed leukocyte reaction represents polyclonal activation of antigen-specific T lymphocytes with receptors for self-Ia antigens. J. Immun. *127:* 2456 (1981).

72 Bensussan, A.; Meuer, S. C.; Schlossman, S. F.; Reinerz, E. L.: Delineation of an immunoregulatory amplifier population recognizing autologous Ia molecules. J. exp. Med. *159:* 559 (1984).

73 Faherty, D. A.; Johnson, D. R.; Zauderer, M.: Origin and specificity of autoreactive T cells in antigen-induced populations. J. exp. Med. *161:* 1293 (1985).

74 Tomonari, K.: In vivo helper activity of autoreactive T cell clones. J. Immun. *135:* 1598 (1985).

75 Stephenson, S. P.; Roser, B.: The molecular basis of transplantation tolerance. Transplant. Proc. *17:* 1145 (1985).

76 Dorsch, S.; Roser, B.: Suppressor cells and transplantation tolerance. Transplantation *33:* 518 (1982).

77 Kimura, H.; Wilson, D. B.: Anti-idiotypic cytotoxic T cells in rats with graft versus host disease. Nature, Lond. *308:* 463 (1984).

78 Lancaster, F.; Chui, Y. L.; Batchelor, J. R.: Anti-idiotypic T cells suppress rejection of renal allografts in rats. Nature, Lond. *315:* 336 (1985).

79 Miller, R. G.: In Sercarz, Cunningham, Strategies of immune regulation (Academic Press, New York 1980).

80 Rammensee, H. G.; Nagy, Z. A.; Klein, J.: Suppression of cell-mediated lymphocytotoxicity against minor histocompatibility antigens mediated by Lyt1+Lyt2+ T cells of stimulator strain origin. Eur. J. Immunol. *12:* 930 (1982).

81 Fink, P. J.; Weissman, I. L.; Bevan, M. J.: Haplotype-specific suppression of cytotoxic T cell induction by antigen inappropriately presented on T cells. J. exp. Med. *157:* 141 (1983).

82 Fink, P. J.; Rammensee, H. G.; Bevan, M. J.: Cloned cytolytic T cells can suppress primary cytotoxic responses directed against them. J. Immun. *133:* 1775 (1984).

83 Claesson, M. H.; Miller, R. G.: Functional heterogeneity in allospecific cytotoxic T cell clones. I. CTL clones express strong anti-self suppressive activity. J. exp. Med. *160:* 1702 (1984).

84 Meuer, S. C.; Schlossman, S. F.; Reinerz, E. L.: Clonal analysis of human cytotoxic T lymphocytes: T4+ and T8+ effector cells recognize products of different major histocompatibility complex regions. Proc. natn. Acad. Sci. USA *79:* 4395 (1982).

85 Rabin, H.; Hopkins, R. F.; Ruscett, F. W.; Neubauer, R. H.; Brown, R. L.; Kawzkami, T. G.: Spontaneous release of a factor with properties of T cell growth factor from a continuous line of primate tumor T cells. J. Immun. *127:* 1852 (1981).

Dr. Neal Flomberg, Assistant Attending Physician and Assistant Member, Memorial Sloan-Kettering Cancer Center, 1275 York Avenue, New York, NY 10021 (USA)

Concepts Immunopathol., vol. 4, pp. 42–76 (Karger, Basel 1987)

Origin and Significance of Autoantibodies

G. Dighiero, A. Kaushik, P. Poncet, X.R. Ge[1]

Unité Immunohématologie et Immunopathologie, Institut Pasteur, Paris, France

Introduction

According to Burnet's [1] clonal selection theory, explanations for tolerance and autoimmunity were attractively simple and clear. Autoreactive lymphocytes are purged during embryonic life to provide self tolerance, and autoantibodies, always noxious, correspond to the expression of mutant forbidden clones which are able to circumvent the process of immunological regulation. During the last several years, however, a considerable amount of data has succeeded in raising doubts concerning the clonal deletion theory as a general explanation for tolerance [2], since (a) autoimmune diseases can be induced by injecting organ extracts; (b) the presence of numerous autoantibodies in the serum have been demonstrated in the normal population [3]; (c) evidence exists for the presence of normal autoreactive B cells [4]; (d) the expression of autoantibodies in normal animals occurs upon mitogenic stimulation.

The first description of natural autoantibodies was reported by Landsteiner in 1900, when he discovered the presence of natural hemaglutinins in serum directed against blood group determinants of the ABO system. In 1964, Boyden [5] defined natural antibodies as a family of molecules present in the body fluids of normal animals which are able to specifically combine with antigens but not with the immunologically acceptable molecules normally present in the body fluids. Nevertheless, natural antibodies directed against various antigens, and often against self antigens, have been described in different animal species. Indeed, a clear distinction between autoantibodies and natural antibodies is difficult to establish.

[1] The skillful secretarial assistance of Miss Francine Auzeloux is acknowledged.

Furthermore, the distinction between physiological natural autoantibodies and noxious autoantibodies remains unclear until now. Even though, the pathogenic role of autoantibodies directed against red blood cells in the case of autoimmune hemolytic anemias and the role of autoantibodies directed against intercellular substances in the case of pemphigus vulgaris are well defined, the responsibility of autoantibodies in the pathogenesis of several autoimmune diseases is presently a matter of discussion. Certain results from clinical trials, indicating an absence of good correlation between the level of autoantibodies against DNA and the clinical course of systemic lupus erythematosus (SLE), as well as the level of autoantibodies against the acelylcholine receptor and the course of myasthenia gravis raise some doubts concerning the pathogenic role of these autoantibodies [6]. It can be argued that noxious autoantibodies constitute only a subpopulation of the detected autoantibodies and methods employed for their detection may overestimate nonpathogenic autoantibodies.

Even though autoantibodies constitute an important issue in the comprehension of autoimmunity, increasing evidence concerning the role of T cells and the major histocompatibility complex has accumulated. Besides the classical model of experimental allergic encephalomyelitis, it has recently been claimed that T cells may inhibit the secretion of insulin by Langerhans cells in the case of murine diabetes [7]. The predisposing role of certain haplotypes like HLA A1, B8, DR3, in the case of autoimmune diseases is well established. Recent work, showing aberrant expression of HLA-DR antigens on thyrocytes from Graves' disease [8], and now extended to other autoimmune diseases, raises the question of the role of this aberrant expression in the stimulation of autoreactive T cells. Finally, the role of sexual hormones has also been well defined.

In this article, we shall discuss the currently available data on autoantibodies which could help elucidate their origin and significance. We have chosen the following two well-documented models of autoimmunity in the studies with which we have been involved. Besides being diverse in their molecular characteristics, ontogeny and physiological or pathological manifestations, these models are representative of natural autoimmunity and autoimmune diseases.

(A) Autoantibodies against mouse erythrocytes in physiological and pathological conditions.

(B) Autoantibodies against DNA and cytoskeletal proteins in physiological and pathological conditions in mouse and humans.

The importance of autoreactive B cell repertoire and role of natural autoantibodies and their relationship with pathogenic autoantibodies will be discussed.

Autoantibodies against Mouse Erythrocytes

In both normal and autoimmune strains of mouse, a number of spontaneously occurring autoantibodies against different erythrocyte antigens, i.e. X, HB, HOL and I, have been described. In the NZB mouse, anti-X autoantibody is involved in the characteristic autoimmune hemolytic anemia. However, anti-HB autoantibodies ubiquitous in all mouse strains do not seem to be associated with the pathological syndrome, and, hence, are of physiological significance with no specific role prescribed as yet. Here, we shall present data on antimouse erythrocyte autoantibodies of the aforesaid categories.

Natural Autoantibodies against Bromelin-Treated Mouse Erythrocytes (HB)

Bromelin Treatment of Erythrocytes and Autoimmunity. A normal unimmunized mouse possesses B cells secreting antibodies against its own erythrocytes, pretreated with the proteolytic enzyme bromelin [9, 10] which are demonstrable by direct plaque forming cell (PFC) assay and seric hemolytic titer. This autoimmune phenomenon was first described in the autoimmune prone NZB strain, in 1973, by Linder and Edgington [11] but was soon extended to normal strains including CBA/J, C57bl/6, Balb/c, nude and germ-free mice at the level of spleen [12, 13] and peritoneal cells (PerC) [14, 15].

The antigen unmasked by bromelin enzyme treatment is not a newly created antigen but represents a normal hidden autoantigen (auto-Ag), called HB auto-Ag, since: (1) injection of bromelinized mouse red blood cells (BrMRBC) in mice does not induce any increase in PFC (without any higher clearance of BrMRBC than sheep RBC which are highly immunogenic) [12, 13, 15, 17]; (2) injection of normal mouse red blood cells to rats induces antibodies to both normal and enzyme-treated mouse erythrocytes [12]; (3) a soluble erythrocyte analogue of the cryptic membrane autoantigen (SEA-HB) is present in the serum of normal mice [18].

The Anti-BrMRBC Autoantibody. An important characteristic of this autoimmune model is that anti-HB Ig is mainly restricted to the IgM class [9, 13, 15, 18–21]. This autoantibody (auto Ab) secretory activity has been found in all mouse strains with quantitative differences in its expression as number of PFC [9, 13, 15, 16, 22] and such variations are not under the control of H-2 locus [22, 23]. Murine hybridomas secreting IgM monoclonal autoAb against BrMRBC (CP hybridomas) have been established [23, 25] from PerC of NZB and CBA/J mice and secreted autoantibodies have been shown to recognize the same HB determinant [26].

A rabbit polyclonal anti-idiotype reagent was raised against Fab fragments of one of these CP IgM [23]. This reagent inhibited anti-BrMRBC PFC from all CP hybridomas irrespective of clones as well as PFC from polyclonal PerC populations of different strains. These results indicate a structural V region relatedness among anti-BrMRBC auto-Ab secreted by different cells [23].

The cross-reactive idiotype borne by anti-BrMRBC auto-Ab (CP idiotype) was detected in normal mouse sera. Ontogenic studies indicated that CP idiotype levels increased as a function of age and reached a maximum in adult, but were not detectable in newborn [23]. Furthermore, there exists a good correlation at the strain level, between differential quantitative expression of anti-BrMRBC PFC and corresponding seric serum CP idiotype [27]. Moreover, peritoneal cell autoimmune phenomenon is markedly expressed in CBA/J, a normal mouse strain based on highest CP idiotype over serum IgM ratio observed in all the strains tested.

The first 35 amino acids of light and heavy chains for 4 monoclonal auto Ab (3 from NZB, 1 from CBA) have, recently, been sequenced which show a high degree of homology (1 substitution on one H chain, 1 substitution on 2 L chains). These results are in agreement with those obtained with anti-idiotypic studies [23].

Idiotypic and structural data considered with the fact that anti-BrMRBC belong to the IgM class, suggest that anti-BrMRBC autoantibodies have a restricted level of V region diversity.

The Autoantigen. Bromelin acts principally on band III of erythrocyte membrane and does not involve any activation of membrane endogenous enzyme for exposure of the antigenic site [28]. After double-dimension gel electrophoresis of iodinated surface proteins of bromelin-treated erythrocytes, an intense interference in labelling due to phospholipids was observed in contrast to the pattern obtained with non-bromelin-treated erythrocytes [Poncet et al., unpubl. observations]. Hence, it can be postulated that digestion of band III with bromelin may induce a structural reorganization of the membrane and results in exposure of polar heads of phospholipids. The involvement of phospholipids in the antigenic determinants recognized on BrMRBC is supported by several findings.

In 1973, Linder and Edgington [18, 29] described a soluble erythrocyte analogue of HB auto-Ag SEA-HB, present in a high molecular weight plasma fraction (approximatively $3 \cdot 10^6$ daltons) and was associated with low density lipoprotein (LDL).

Serban et al. [30] showed that trimethyl ammonium (TMA) containing compounds can inhibit complement dependent lysis of BrMRBC by monoclonal anti-BrMRBC auto-Ab. TMA is a moiety present on phosphorylcholine (PC), an ubiquitous molecule, which is included in the phosphatidyl choline component of membrane. However, anti-BrMRBC auto-Ab are not identical to anti-PC Ab since their affinity for PC is 100 times lower than a 'true' anti-PC Ab (1–5 $10^3 M^{-1}$ v. $2 \cdot 10^5$ M^{-1}) [23]. Hence, TMA is likely to constitute a part of the antigenic determinant. More recently, Cox and Hardy [31] demonstrated that phosphatidylcholine in a certain configuration on liposomes is recognized by anti-BrMRBC autoAb. Similarly, cholesterol particles covered with phosphatidylcholine are specifically agglutinated by monoclonal auto-Ab [Poncet et al., unpubl. observations].

B Cells Involved in Secretion of Anti-BrMRBC Autoantibody. The anti-BrMRBC secreting cells in normal mice were first observed in spleen [9, 10] and subsequently among PerC [14, 15]. In fact, Bussard [19] had already demonstrated that B cells from the peritoneal cavity of a normal unimmunized mouse secreted antisheep erythrocyte IgM antibodies. Hence, these results were interpreted as a consequence of a cross-reactivity between SRBC and BrMRBC [14]. After 4 days of in vitro culture, the PerC anti-BrMRBC plaque forming activity (PFA) dramatically increases without involving cell division [15, 16, 20, 32, 33]. The cells secreting this antibody are already differentiated and are only repressed for secretion without in vitro culture [33, 34]. A large number of peritoneal B cells are engaged in synthesising anti-BrMRBC IgM auto-Ab [32] which undergo curious morphological modifications during in vitro culture [35].

Why the peritoneal cavity is the preferential site of localisation of anti-BrMRBC secreting cells and why cells are repressed for secretion at the onset of the culture is still obscure, however.

The limiting dilution experiments led Cox et al. [36] to suggest that derepression in culture is under the control of a factor released by other cells. Collizzi et al. [37] proposed IL-1 as a possible factor.

A subpopulation of B cells, Ly 1B, that bears both IgM and Ly1 markers sorted out by cytofluorometry [38] has been reported to be engaged in secretion of IgM autoAb against T cells, DNA and BrMRBC [39]. Interestingly, Ly 1B cells constitute 40–80% of IgM-bearing PerC in NZB, 20–40% in Balb/c, 1–5% in SJL and lack totally in CBA/N [40]. This subset represents 1–2% of splenic cells in normal mouse strains and 5–10% of NZB splenocytes. These results are in agreement with regard to anti-BrMRBC PerC PFA and amount of circulating CP idiotype [27]. However, it remains unclear whether the Ly1B cell subpopulation includes all auto-Ab secreting cells. More recently, the Herzenberg group [41] employing cell transfer studies has shown that Ly1B cells seem to correspond to a distinct developmental lineage, and the peritoneal cavity could constitute the unique location of progenitors of Ly1B in adult.

Autoantibodies against Other Erythrocyte Antigens

The characteristic autoimmune type of Coombs'-positive hemolytic anemia observed in NZB is associated with the appearance of autoantibodies which increase with age [42] and react with an exposed labile glycoprotein erythrocyte surface autoantigen [13]. Certain characteristics of hemolytic anemia, namely spherocytosis, reticulocytosis, enhanced osmotic fragility of red blood cells, decreased red blood survival in vivo and splenomegaly [43] are similar to hemolytic anemia observed in humans. A soluble analogue of erythrocyte bound X antigen, termed SEA-X (molecular weight approximately 2×10^5 daltons), has been detected in plasma of all mouse strains with different H-2 haplotypes [13, 18]. However, anti-X autoantibody is restricted to the NZB strain which is because of the exclusive presence of X-binding T helper cells in these mice, though X-autoantigen binding B cells are present in all mouse strains examined [44]. The anti-X autoantibodies are predominantly of the IgG class, and are equally distributed among IgG1, IgG2a and IgG2b subclasses [13].

Holborow et al. [45] have described an autoantibody, predominantly of IgG class, in NZB directed against antigens exposed in dried red cell smears and on erythrocyte stromata but are inaccessible to autoantibody on intact erythrocytes. It has been suggested that this autoantigen may be the murine analogue of spectrin, a component of the internal aspect of red cell membrane [46]. Another cold-reactive IgM autoantibody directed against cryptic murine erythrocyte autoantigen (I) but exposed on human erythrocytes has been reported [47]. These autoantibodies are found in several murine strains but their pathogenic significance has not been elucidated [45, 47].

Lewis et al. [48] produced eleven monoclonal antimouse erythrocyte autoantibodies from unimmunized NZB mice which differed in their antigenic reactivities and immunoglobulin isotypes. All of them reacted with intact mouse red cells while two of them cross-reacted with sheep erythrocytes and bromelin-treated mouse erythrocytes.

Recently, Ozaki et al. [49] obtained two monoclonal IgM autoantibodies from a nonimmunized NZB mouse which reacted with exposed erythrocyte autoantigens but were distinct from anti-X, anti-HB, anti-HOL, and anti-I autoantibodies. Interestingly, implantation of these hybridoma cells induced hemolytic anemia associated with marked splenomegaly. The authors proposed that varieties of erythrocyte autoantibodies may be involved in the development of naturally occurring hemolytic anemia in NZB.

Normal Autoantibodies against DNA and Cytoskeleton Proteins in Humans and Mice:

During preparation of specific antisera against tubulin, Karsenti et al. [50] detected the presence of natural antitubulin antibodies in the sera of normal human and several species of normal nonimmunized animals. They subsequently isolated and characterized these antibodies, which were able to bind with tubulin. For several years at the Unité d'Immunocytochimie of the Pasteur Institute, we have tried to confirm and extend these results. Our results, together with the results of other groups, will be presented here under five main topics.

Natural Autoantibodies Constitute an Important Fraction of Normal Circulating Human Serum Ig. In order to demonstrate natural autoantibodies in normal human serum, we, in collaboration with Brigitte Guilbert and Stratis Avrameas [51], immobilized nine different antigens (tubulin, actin, thyroglobulin, myoglobin, fetuin, albumin, transferrin, collagen and cytochrome C) on ACA 34 beads. Sera from normal donors were successively passed through the nine immunoadsorbents. The eluted proteins, composed mainly of IgG (about 70%) but also IgA and IgM (about 15% each), as well as their Fab fractions, were tested by noncompetitive and competitive Elisa against the nine antigens. The competitive enzyme immunoassays enabled classification of the isolated antibodies into three groups: (1) Composed of antitubulin and antithyroglobulin antibodies, which could only be inhibited by the homologous antigen. (2) Consisting of antiactin, antifetuin and antimyoglobin antibodies which were chiefly inhibited by their homologous antigens, but also and to a significant degree, by two or three additional antigens. Thus, the binding of antiactin antibodies to immobilized actin was mainly inhibited by actin; however, tubulin and thyroglobulin also inhibited the reaction to a certain extent. (3) Comprised of antialbumin, antitransferrin, anticollagen and anticytochrome 'C' antibodies which clearly reacted by their Fab portions, but failed to exhibit significant levels of inhibition, when preincubated with the homologous antigen. Additional proof concerning the specificity of the binding was afforded by immunocytochemical staining of human cultured hepatocytes. Subsequently, Lutz and Wipf [52] demonstrated the constant presence of natural autoantibodies against skeletal proteins of red blood cells among the IgG fractions of sera of healthy human subjects. These results conform to those from other groups, who succeeded in showing the presence in normal serum of natural antibodies directed against brain antigens [53], thymus cells [54], carbohydrate components [55], denatured human collagen, elastin, collagen, gelatin, normal erythrocytes, thyroid components, gammaglobulin and gastric parietal cells [56], lymphocytes [57, 58] and IgG [59].

Human Monoclonal Ig (MIg), Frequently Correspond to Expansion of a Clone Normally Producing a Natural Autoantibody. MIg were considered as abnormal immunoglobulins without known functional antibody activity for a long time. Structural studies carried out during the last two decades have indicated that MIg correspond to normal synthetic products whose counterparts can be found in the heterogeneous normal Ig population. Some MIg have been shown to possess antibody activity directed against autoantigens, bacterial antigens and haptens. Kritzman et al. [60] reported the first case of monoclonal IgM with anti-Fc activity and Williams et al. [61] reported the first case of monoclonal IgM with an antibody activity directed against the Ii blood group, in cases of cold agglutinin disease. Although these reactivities, mostly confined to the IgM isotype, appear to occur frequently, yet the incidence of other auto- and heteroantigen antibody activities appear to be negligible.

The results obtained with normal human serum prompted us, together with Brigitte Guilbert, Peggy Lymberi, Stratis Avrameas, Jean-Paul Fermand and Françoise Danon, to examine whether some MIg possessed antibody activity against actin, tubulin, myosin, thyroglobulin, dsDNA, myoglobin, fetuin, albumin and transferrin [62, 63].

Serum samples comprising a total of 612 different MIg (273 IgG, 136 IgA, 158 IgM, 30 Bence-Jones proteins, 31 IgD and 13 double MIg) were tested by Elisa methods. Five hundred and seventy-six sera out of the 612 examined, did not exhibit binding in excess of normal values. The remaining 36 sera were found to display antibody activity against one or more antigen. One MIg (IgM) bound to dsDNA only, one (IgAK) mainly to myosin and, to a lesser extent, to actin and tubulin. The 32 other MIg (7 IgGK, 6 IgG, 10 IgMK, 5 IgM, 2 IgAK and 1 IgA) reacted chiefly with actin, but also constantly and significantly with tubulin and thyroglobulin. Furthermore, 5 of these 32 MIg also displayed binding against myosin.

The specificity of the interaction of these MIg with the respective antigen was demonstrated by competitive and noncompetitive Elisa and immunocytologic and immunoblotting experiments. Furthermore, it was demonstrated that the binding was mediated by the dynamic fragment (F(ab')2 of the MIg.

Interestingly, retrospective clinical analysis was possible for 31 out of the 36 patients. Twenty-six patients displayed malignant lymphoplasmocytic disorders. The five others were followed for miscellaneous disorders without signs of multiple myeloma or Waldenström's macroglobulinemia. The data for the 31 patients were analyzed in order to determine whether there was any relationship between the antibody activity of the MIg and the symptoms shown by the patient. No such relationship was, however, demonstrable. Indeed, the patient with a monoclonal anti-dsDNA did not show any symptoms related to systemic lupus erythematosus, and no symptoms could be related to the presence of anticytoskeleton antibodies in the 30 other patients examined.

Studies on Autoreactive B Cell Repertoire by Production of Hybridoma Cell Lines Secreting Natural Monoclonal Autoantibodies. The presence of natural autoantibodies under normal physiological conditions implies necessarily the presence of autoreactive B lymphocytes. In order to demonstrate their presence, in collaboration with Peggy Lymberi, Jean-Claude Mazié, R. Whalen, G. Butler-Browne and S. Avrameas, we employed hybridoma technology to fuse unimmunized BALB/c splenocytes with nonsecreting myelomas. The Ig-secreting hybrids were tested for antibody activity against the cytoskeleton proteins, DNA and TNP. From 161 Ig-secreting cases (IgM in most cases), obtained from unimmunized 12-week-old BALB/c mice, 2 were found to react exclusively with DNA, 1 with DNA and cytoskeleton proteins, 1 exclusively with thyroglobulin and 1 mainly with myosin, but also significantly with actin, tubulin, spectrin and dsDNA [64].

Two of the clones reacting with DNA and the clone binding to thyroglobulin were lost during the first week of culture. The two remaining clones were subcloned and injected into BALB/c mice to induce ascites. The first one corresponded to an IgM (D23), which reacted mainly with dsDNA and exhibited important reactivity with cytoskeleton proteins in direct binding experiments. However, only significant inhibition was obtained with dsDNA during competitive enzyme immunoassays. The second clone (E7) was also an IgM, mainly binding to myosin, but also reacting significantly with actin, tubulin, myosin, spectrin, TNP and dsDNA. Competition experiments indicated that the binding to myosin was specifically inhibited by mouse myosin, but also (to a lesser but significant extent) by actin, tubulin, spectrin, TNP and dsDNA. Blotting experiments, as well as immunocytochemical analysis confirmed the reactivity with cytoskeleton proteins. Furthermore, the binding to myosin could be more clearly defined. It was thus demonstrated that E7 was reacting with rat, rabbit, mouse and chicken myosin, and although it was found to bind with light meromyosin, heavy meromyosin, S2, S1 and rod fragments, no reaction was observed with the light chain of myosin. The reactivity with dsDNA, was further substantiated by the fact that E7 reacted to purified dsDNA obtained from PBR 322 plasmid.

To gain insight into the ontogeny of autoreactive B cell repertoire, together with P. Lymbery, D. Holmberg, I. Lundquist, A. Coutinho and S. Avrameas, we tested a large collection of Ig-secreting natural hybridomas, obtained from 6-day-old BALB/c and BALB.B10 unimmunized mice [65]. Results indicated: (1) A high frequency of the auto-reactive

B-cell repertoire in newborn mice. This frequency, in the case of BALB/c mice approached 10%. (2) The clones obtained displayed, in most cases, a broad polyspecific reactivity.

Similar results with BALB/c mice, were recently reported by Monier et al. [66]. Cairns et al. [67] also obtained anti-DNA autoantibodies with a spectrum of nucleic acid specificities similar to systemic lupus erythematosus, with hybridomas obtained from normal human tonsillar lymphoid cells. Prabhakar et al. [68] were also able to obtain hybridomas from B lymphocytes of SJL/J or BALB/cJ mice, which showed multiple organ reactivity.

A High Incidence of Cross-Reactive Idiotypes Among Murine Natural Autoantibodies. Since natural autoantibodies are present in significant amounts in normal physiological conditions, we were interested in analyzing the idiotype of these antibodies. Anti-idiotypic (id) antibodies, against the two D23 and E7 clones of adult BALB/c origin and exhibiting a widespread binding, were induced in rabbits. These anti-id reagents were used to explore the binding of 12 natural monoclonal autoantibodies, obtained from adult and newborn unimmunized mice. Both anti-id reagents (anti-E7 and anti-D23) recognized cross-reactive idiotopes frequently shared by natural monoclonal autoantibodies. All the antibodies exhibiting cross-reactive idiotopes displayed widespread reactivity with structurally dissimilar self and non-self antigens. Both anti-D23 and anti-E7 recognized idiotopes localized next to the paratope, since their binding to the homologous id was inhibited by the antigen. On the contrary, the cross-reactive idiotopes seemed to be located outside their antigen-binding sites. Finally, these idiotopes were also detected in normal mouse BALB/c serum [69].

B Lymphocyte Subset Involved in the Production of Autoantibodies. As pointed out earlier, virtually all IgM autoantibody secreting activity against DNA and BrMRBC [39] resides in Ly1B cells ($Ly1^+$, $thy1^-$, high IgM^+, low IgD^+ and Ia^+). An alternative approach has emerged with the availability of CBA/N mice, a sex-linked immunodeficient mouse strain defined by the presence of a gene or closely linked group of genes (known as Xid genes). This strain is mainly characterized by the absence of a subset of B lymphocytes defined by the presence of the Lyb-5 surface marker, low density surface membrane IgM and the absence of complement receptors [70]. The main immunologic abnormality of these mice is evident by their failure to respond to TI-2 antigens [70, 71]. When challenged with LPS or poly (IC), CBA/N mice or male hybrids obtained from CBA/N mothers with normal strains, secrete little or no anti-DNA and anti-altered erythrocyte autoantibodies, whereas normal strains or F1 females obtained from CBA/N mothers produce large amounts of these autoantibodies. The latter results along with those obtained with (CBA/N × NZB)F1 mice and especially with congenic NZB-Xid, which do not manifest the autoimmune syndrome characteristic of NZB mice, led some authors to propose that the $Lyb3^+$ 5^+ cells lacking in Xid mice may be important in autoantibody production and that in their absence autoantibody production is markedly reduced [71].

To explore this problem, we recently fused spleen cells from 6-day-old (CBA/N × BALB/c)F1 male and female mice, to a nonsecreting myeloma. According to the X-linked recessive inheritance of the Xid gene, the mating of a CBA/N female with a male from a normal strain yields male offspring expressing the Xid defect, whereas the female offspring are heterozygous and phenotypically normal [70]. Hence, we compared the MIg secreted by males to those secreted by females, for their ability to react with DNA, cytoskeletal proteins and TNP. Our results failed to show any significant differences between males and females [72]. Thus, it seems that CBA/N mice carry the genetic information for the production of natural autoantibodies against these antigens. Recently, Smith et al. [73], tried to integrate both approaches by studying in NZB and NZB-Xid mice, the frequencies of $Lyb5^+$ and $Lyb5^-$ B cells, within the $Ly1^+$ B subset. Even though they concluded that most of the $Ly1^+$ B cells fell largely in the $Lyb5^+$ compartment and that autoantibody-producing $Ly1^+$ B cells were predominantly $Lyb5^+$; they could, however, demonstrate that a small percentage of $Lyb5^-$ $Ly1^+$ B cells could produce autoantibodies against DNA and bromelin-treated mouse red blood cells.

Lupus Autoantibodies against DNA and Cytoskeleton Proteins

Human and mouse systemic lupus erythematosus (SLE), an organ nonspecific autoimmune manifestation characterized by B cell hyperactivity resulting in gross serological abnormalities, offers a useful model to gain insight into the etiopathogenesis of this disorder, besides understanding immunoregulation and autoimmunity in general. These studies on SLE offer a useful approach in delineating the aforesaid aspects as defective humoral self reactivity in this disorder which is initiated without any known external agent. The availability of a variety of mouse inbred strains like NZB, NZW, MRL, BXSB, Palmerstrom North and Motheaten, which spontaneously develop a disease similar to human SLE has allowed considerable progress in the comprehension of the complex pathogenetic mechanisms leading to this disorder. Possible analogies between human and murine lupus and the complete histopathologic, serologic, lymphocytic, virologic, hormonal and genetic characteristics of immune lupus have been reviewed earlier [71, 74, 75]. Hence, a detailed description of the above-mentioned subjects is excluded.

In this section, only recent information resulting mainly from studies performed with monoclonal autoantibodies, obtained with lymphocytes from autoimmune lupus mouse strains and from human SLE patients will be considered. This information will relate essentially to the following three topics.

(a) Polyspecificity among lupus anti-DNA autoantibodies. (b) Idiotypic and structural analysis of lupus monoclonal autoantibodies. (c) The stimulating immunogen in lupus.

Polyspecificity among Lupus Anti-DNA Autoantibodies. The development of SLE in mouse and man is accompanied by the appearance of autoantibodies exhibiting multiple binding specificities against a number of (a) intracellular antigens (DNA, RNA, Sm, RNP, histones, nucleolus, mitochondrias, lyzosomes, ribosomes, etc.); (b) cell membrane (determinants on erythrocytes, lymphocytes, neutrophils, neurones, platelets, muscles, etc.); (c) extracellular plasma components (immunoglobulins, complement components, clotting factors, etc.).

The most conspicuous among these lupus autoantibodies are those recognizing nuclear antigens, i.e. DNA, RNA, nuclear proteins and protein-nucleic acid complexes [76, 77]. The autoantibodies selectively reacting with double-stranded DNA (dsDNA) are considered to be the most pathogenic [74, 78]. Conventionally, these autoantibodies are believed to form DNA-anti-DNA immune complexes which fix complement and initiate inflammatory reaction resulting in tissue destruction. Such a befittingly simple description becomes complex because of the wide spectrum of reactivities of anti-DNA autoantibodies including their diversity of reaction with nuclear antigens alone. A majority of the lupus autoantibodies react with single stranded DNA and not with the native helical structure [79]. Some of them react with nucleosides [80] including cytidine and guanosine [81] while others specific for single-stranded DNA (ssDNA) recognize short base sequences [82, 83]. The nucleoside-protein-Sepharose conjugate containing nucleosides of all the four DNA bases has been shown to absorb all anti-ssDNA activity from serum of MRL-lpr/lpr, NZB and NZW strains in contrast to anti-dsDNA activity. A conjugate with guanosine alone removes 60% anti-ssDNA activity while thymidine eliminates 25% of this reactivity [84]. A similar heterogeneity among these lupus serum autoantibodies is revealed by their varying activity towards synthetic polynucleotides [78]. The lupus autoantibodies also exhibit reactivity to poly (A) [85], ssRNA [86], dsRNA [87], RNA-DNA hybrid [88] and poly (ADP ribose) [89]. Some lupus autoantibodies react with both ssDNA and Z helical DNA or the Z form alone [90]. The majority of patients with active SLE possess serum autoantibodies reacting with cardiolipin [91] which cause a biologically false-positive test for syphilis. Moreover, the reactivity towards cardiolipid resides in the DNA binding fraction of lupus serum [92]. Nevertheless, most of the high-titered anti-DNA sera from patients with active SLE have a stronger binding to DNA than cardiolipin [93].

The lupus-derived monoclonal anti-DNA autoantibodies from mice and humans show a parallel pattern of reactivity as observed from serum autoantibodies and, hence, have been of immense value in understanding the wide array of polyspecificity of lupus autoantibodies [94–103]. Many monoclonal anti-DNA autoantibodies are multispecific since they react with a number of unrelated antigens such as phospholipids [96, 100, 104, 105], vimentin [99, 106], rheumatoid factor [107], proteoglycan [108], cell surface proteins [109], platelets [95], nucleosome subunits of chromatin [107] and klebsiella antigens [110]. Most of the monoclonal anti-DNA autoantibodies exhibit better binding specificity towards ssDNA compared to native DNA. Some of these autoantibodies possess specific reactivity for individual bases or nucleotides with guanine and oligo (dt) sequences being predominant determinants [84, 111–113] while others exhibit preferential specificity for dsDNA [96, 114, 115]. The reactivity of a single antibody molecule with multiple polynucleotides in some cases, has been believed to be caused by an antigenic determinant residing in a phosphodiester-linked phosphate structure which is common to all polynucleotides. These phosphodiester containing epitopes are also responsible for the ability of some monoclonal anti-DNA autoantibodies to react with certain phospholipids including cardiolipin [105, 106]. Ten of 21 human monoclonal anti-DNA autoantibodies have been shown to react with cardiolipin [113]. Moreover, hybridomas derived from cardiolipin immunized mice produced monoclonal antibodies that bound not only to cardiolipin but also to ssDNA and even to dsDNA [104]. However, Shoenfeld et al. [96] have demonstrated that only about 30% of monoclonal anti-DNA antibodies competed with cardiolipin. Furthermore, cardiolipin failed to compete with the DNA binding of NZB/NZW derived monoclonal antibodies [117]. Recent trends indicate that only a minor subset of anti-DNA autoantibodies cross-react with cardiolipin [118]. Morgan et al. [103] have employed lupus-derived monoclonal anti-DNA autoantibodies to define five antigenic determinants based on their reaction pattern in Elisa, precipitation assay and indirect immunofluorescence assay on cells. The first group of monoclonal autoantibodies recognizes conformational determinants expressed on dsDNA only; the second group reacts with backbone dependent sugar phosphate determinants on both ssDNA and dsDNA; the third group recognizes antigenic determinants predominantly expressed on ssDNA and weakly present on dsDNA; the fourth group reacts with base dependent determinants on ssDNA; the fifth group reacts with determinants on ssDNA which are also expressed weakly on dsDNA and RNA.

These observations suggest that monoclonal anti-DNA autoantibodies are collectively of limited heterogeneity with regard to their specificity. The minor correlation observed between different assays for anti-DNA antibodies could be because of the varying range of affinities and cross-reactivities measured by each system. Moreover, some of the cross-reactivities could be a result of interaction between the polyanionic structure of DNA and positively charged immunoglobulin molecules. Similar cross-reactions with dextran sulfate and heparan sulfate both of which contain repeating anionic groups have been reported [108].

Idiotypic and Structural Analysis of Lupus Monoclonal Autoantibodies. Rauch et al. [119] employing a polyclonal rabbit antiDNA monoclonal autoantibody idiotype (H130) from MRL lpr/lpr mouse detected cross-reactions with 8 of 12 other MRL derived monoclonal anti-DNA autoantibodies and showed its presence in all the 40 MRL sera tested. These findings were substantiated by Tron et al. [120] who employed a monoclonal anti-idiotypic reagent against NZB/NZW F1 anti-DNA antibody (F227) to demonstrate the presence of F227 idiotype in all the 24 NZB/NZW F1 mice examined. Marion et al. [121] made similar observations using rabbit antiserum against NZB/NZW F1 derived monoclonal anti-DNA antibody to detect a common idiotype on 8 of 13 monoclonal autoantibodies possessing similar binding specificities.

Shoenfeld et al. [96] employing three anti-idiotypic reagents against monoclonal human anti-DNA autoantibodies, each recognizing distinct idiotypic structures, demonstrated extensive cross-reactivities among 60 human anti-DNA monoclonal autoantibodies. The screening of serum from 9 lupus patients by these 3 reagents revealed that 54% of them possessed a common or shared idiotype (16/6). Moreover, the idiotype profile correlated well with the clinical status of 12 patients examined serially [122]. Similarly, Soloman et al. [123] prepared an anti-idiotypic reagent related to anti-dsDNA antibody purified from lupus patient serum and demonstrated cross-reacting idiotype in 8 of 9 patients' serum.

Four idiotypically related monoclonal anti-DNA autoantibodies from different patients have been found to have identical amino terminal light chain and similar amino terminal heavy chain sequences [124]. Eilat et al. [117] have sequenced heavy and light chains of anti-RNA and anti-DNA monoclonal autoantibodies from NZB/NZW F1 mice and shown that most of the heavy chains were from the V_HII gene group with some base substitutions. One of the anti-DNA antibodies was from the V_HIII group and had only one base substitution compared to a germline anti-phosphorylcholine antibody. In this context, even more remarkable is the finding that a point mutation in the V_H gene of mouse myeloma changed the antigenic specificity of its immunoglobulin from antiphosphorylcholine to anti-DNA [125]. The nucleotide sequence data on monoclonal anti-DNA autoantibodies from MRL/1 mouse [126] have shown that the heavy chain 5, untranslated region, leader peptide and amino acids (1–94) were encoded by a V gene closely related to C57 BL/6 nitrophenyl antibody family. More recently, Naparstek et al. [127] have presented evidence indicating that autoantibodies encoded by germline V genes may be the precursors of antibodies that are induced by exogenous antigens since $V_H Id^{CR}$ gene segment encoding a large proportion of anti-arsonate antibodies in A/J mice in its unmutated form encodes antibodies with auto-reactivity.

The Stimulating Immunogen in Lupus. The diverse ligand-binding properties of lupus monoclonal anti-DNA autoantibodies show that DNA might not be the preferred target antigen for some of them. This has led to an intense search for the stimulating immunogen especially because of low immunogenicity of DNA, though it is immunogenic in modified form. Schwartz and Stollar [79] have reviewed the antigenicity of DNA and its possible implications in the onset of production of anti-DNA autoantibodies, while Eilat [93] has evaluated experimental evidence suggesting that the target antigen for anti-DNA autoantibodies may be other than DNA. Nevertheless, the stimulating immunogen in SLE remains an unresolved enigma until now. At the same time, the major immunological event in SLE is that all the nuclear constituents may serve as antigen [74]. Interestingly, hybridomas derived from cardiolipin-immunized mice produced monoclonal autoantibodies that bound not only to cardiolipin but ssDNA and dsDNA as well [104].

Scott [118] has proposed that B cells could be stimulated by: (i) DNA released during natural cell turnover either naked or, probably, complexed with chromatin proteins; (ii) DNA complexed with foreign protein, e.g. virus or other pathogen; (iii) a self or non-self cross-reacting antigen. Hahn [128] and Dang and Harbeck [129] have earlier shown that the anti-DNA populations found in glomerular eluates of SLE patients and NZB/NZW mice are restricted to alkaline antibodies with high isoelectric points. Faaber et al. [108] have shown SLE patient serum reactivity with negatively charged glucosaminoglycans, such as hyaluronic acid and chondroitin sulphate which paralleled serum anti-DNA activity. These authors proposed that several compounds could serve as antigenic targets for anti-DNA autoantibodies provided their structure contained repeating negatively charged groups. The cross-reactions with dextran sulfate and heparan sulfate both of which contain repeating anionic groups have been reported though the exact nature of their interaction remains unclear. The cross-reaction with heparan sulfate is especially important since this is the major glycosaminoglycan of glomerular basement membrane. The half-life of radiolabelled mouse monoclonal anti-DNA autoantibody in the circulation of Balb/c or NZB/NZW has been shown to be much shorter compared to myeloma proteins of the same immunoglobulin class and subclass [Chetset et al., unpubl.] This experimental evidence led Eilat [93] to hypothesise that a negatively charged cross-reactive antigen, possibly a proteoglycan, especially, heparan sulfate may be responsible for tissue damage in SLE by serving as an antigen for anti-DNA autoantibodies in the glomerulus. Such a scheme may operate in the pathogenesis of SLE in a nonspecific manner and does not invalidate the classical serum sickness models for immune complex glomerulonephritis [130, 131].

These extensive data raise several questions which we shall subsequently discuss.

(1) What is the extent of the natural autoreactive B cell repertoire?

(2) What is the epitope recognized by these autoantibodies?

(3) What is the origin and possible significance of these natural autoantibodies?

What Is the Extent of the Natural Autoreactive B Cell Repertoire? Natural autoantibodies against different autoantigens including DNA, cytoskeletal proteins and isologous erythrocytes share certain common features. Most of these autoantibodies possess common cross-reactive idiotypes, constitute a significant fraction of normal circulating serum Ig, and some of them have been reported to be secreted principally by Ly1B cells. Moreover, the antigen(s) against which these antibodies are directed seem to be of TI-2 type as CBA/N mice lack these autoantibodies in their serum, in general, though the stimulating immunogen remains an unresolved puzzle. Indeed, the existence of natural antibodies directed against autoantigens raises doubts concerning the distinction between a self and non-self antigen. It has been postulated that B lymphocytes bearing surface Ig for a given foreign structure are responsible for the synthesis of specific antibodies when challenged by that particular antigen. However, it is improbable that a similar structure is not present within the host itself, especially if certain idiotypes are believed to sterically represent mirror images of antigens which through complimentary idiotype and anti-idiotype circuits are likely to make the immune system accept structural diversity in the universe as nothing new. It has also been argued that most of such antigens are hidden and, hence, unable to challenge the immune system. On the contrary, autoantibodies against circulating proteins like Fc fragment of IgG, albumin and transferrin have been detected. Moreover, body tissues are continuously undergoing destruction and regeneration in all individuals.

Taken together, these results challenge the clonal deletion theory as a general and unique explanation for self tolerance. At the same time, clonal deletion mechanisms cannot be completely excluded because autoantibodies directed against certain specific and critical antigens like the A group, in the case of a subject belonging to the A group, or against polymorphic antigens of the major histocompatibility system have not been reported, at least not to our knowledge. The experiments with unimmunized mice clearly indicate that these autoantibodies are produced by autoreactive B cell clones and the frequencies of B lymphocytes binding to DNA, TNP, cytoskeletal proteins and BrMRBC are very high. These results conform to those observed among clonal precursor cells after stimulation with LPS, where high frequencies of B cell clones reactive for haptens like NIP, TNP and, more recently, for phosphorylcholine were found [132, 133]. Further, an important percentage of the clones reacting with TNP also bind to cytoskeletal proteins. A preliminary study [Lymberi et al., unpubl. data] has indicated that an important number of clones reacting with cytoskeletal proteins also bind to other haptens, suggesting that there might be an overlap between these repertoires.

Cox et al. [36] have shown by limited dilution cell culture technique that there exists one anti-BrMRBC autoantibody precursor cell for every 150–200 PerC, and their frequencies could be increased to 1 to 50 PerC by addition of LPS and dextran sulfate. Interestingly, in vitro culture of PerC for 4 days leads to a dramatic increase in anti-BrMRBC PFA without involving cell division. Hence, these autoantibody secreting cells are already differentiated but repressed for secretion.

A definitely high frequency of clones binding to the panel of antigens tested was also found for splenocytes from 6-day-old compared to 12-week-old mice. This indicates that a part of the repertoire is, perhaps, deleted or diluted during postnatal development. The results observed with adult mice have shown that this group of antibody specificities constitutes, at least 2% of the natural antibody repertoire, though the frequency of the clones probably decreases with age. Alternatively, these B cells might be present at the same frequencies, but a strict control is exerted on them precluding their activation. Thus, it is not surprising to find that these natural monoclonal antibodies exhibit a high frequency of cross-reactive idiotypes. The two anti-id antibodies, raised against D23 (an IgMk recognizing mainly dsDNA, but also actin, tubulin, myosin and TNP) and E7 (an IgMk binding mainly to myosin, but also significantly to actin, tubulin, spectrin, TNP and dsDNA), have been shown to recognize a cross-reacting idiotype which seems to be located near the antigen combining site [69].

A polyclonal rabbit anti-CP idiotype recognized a common cross-reactive idiotype on anti-BrMRBC hybridomas from different mouse strains and was used to demonstrate the presence of this idiotype in most mouse strains which increased as a function of age. Surprisingly, CP idiotype is preferentially expressed in CBA/J, a normal mouse strain [27].

The presence of D23, E7 and CP idiotypes in normal mouse sera, indicates that these natural monoclonal antibodies are secreted by autoreactive B clones. It seems likely that antibodies exhibiting these specificities correspond to recurrent and frequent idiotypes, and that restricted families of germ-line genes encode for them [23, 69]. This hypothesis gains support from the fact that a high degree of homology exists between the first 35 amino acids of light and heavy chains in 4 anti-BrMRBC monoclonal antibodies derived from NZB and CBA/J mouse. Coutinho and his colleagues have also reported a very high degree of idiotypic connectivity among newborn natural autoantibodies [134], based on comparative analysis of unselected IgM secreting hybridomas derived from unprimed naturally activated newborn splenocytes and mitogen-stimulated adult B cells. Similar indications of high connectivity and autoreactivity have also been obtained from hybridomas derived from fetal liver or newborn spleen. [Kearny, cit. by Holmberg and Coutinho, 135]. Holmberg and Coutinho [135] have suggested that this naturally activated lymphocyte compartment represents an internal activity set and is constituted by 10–15% of all lymphocytes. The activated cells in this repertoire are under stringent control by other members of the same set. Pathological autoimmune consequences might be the result of perturbation in the physiological dynamic equilibrium in this autoreactive set. Interestingly, precursor lymphocytes involved in production of anti-DNA as well as anti-BrMRBC autoantibodies are present in both lupus prone and normal mice [12, 64, 79]. It may be recalled that extensive idiotypic cross-reactivities exist among lupus monoclonal anti-DNA autoantibodies in mice and humans [79]. More recently, Morgan et al. [136] have reported the sharing of idiotype (16/6) on monoclonal mouse and human anti-DNA autoantibodies. These observations have profound implications and, as suggested by various authors, indicate structural similarities between the combining sites of antibodies in these two species and evolutionary conservation of V genes coding for primitive ancestral antibodies reacting with DNA which become diversified through somatic mutation.

The natural autoantibodies against BrMRBC differ from anti-DNA autoantibodies since no idiotypic relationship exists in these two categories of natural autoantibodies [Poncet et al., unpubl. observations] though cross-reactive idiotype (CP) is also ubiquitous in most mice strains [27]. In contrast to polyspecific natural autoantibodies whose repertoire is diluted out in adult mice, the anti-BrMRBC autoantibody repertoire seems to expand as a function of age [12, 23]. It seems likely that these natural autoantibodies are an extension of different autoreactive B cell repertoires or that such discrepancies exist because of different ontogenic or lineage relationships between these natural autoantibodies.

A high incidence of MIg with autoantigen activity in our study (5.75%), especially, against cytoskeleton proteins (5.22%) is not surprising considering the consistent presence of natural autoantibodies in normal serum and a high frequency of autoantibody precursor cells obtained by somatic hybridization. Moreover, the antibody specificities in both cases appear to be similar, implying that, for some patients at least, MIg might reflect the expansion of a clone normally programmed to secrete natural autoantibody [62, 63]. Assuming that certain malignant monoclonal gammopathies arise from the proliferation of such a clone, it may be hypothesized that this might be the consequence of dysfunction of the system that normally regulates this antibody production.

What Is the Epitope Recognized by These Autoantibodies? Anti-DNA, antithyroglobulin, antitubulin and antierythrocyte natural autoantibodies display a varying range of binding specificity and the precise antigenic determinant recognized by them remains undefined. In contrast to induced antibodies and antierythrocyte autoantibodies which exhibit a restricted specificity, most natural antibodies, like lupus autoantibodies, frequently show polyspecific binding. A simultaneous binding of these autoantibodies to several cytoskeleton proteins, to cytoskeleton proteins and TNP, to cytoskeleton proteins and thyroglobulin, and in some cases to cytoskeleton proteins, TNP and DNA, is commonly observed. The specificity of the binding [51, 62–65] has been clearly demonstrated by the fact that: (a) the binding is mediated by both Ig and its $F(ab)'_2$ fragment; (b) reactivity is inhibited by pre-incubation with the different antigen – in the case of antibodies exhibiting widespread binding, a major inhibition is found for one antigen, but a significant inhibition is also observed with other antigens; (c) the binding is demonstrable by immunoenzymatic methods, as well as immunocytological and immunoblotting techniques; (d) in some cases, the antibody can be isolated by affinity chromatography on a TNP immunoadsorbent and affinity isolated antibody still exhibits its initial widespread reactivity. Since no evident homologies exist among actin, tubulin, myosin, TNP and DNA, the cross-reactive structures among these antigens remain difficult to be assessed. The cross-reaction of anti-DNA antibodies with cytoskeleton proteins was recently confirmed by André-Schwartz et al. [99]. More recently, we have obtained preliminary results indicating that some of these monoclonal anti-DNA natural autoantibodies may exhibit cross-reactivity towards cardiolipin. These observations await final confirmation. Similar puzzling cross-reactions with other monoclonal antibodies have now been widely described and, in most cases, no satisfactory explanation for these cross-reactions is available [51, 62–65, 68, 79, 96, 100, 107, 137]. Therefore, the physicochemical basis of such cross-reactions needs to be delineated and the identification of an autoantibody as 'anti-myosin' may only partially describe the range of its binding abilities.

Alternative explanations for the molecular basis underlying polyspecific antibodies have been postulated [138], based on the notion that antibody-combining sites are considerably larger than those needed to be complementary to a single epitope. Thus, a relatively large binding site may consist of separate subregions with a capacity to react with different epitopes. In that case, co-inhibition displayed by antigens may be explained by overlapping spatial requirements rather than the same amino acid contact within the antibody-combining site [107].

These results indicate that polyspecific antibodies are able to recognize similar structures present on many antigens. This hypothesis would imply that B cells carry a polyspecific receptor capable of fixing many different antigens. Varga et al. [138] proposed that when such a clone displaying a multispecific cell surface receptor is induced by one of the binding antigens, the antibody produced by this clone would keep its capacity to bind several different antigens. Alternatively, as we postulated earlier, upon active immunization, B cells are stimulated after binding to a given antigen into a series of divisions and mutations which under the selective pressure of the antigen would induce the production of highly specific antibodies for a given epitope of that antigen [64, 139]. Recent data, indicating a high frequency of point mutations around rearranged antibody variable genes [140], would be compatible with the rapid generation of a large number of variants and intraclonal diversity. Polyspecificity has been well analyzed among monoclonal lupus autoantibodies against DNA and cytoskeletal proteins and are presently believed to be of limited heterogeneity. Some of the cross-reactivities of these lupus autoantibodies have been ascribed to their high isoelectric points which are responsible for their interaction with polyanionic structures like DNA, dextran sulfate and heparan sulfate [108]. Similar studies should be performed with natural autoantibodies and their precise heterogeneity should be defined taking into consideration the range of specificities measured by each assay system employed.

As pointed out earlier, all natural autoantibodies do not seem to exhibit multispecific binding. The autoantibodies against BrMRBC seem to monospecifically recognize an autoantigen on mouse erythrocytes exposed after bromelain treatment which is partly constituted by TMA. Despite the availability of a soluble analogue of this antigen, SEA-HB in the high molecular weight fraction of plasma, a precise structural analysis of this autoantigen remains unexplored. Only limited information is available about binding specificities of autoantibodies against other erythrocyte antigens. The recent demonstration of monoclonal IgM autoantibodies from the NZB mouse which recognize an autoantigen other than X, HB, HOL and I but are capable of inducing hemolytic anemia seems to indicate that a variety of antigenic determinants may be involved in the etiopathogenesis of this disease [49].

What Is the Origin and Possible Significance of These Natural Autoantibodies? It has been postulated that natural antibodies arise as a consequence of continuous polyclonal stimulation induced by intestinal flora, food, external aggression, etc. The antibodies against BrMRBC recognize an antigenic determinant partly constituted by TMA, a moiety present on phosphorylcholine. However, these autoantibodies have also been demonstrated in germ-free mice. Although natural hybridomas obtained from germ- and antigen-free animals are further needed to prove this hypothesis, our results showing significantly high frequencies of clones producing natural autoantibodies at 6 days compared to adult mice indicate that these clones are indeed a result of internal stimulation and are actually diluted out in mature mice, as a result of responses to environmental antigens [65]. Nevertheless, the presence of these natural autoreactive clones in infant mice is compatible with germline origin of natural autoantibodies. The possibilities, however, exist for the occurrence of natural autoantibodies in either physiological conditions as a result of stimulation by liberated self constituents (normally hidden) during normal cell turnover or autoantigens complexed with foreign protein or a self or foreign cross-reacting antigen. Certain clues with regard to origin of autoantibodies emerge from idiotypic and structural analysis of monoclonal lupus autoantibodies against DNA. Eilat observed one monoclonal anti-DNA autoantibody derived from the NZB/NZWF1 mouse which had only one base substitution compared to germ line antiphosphorylcholine, an important bacterial antigen. More remarkable is the demonstration that a point mutation in the mouse myeloma V_H region changed the antigen specificity of its immunoglobulin from antiphosphorylcholine to anti-DNA [125]. A monoclonal antibacterial antibody (Waldenström IgM paraproteins, WEA) also binds to DNA and poly (G) and bears the same idiotypic marker as the monoclonal lupus autoantibodies to which it is structurally related [124]. More recently, evidence has accumulated in support of the hypothesis that autoantibodies are present in the pre-immune repertoire, encoded by germ line genes, and somatic mutation under selective pressure of foreign antigen results in the loss of autoantibody phenotype giving rise to monospecific foreign reactivity. The direct clues in support of these ideas emerge from the recent demonstration by Naparstek et al. [127] who showed that genes encoding for autoantibodies mutate upon arsonate immunization leading to loss of pre-immune reactivity and an increase in antibody affinity for the hapten. All these observations imply that the same germ line genes may encode for both autoantibodies and antibodies to foreign antigens in, at least, certain instances.

In the recent past, two different approaches have been employed to define the B cell subpopulations implicated in the production of autoantibodies. Hayakawa et al. [38, 39] have shown that Ly1 B cells which account for 1–2% of BALB/c splenocytes and 5–10% of NZB spleen cells are mainly involved in the secretion of IgM autoantibody directed against DNA and bromelain-treated mouse erythrocytes. The CBA/N mice carrying Xid gene lack the ability to respond to TI-2 antigens [70]. These mice secrete negligible anti-DNA or anti-BrMRBC autoantibodies even upon mitogenic stimulation. More recently, we have observed an absence of detectable levels of serum CP idiotype related to anti-BrMRBC autoantibody in CBA/N mice which totally lack the Ly1 B cell population in their peritoneal cavity [40]. Further similar observations on congenic NZB-Xid mice have clearly shown that $Lyb5^+$ cells lacking in Xid mice are important for natural autoantibody production [71]. Smith et al. [73] studied the relationships among splenic Xid $Ly1^+$ and $Lyb5^+$ B cells by flow cytometry and demonstrated that the autoantibody producing $Ly1^+$ B cells were predominantly $Lyb5^+$. To further analyze this problem, we fused splenocytes from 6-day-old (CBA/N×BALB/c)F1 male and female mice to a nonsecreting myeloma and compared the binding specificities to DNA, cytoskeletal proteins and TNP by the MIg originating from defective males and phenotypically normal females. Even though somatic hybridization has to be employed carefully to evaluate the expressed versus potential repertoire of antibody-forming cells, our results demonstrate, contrary to previously cited observations, that B cells from infant Xid mice carry the genetic information [72] for the production of autoantibodies against DNA and cytoskeletal proteins. These results suggest, but do not prove, in the absence of fusions performed with Lyb^{5-} cells, that this latter population of cells which largely predominates in Xid mice may be involved in the production of natural autoantibodies against the above-mentioned specificities. If so, the Xid gene may act as a regulatory gene, as Xid mice in contrast to normal strains are unable to secrete anti-DNA autoantibodies upon mitogenic stimulation despite carrying the genetic information. This regulatory mechanism may also account for the failure of NZB-Xid mice to fully manifest the autoimmune syndrome characteristic of NZB mice [71]. Since the Xid gene has recently been cloned [141], this hypothesis may be easily tested in the near future.

The presence of antibodies exhibiting a wide specificity may constitute an advantage for the animal. They may constitute the first barrier of defence against external aggression while more specific antibodies are in the process of being elicited. They may also play an important role in the elimination of dead tissues as suggested by Grabar [142]. Furthermore, it cannot be excluded that these antibodies play a role in 'self tolerance', by binding to selfantigens and, thus, precluding the activation of other self-reactive B cells or through interactions within the idiotypic network. Holmberg and Coutinho [135] have proposed that the high idiotypic connectivity within natural autoantibodies, may be a simple general strategy to avoid self-aggression by bringing self reactive lymphocyte within this network as they will be under continuous stingent control by other members of the set. Blocking by natural auto-antiidiotype can be another possibility which fits well within the 'network theory'. Schraber et al. [143, 144] described a method to reveal auto-anti-idiotype by incorporation of very low concentrations of antigen in a local hemolytic plaque assay which will dissociate idiotype anti-idiotype blocking complex on the cell surface allowing antibody secretion. In the anti-BrMRBC model, Wieties and Moticka [145] demonstrated such antigen augmentable plaques using 3 *M* KCl extract of Br MRBC or cross-reactive hapten phosphoryl choline as antigen and recovered in the elute an 'auto-anti-idiotype' (likely to be IgM isotype) which could specifically suppress anti-BrMRBC plaques. These hapten augmentable plaques could also be observed in heterogenous PerC population by incorporating choline bromide at a concentration of 10^{-6}–10^{-7} *M* in the hemolytic plaque detection system [Poncet et al., unpubl. observations].

The wider presence of these autoantibodies, and the ease with which they can be obtained, supports the idea that they constitute a major component of the B cell repertoire. Our results with normal human serum [51] indicate that this repertoire is actually expressed at low concentrations in normal serum. As these normal autoantibodies appear to share antibody specificities with autoantibodies obtained from lupus patients and autoimmune mice [64], it has been hypothesized that these diseases may arise as a consequence of the perturbation of the immunoregulatory system by environmental factors which can induce lymphocytes to circumvent the normal regulatory pathway [146]. However, we have failed to find clinical symptoms related to the presence of the MIg in 31 patients with MIg displaying high levels of autoantibody specificities. Interestingly, the patients whose MIg exhibited anti-native DNA activity did not show clinical features suggestive of systemic lupus erythematosus [63]. This suggests that the problems may be rather more complex and that inside these autoantibodies may coexist a population with a physiological role accounting for the majority of autoantibodies, besides a subpopulation with a noxious role. The distinction between autoantibodies with a pathological or nonpathological role remains an unresolved enigma until now. The high isoelectric point of anti-DNA autoantibodies in SLE patients seems to be a pathogenesis-determining factor based on their reactivity with polyanionic structures, especially, heparan sulfate which is a major glycosaminoglycan of glomerular basement membrane. The large collections of monoclonal autoantibodies, now available, obtained from normal and autoimmune mouse and human lymphocytes, should allow the elucidation of this problem at the molecular level.

References

1 Burnet, F. M.: The clonal selection theory of acquired immunity (Cambride University Press, London, New York 1959).

2 MacKay, I. R.: Natural autoantibodies to the forebidden clones to the rear? Immunol. Today *4:* 340–342 (1983).

3 Hooper, B.; Whittingham, S.; Mathews, J. D.: Auto-immunity in a rural community. Clin. exp. Immunol. *12:* 79–87 (1972).

4 Roberts, I. M.; Whittingham, S.; Mackay, I. R.: Tolerance to an

autoantigen-thyroglobulin. Antigen-binding lymphocytes in thymus and blood in health and auto-immune disease. Lancet *ii:* 936–940 (1973).
5 Boyden, S.V.: Autoimmunity and inflammation. Nature, Lond. *201:* 200–201 (1964).
6 Bach, J.F.: Auto-immunité une révolution conceptuelle. Méd. Sci. *1:* 176–177 (1985).
7 Assan, R.; Debray-Sachs, M.; Laborie, C.: Metabolic and immunological effects of cyclosporin in recently diagnosed type I diabetes mellitus. Lancet *i:* 67–71 (1985).
8 Hanafusa, T.; Pujol-Borrell, R.; Chiovato, L.; Russell, R.C.G.; Doniach, D.; Bottazzo, G.F.: Aberrant expression of HLA-DR antigen on thymocytes in Graves' disease Relevance for autoimmunity. Lancet *ii:* 1111–1115 (1984).
9 Cunningham, A.J.: Large numbers of cells in normal mice produce antibody components of isologus erythrocytes. Nature, Lond. *252:* 749–751 (1974).
10 De Heer, D.H.; Edgington, T.S.: Identification of derepressed auto immunocompetent B lymphoïd cells in NZB mice. Clin. exp. Immunol. *16:* 431-443 (1974).
11 Linder, E.J.; Edgington, T.S.: Antigenic specificity of anti-erythrocyte autoantibody responses by NZB mice. Identification and partial characterization of two erythrocyte surface antigens. J. Immun. *108:* 1615–1623 (1972).
12 Cunningham, A.J.: Self-tolerance maintained by active suppressor mechanisms. Transplant. Rev. *31:* 23–43 (1976).
13 De Heer, D.H.; Edgington, T.S.: Cellular events associated with the immunogenesis of anti-erythrocyte autoantibody responses of NZB mice. Transplant. Rev. *31:* 116–155 (1976).
14 Pages. J.M.; Bussard, A.E.: Precommitment of normal mouse peritoneal cells by erythrocyte antigens in relation to auto-antibody production. Nature, Lond. *257:* 316–317 (1975).
15 Lord, E.; Dutton, R.W.: The properties of plaque forming cells from auto-immune and normal strains of mice with specificity for autologous erythrocyte antigens. J. Immun. *115:* 1199–1205 (1975).
16 Gisler, R.H.; Pages, J.M.; Bussard, A.E.: Spontaneous development of plaque-forming cells against sheep erythrocytes by mouse peritoneal cells in culture. Ann. Immunol., Paris *126C:* 231–238 (1975).
17 Cox, K.O.; Baddams, H.; Evans, A.: Studies of the antigenicity and immunogenicity of bromelain pretreated red blood cells. Aust. J. exp. Biol. med. Sci. *55:* 27–37 (1977).
18 Linder, E.J.; Edgington, T.S.: Immunobiology of the autoantibody response. I. Circulating analogues of erythrocyte autoantigens and heterogeneity of the autoimmune response of NZB mice. Clin. exp. Immunol. *13:* 279–292 (1973).
19 Bussard, A.E.: Antibody formation in non-immune peritoneal cells after incubation in gum containing antigen. Sciences *153:* 887–888 (1966).
20 Cox, K.O.; Evans, D.; Brooks, D.; Cunliffe, D.A.: In vitro investigation of autoantibody secreting peritoneal cells and their regulation. Immunology *38:* 355–365 (1979).
21 Bussard, A.E.; Vinit, M.A.; Pages, J.M.: Immunochemical characterization of the autoantibodies produced by mouse peritoneal cells in culture. Immunochemistry *14:* 1–9 (1976).

22 Cox. K.O.; Samcewicz, B.: Non H-2 genes involved in suppressing autoimmunity. Cell. Immunol. *77:* 357–362 (1983).

23 Poncet, P.; Kocher, H.P.; Pages, J.; Jaton, J.C.; Bussard, A.E.: Monoclonal autoantibodies against mouse red blood cells. A. family of structurally restricted molecules. Mol. Immunol. *22:* 541–551 (1985).

24 Pages. J.M.; Bussard, A.E.: Establishment and characterization of permanent murine hybridoma secreting monoclonal autoantibodies. Cell. Immunol. *41:* 188–194 (1978).

25 Pages. J.; Poncet, P.; Serban, D.; Witz, I.; Bussard, A.E.: Relationship between choline derivatives and mouse erythrocyte membrane antigens revealed by mouse monoclonal antibodies. I. Anticholine activity of antimouse erythrocyte monoclonal antibodies. Immun. Lett. *5:* 167–173 (1982).

26 De Heer, D.H.; Pages. J.M.; Bussard. A.E.: Specificity of anti-erythrocyte autoantibodies secreted by a NZB-derived hybridoma and NZB peritoneal cells. Cell. Immunol. *49:* 135–141 (1980).

27 Kaushik, A.; Poncet, P.; Bussard, A.: Autoantibodies against bromelainized mouse erythrocyte: Strain distribution of serum idiotype expression and relative peritoneal cell activity Cell. Immunol. (in press).

28 Cunliffe, D.A.; Cox, K.O.: Effects of bromelain and pronase on erythrocyte membranes. Mol. Immunol. *16:* 427–433 (1979).

29 Linder, E.J.; Edgington, T.S.: Immunobiology of the auto-antibody response. II. The lipoprotein-associated soluble HB erythrocyte autoantigen of NZB mice. J. Immun. *110:* 53–62 (1973).

30 Serban, D.; Pages, J.M.; Bussard, A.E.; Witz, I.P.: The participation of trimethylammonium in the mouse erythrocyte epitope recognized by monoclonal autoantibodies. Immun. Lett. *3:* 315–319 (1981).

31 Cox, K.O.; Hardy, S.J.: Autoantibody against mouse bromelain-modified RBC are specifically inhibited by a common membrane phospholipid, phosphatidylcholine. Immunology *55:* 263–269 (1985).

32 Steele, E.J.; Cunningham, A.J.: High proportion of Ig-producing cells making autoantibody in normal mice. Nature, Lond. *274:* 483–484 (1978).

33 Garzelli, C.; Campa, M.; Forlani, A.; Colizzi, V.; Falcone, G.: LPS-induced enhancement of PFC response to bromelain treated syngeneic erythrocytes in mouse peritoneal cell cultures. Int. Archs Allergy appl. Immun. *69:* 143–147 (1982).

34 Pages, J.; Gisler, R.; Arnaud, D.; Bussard, A.E.: Spontaneous conversion of precursor cells into anti sheep erythrocyte antibody producing cells in culture of mouse peritoneal cells. Ann. Immun., Pairs *1276:* 31–41 (1976).

35 Pages, J.; Thiernesse, N.; Bernard, J.; Jeannesson, P.; Arnaud, D.; Bussard, A.E.: Ultrastructure of mouse peritoneal cells engaged in spontaneous secretion of antibody against mouse and sheep erythrocytes and evolution of cell types during culture. Cell. Immunol *35:* 289–302 (1978).

36 Cox, K.O.; Daenke, S.; Samcewicz, B.: Peritoneal B cells differentiate without proliferation into autoantibody secretors under the influence of factors released by other cells. Scand. J. Immunol. *20:* 527–532 (1984).

37 Colizzi, V.; Forlani, A.; Bazziachi, L.: Interleukin-1 increases the autoantibody production to bromelain treated mouse red cells (BR-MRC) in vitro. Autumn Meeting British Society for Immunology. Po *49:* 95–96 (1984).

38 Hayakawa, K.; Hardy, R.R.; Parks, D.R.; Herzenberg, L.A.: The 'Ly-1 B' cell subpopulation in normal, immunodefective, and autoimmune mice. J. exp. Med. *157:* 202–218 (1983).
39 Hayakawa, K.; Hardy, R.R.; Honda, M.; Herzenberg, L.A.; Steinberg, A.D.; Herzenberg, L.A.: Ly1-B cells: functionally distinct lymphocytes that secrete IgM autoantibodies. Proc. natn. Acad. Sci. USA *81:* 2494–2498 (1984).
40 Hayakawa, K.; Hardy, R.R.; Herzenberg, L.A.; Steinberg, A.D.; Herzenberg, L.A.: Ly-1 B: A functionally distinct B cell subpopulation. Prog. Immunol. *5:* 661–665 (1983).
41 Hayakawa, K.; Hardy, R.R.; Herzenberg, L.A.; Herzenberg, L.A.: Progenitors for Ly1-B cells are distinct from progenitors for other B-cells. J. exp. Med. *161:* 1554–1568 (1985).
42 Howie, J.B.; Helyer, B.J.: The immunology and pathology of NZB mice. Adv. Immunol. *9:* 215–266 (1968).
43 Pirofsky, B.: Autoimmunization and the autoimmune hemolytic anemia (Williams & Wilkins, Baltimore 1969).
44 Deheer, D.H.; Edgrington, T.S.: Specific antigen-binding and antibody secreting lymphocytes associated with erythrocyte autoantibody responses of NZB and genetically unrelated mice. J. Immun. *116:* 1051–1058 (1976).
45 Holborrow, E.J.; Barnes, R.D.S.; Tuffrey, M.: A new red cell autoantibody in NZB mice. Nature, Lond. *207:* 601–604 (1965).
46 Linder, E.: Autoantibodies against the inner aspect of erythrocyte membrane in NZB mice. Clin. exp. Immunol. *27:* 531–537 (1977).
47 Costa, N.; Yakulis, V.; Heller, P.: Cold-reacting antibody in NZB/B1 mice. Blood *35:* 583–590 (1970).
48 Lewis, D.E.; Griswold, S.; Warmer, N.L.: Monoclonal anti-erythrocyte auto-antibodies from unimmunized NZB mice. Hybridoma *1:* 71–76 (1981).
49 Ozaki, S.; Nagasawa, R.; Sato, H.; Shirai, T.: Hybridoma autoantibodies to erythrocytes from NZB mice and the induction of hemolytic anemia. Immun. Lett. *8:* 115–119 (1984).
50 Karsenti, E.; Guilbert, B.; Bornens, M.; Avrameas, S.: Antibodies to tubulin in normal nonimmunized animals. Proc. natn. Acad. Sci. USA *74:* 3997–4004 (1977).
51 Guilbert, B.; Dighiero, G.; Avrameas, S.: Naturally occuring antibodies against nine common antigens in normal humans. I. Detection, isolation, and characterization. J. Immun. *128:* 2779–2787 (1982).
52 Lutz, H.U.; Wipf, G.: Naturally occurring auto-antibodies to skeletal proteins from human red blood cells. J. Immun. *128:* 1695–1699 (1982).
53 Martin. S.E.; Martin. W.J.: Interspecies brain antigen detected by naturally occurring mouse anti-brain auto -antibody. Proc. natn. Acad. Sci. USA *72:* 1036–1041 (1975).
54 Martin. W.J.; Martin. S.E.: Thymus reactive IgM auto-antibodies in normal mouse sera. Nature, Lond. *254:* 716–718 (1975).
55 Sela, B.A.; Wang, J.L.; Edelman, G.M.: Antibodies reactive with cell surface carbohydrates. Proc. natn. Acad. Sci. USA *72:* 1127–1132 (1975).
56 Walford, R.L.: The immunologic theory of aging (Munksgaard, Copenhagen 1969).
57 Rogentine, G.N.; Plocinik, B.A.: Carbohydrate inhibition studies of the naturally

human antibody to neuraminidase-treated human lymphocytes. J. Immun. *113:* 848–854 (1974).
58 Winchester, R.J.; Shu Man Fu; Winfield, J.B.; Kunkel, H.G.: Immunofluorescent studies on antibodies directed to a membrane structure present in lymphocytes and erythrocytes. J. Immun. *114:* 410–417 (1975).
59 Shinomiye, T.; Koyame, J.: Naturally occurring antibodies reacting with some buried determinants of homologous IgG exposed by spleen protease digestion. Immunochemistry *11:* 467–473 (1974).
60 Kritzman, J.; Kunkel, H.G.; McCarthy, J.; Mellors, R.C.: Studies of a Waldenström-type macroglobulin with rheumatoïd factor properties. J. Lab. clin. Med. *57:* 905–912 (1961).
61 Williams, R.C.; Kunkel, H.G.; Capra, J.D.: Antigenic specificities related to the cold agglutinin activity of gamma M-globulins. Science *161:* 379–382 (1968).
62 Dighiero, G.; Guilbert, B.; Avrameas, S.: Naturally occuring antibodies against nine common antigens in human sera. II. High incidence of monoclonal Ig exhibiting antibody activity against actin and tubulin and sharing antibody specificities with natural antibodies. J. Immun. *128:* 2788–2792 (1982).
63 Dighiero, G.; Guilbert, B.; Fermant, J.P.; Lymberi, P.; Danon, F.; Avrameas, S.: Thirty-six human monoclonal immunoglobulins (MIg) with antibody activity against cytoskeleton proteins, thyroglobulin and native DNA. Immunological studies and clinical correlations. Blood *62:* 264–270 (1983).
64 Dighiero, G.; Lymberi, P.; Mazié, J.C.; Rouyre, S.; Butler-Browne, G.S.; Whalen, R.G.; Avrameas, S.: Murine hybridomas secreting natural monoclonal antibodies reacting with self antigens. J. Immun. *131:* 2267–2272 (1983).
65 Dighiero, G.; Lymberi, P.; Holmberg, D.; Lundquist, I.; Coutinho, A.; Avrameas, S.: High frequency of natural autoantibodies in normal newborn mice. J. Immun. *134:* 765–771 (1985).
66 Monier, J.C.; Brochier, J.; Moreira, A.; Sault, C.; Roux B.: Generation of hybridoma antibodies to double-stranded DNA from non-autoimmune BALB/c strain: studies on anti-idiotype. Immun. Lett. *8:* 61–68 (1984).
67 Cairns, E.; Block, J.; Bell, D.A.: Anti-DNA autoantibody-producing hybridomas of normal human lymphoïd cell origin. J. Immun. *74:* 880–887 (1984).
68 Prabhakar, B.S.; Saegusa, J.; Onodera, T.; Notkins, A.L.: Lymphocytes capable of making monoclonal autoantibodies that react with multiple organs are a commun feature of the normal B cell repertoire. J. Immun. *133:* 2815–2817 (1984).
69 Lymberi, P.; Dighiero, G.; Ternynck, T.; Avrameas, S.: A high incidence of cross-reactive idiotypes among murine natural autoantibodies. Eur. J. Immunol. *15:* 702–707 (1985).
70 Scher, I.: The CBA/N mouse strain. An experimental model illustrating the influence of the X-chromosome on immunity. Adv. Immunol. *33:* 2–69 (1982).
71 Smith, H.R.; Steinberg, A.D.: Autoimmunity, a perspective. A. Rev. Immunol. *1:* 175–210 (1983).
72 Dighiero, G.; Poncet, P.; Rouyre, S.; Mazié, J.C.: New-born Xid mice carry the genetic information for the production of natural autoantibodies. J. Immun. *136:* 4000–4005 (1986).
73 Smith, H.R.; Taffe, L.J.; Chused, T.M.; Raveche, E.S.; Klinman, D.M.; Stein-

berg, A.D.: Analysis of B-cell subpopulations. I. Relationships among splenic Xid, Ly 1^+, and Lyb 5^+ B cells. Cell. Immunol. *92:* 190–196 (1985).
74 Tan, E.M.: Autoantibodies to nuclear antigens (ANA). Their immunobiology and medicine. Adv. Immunol. *33:* 167–240 (1982).
75 Theofilopoulos, A.N.; Dixon, F.J.: Murine models of systemic lupus erythematosus. Adv. Immunol. *37:* 269–390 (1985).
76 Stollar, B.D.: Nucleic acids as antigens; in Sela, The antigens, vol. 1, pp. 1–85 (Academic press, New York 1973).
77 Andrews, B.; Eisenberg, R.A.; Theofilopoulous, A.D.; Isui, S.I.; Wilson, C.B.; McConahey, P.J.; Murphy, E.D.; Roths, J.B.; Dixon, F.J.: Spontaneous murine lupus like syndromes. Clinical and immunopathological manifestations in several strains. J. exp. Med. *148:* 1198–1215 (1978).
78 Koffler, D.; Carr, R.; Agnello, V.; Thoburn, R.; Kunkel, H.G.: Antibodies to polynucleotides in human sera: antigenic specificity and relation to disease. J. exp. Med. *134:* 294–312 (1971).
79 Schwartz, R.S.; Stollar, B.D.: Origins of anti-DNA autoantibodies. J. clin. Invest. *75:* 321–327 (1985).
80 Alarcon-Segovia, D.; Fishbain, E.; Alcala, H.; Oliguin-Palacios, E.; Estrada-Parra, S.: The range and specificity of antinuclear antibodies in systemic lupus erythmatosus. Clin. exp. Immunol. *6:* 557–571 (1970).
81 Weisbart, R.M.; Garrett, R.A.; Liebling, M.R.; Barnett, E.V.; Paulus, H.E.; Katz, D.H.: Specificity of antinucleoside antibodies in systemic lupus erythematosus. Clin. Immunol. Immunopathol. *27:* 403–411 (1983).
82 Stollar, B.D.; Levine, L.; Lehrer, M.I.; Vunakis, H.V.: The antigenic determinants of denaturated DNA reactive with lupus erythematosus serum. Proc. natn. Acad. Sci. USA *48:* 874–880 (1962).
83 Stollar, B.D.; Levine, L.; Marmur, J.: Antibodies to denatured deoxyribonucleic acid in lupus erythematosus serum. II. Characterization of antibodies in several sera. Biochim. biophys. Acta *61:* 7–18 (1962).
84 Munns, T.W.; Liszewski, M.K.; Hahn, B.H.: Antibody-nucleic acid complexes. Conformational and base specificities associated with spontaneously occuring poly- and monoclonal anti-DNA antibodies from autoimmune mice. Biochemistry *23:* 2964–2970 (1984).
85 Dehoratius, R.J.; Pillarisetty, R.; Messner, R.P.; Talal, N.: Anti-nucleic acid antibodies in systemic lupus erythematosus patients and their families. J. clin. Invest. *56:* 1149–1154 (1975).
86 Eilat, D.; Steinberg, A.D.; Schechter, A.: The reaction of SLE antibodies with native, single stranded RNA: Radioassay and binding specificities. J. Immun. *120:* 550–557 (1978).
87 Schur, P.H.; Monroe, M.: Antibodies to ribonucleic acid in systemic lupus erythematosus. Proc. natn. Acad. Sci. USA *63:* 1108–1112 (1969).
88 Talal, N.; Gallo, R.C.: Antibodies to DNA: RNA hybrid in systemic lupus erythematosus measured by a cellulose ester filter radioimmunoassay. Nature New Biol. *240:* 240–242 (1972).
89 Yokohari, R.: Naturally occurring antibodies to poly (ADP-ribose) in patients with lupus erythematosus. Nature, Lond. *265:* 175–177 (1977).
90 Lafer, E.M.; Valle, R.P.C.; Moller, A.; Nordheim, A.; Schur, P.S.; Rich, A.;

Stollar, B.D.: Z-DNA specific antibodies in human systemic lupus erythematosus. J. clin. Invest. *71:* 314–321 (1983).

91 Harris, E.N.; Gharavi, A.E.; Boey, M.L.; Patel, B.M.; Mackworth-Young, C.G.; Loizon, S.; Hughes, G.R.V.: Anti-cardiolipin antibodies: detection by radioimmunoassay and association with thrombosis in systemic lupus erythematosus. Lancet *ii:* 1211–1214 (1983).

92 Koike T.; Tomioka, H.; Kumagai, A.: Antibodies cross-reactive with DNA and cardiolipin in patients with systemic lupus erythematosus. Clin. exp. Immunol. *50:* 298–302 (1982).

93 Eilat, D.: Cross-reactions of anti-DNA autoantibodies and the central dogma of lupus nephritis. Immunol. Today *6:* 123–127 (1985).

94 Andrzewski, C.; Stollar, B.D.; Lalor, T.M.; Schwartz, R.S.: Hybridoma autoantibodies to DNA. J. Immun. *124:* 1499–1502 (1980).

95 Schoenfeld, Y.; Hsu-lin, S.C.; Gabriels, J.E.; Silberstein, L.E.; Furie, B.C.; Furie, B.; Stollar, B.D.; Schwartz R.S.: Production of autoantibodies by human-human hybridomas. J. clin. Invest. *70:* 205–208 (1982).

96 Shoenfeld, Y.; Rauch, J.; Massicotte, H.; Datta, S.K.; André-Schwartz, J.; Stollar, B.D.; Schwartz R.S.: Polyspecificity of monoclonal lupus autoantibodies produced by human-human hybridomas. New Engl. J. Med. *308:* 414–420 (1983).

97 Billings, P.B.; Allen, R.W.; Jensen, F.C.; Hoch, S.O.: Anti-RNP monoclonal antibodies derived from a mouse strain with lupus-like autoimmunity. J. Immun. *128:* 1176–1180 (1982).

98 Isenberg, D.A.; Shoenfeld, Y.; Schwartz, R.S.: The use of hybridomas to analyse autoimmunity. Br. med. Bull. *40:* 262–266 (1984).

99 André-Schwartz, J.; Datta, S.K.; Shoenfeld, Y.; Isenberg, D.A.; Stollar, B.D.; Schwartz, R.S.: Binding of cytoskeletal proteins by monoclonal anti-DNA lupus autoantibodies. Clin. Immunol. Immunopathol. *31:* 261–271 (1984).

100 Rauch, J.; Massicotte, H.; Tannenbaum, H.: Hybridoma anti-DNA autoantibodies from patients with rheumatoid arthritis and systemic lupus erythematosus demonstrate similar nucleic acid binding characteristics. J. Immun. *136:* 180–186 (1985).

101 Jacob, L.; Lety, M.; Louvard, D.; Bach, J.F.: Binding of a monoclonal anti-DNA autoantibody to identical protein(s) present at the surface of several human cell types involved in lupus pathogenesis. J. clin. Invest. *75:* 315–317 (1985).

102 Elkon, K.B.; Parnassa, A.P.; Cora, L.F.: Lupus autoantibodies target ribosomal P proteins. J. exp. Med. *162:* 459–471 (1985).

103 Morgan, A.; Buchanan, R.R.C.; Lew, A.M.; Olsen, I.; Staines, N.A.: Five groups of antigenic determinant on DNA identified by monoclonal antibodies from (NZB×NZW)F1 and MRL/Mp-lpr/lpr mice. Immunology *55:* 75–83 (1985).

104 Rauch, J.; Tannenbaum, H.; Stollar, B.D.; Schwartz, R.S.: Monoclonal anticardiolipin antibodies bind to DNA. Eur. J. Immunol. *14:* 529–534 (1984).

105 Lafer, E.M.; Rauch, J.; Andrzewski, C.; Mudd, D.; Furie, B.; Furie, B.; Schwartz, R.S.; Stollar, B.D.: Polyspecific monoclonal lupus auto-antibodies reactive with both polynucleotides and phospholipids. J. exp. Med. *153:* 897–909 (1981).

106 Haskard, D.O.; Gul, V.; Morgan, A.; Kataaha, P.; Staines, N.A.; Archer, J.R.:

Human monoclonal autoantibodies from patients with rheumatoid arthritis against cellular constituents. Clin. exp. Immunol. *61:* 496–502 (1985).

107 Rubin, R.L.; Balderas, R.S.; Tan, E.M.; Dixon, F.J.; Theofilopoulos, A.N.: Multiple autoantigen binding capabilities of mouse monoclonal antibodies selected for rheumatoid factor activity. J. exp. Med. *159:* 1429–1440 (1984).

108 Faaber, P.; Capel, P.J.A.; Rijke,, G.P.M.; Vierwindent, G.; Van der Putte, L.B.A.; Koene, R.A.P.: Cross-reactivity of anti-DNA antibodies with proteoglycans. Clin. exp. Immunol. *55:* 502–508 (1984).

109 Jacob, L.; Tron, F.; Bach, J.F.; Louvard, D.: A monoclonal anti-DNA antibody also binds to cell surface proteins. Proc. natn. Acad. Sci. USA *81:* 3843–3845 (1984).

110 Naparstek, Y.; Duggan, D.; Schattner, A.; Madio, M.P.; Goni, F.; Frangione, B.; Stollar, B.D.; Kabat, E.A.; Schwartz, R.S.: Immunochemical similarities between monoclonal antibacterial Waldenström's macroglobulins and monoclonal anti-DNA lupus autoantibodies. J. exp. Med. *161:* 1525–1538 (1985).

111 Munns, T.W.; Liszewski, M.K.; Tellam, J.J.; Ebling, F.M.; Hahn, B.H.: Antibody nucleic acid complexes. Identification of the antigenic determinant of a murine monoclonal antibody specific for single stranded nucleic acids. Biochemistry *21:* 2929–2936 (1982).

112 Weisbart, R.H.; Chan, G.; Kacena, A.; Saxton, R.E.: Characterization of mouse and human monoclonal antibodies cross-reactive with SLE serum antibodies to guanosine. J. Immun. *132:* 2909–2912 (1984).

113 Lee, J.S.; Lewis, J.R.; Morgan, A.R.; Mosmann, J.R.; Singh, B.: Monoclonal antibodies showing sequence specificity in their interaction with single stranded DNA. Nucl. Acids Res. *9:* 1707–1721 (1981).

114 Ballard, D.W.; Woss, E.W.: Monoclonal murine anti-nucleic acid antibody with double stranded specificity. Mol. Immunol. *19:* 793–799 (1982).

115 Jacob, L.; Tron, F.: Monoclonal anti-deoxyribonucleic acid antibodies. I. Isotope and specificity studies. J. Immun. *128:* 895–898 (1982).

116 Koike, T.; Maruyama, N.; Funaki, H.; Tomioka, H.; Yoshida, S.: Specificity of mouse hybridoma antibodies to DNA. II. Phospholipid reactivity and biological false positive serological test for syphilis. Clin. exp. Immunol. *57:* 345–350 (1984).

117 Eilat, D.; Hochberg, M.; Pumphrey, J.; Rudikoff, S.: Monoclonal antibodies to DNA and RNA from NZB/NZW F1 mice. Antigenic specificities and NH2 terminal amino acid sequences. J. Immun. *133:* 489–494 (1984).

118 Scott, D.I.: Autoantibodies and nuclear antigens. Immunol. Today. *6:* 314–315 (1985).

119 Rauch, J.; Murphy, E.; Roths, J.B.; Stollar, B.D.; Schwartz, R.S.: A high frequency idiotypic marker of anti-DNA autoantibodies in MR-lpr/lpr mice. J. Immun. *129:* 236–241 (1982).

120 Tron, F.; Le Guern, C.L.; Cazenave, P.A.; Bach, J.F.: Intrastrain recurrent idiotypes among anti-DNA antibodies of (NZB/NZW)F1 hybrid mice. Eur. J. Immunol. *12:* 761–766 (1982).

121 Marion, T.N.; Lawton, A.R.; Kearney, J.F.; Briles, D.E.: Anti-DNA autoantibodies in (NZB × NZW)F1 mice are clonally heterogenous, but a majority share a common idiotype. J. Immun. *128:* 668–674 (1982).

122 Isenberg, D.A.; Shoenfeld, Y.; Madaio, M.P.; Rauch, J.; Reichlin, M.; Stollar,

B. D.; Schwartz, R. S.: Anti-DNA antibody idiotypes in systemic lupus erythematosus. Lancet *ii:* 417–421 (1984).

123 Soloman, G.; Schiffenbauer, J.; Keiser, H. G.; Diamond, B.: Use of monoclonal auto-antibodies to identify shared idiotypes on human antibodies to native DNA from patients with systemic lupus erythematosus. Proc. natn. Acad. Sci. USA *80:* 850–854 (1983).

124 Naparstek, Y.; Schattner, A.; Duggan, D.; Madio, M.; Schwartz, R.; Stollar, B. D.; Kabat, E.; Frangione, B.; Goni, F.; Atkinson, P.; Furie, B. C.; Lampman, G.; Furie, B.: Structural and immunochemical resemblences between monoclonal and anti-DNA autoantibodies and monoclonal anti-bacterial antibodies (Abstract). Clin. Res. *32:* 507A (1984).

125 Diamond, B.; Scharff, M. D.: Somatic mutation of the T15 heavy chain give rise to an antibody with autoantibody specificity. Proc. natn. Acad. Sci. USA *81:* 5841–5844 (1984).

126 Kofler, R.; Noonars, D. I.; Levy, D. E.; Wilson, M. C.; Moller, N. P. H.; Dixon, F. J.; Theofilopoulos, A. N.: Genetic elements utilized for a murine lupus anti-DNA autoantibody are closely related to those for antibodies to exogenous antigens. J. exp. Med. *161:* 805–815 (1985).

127 Naparstek, Y.; André-Schwartz, J.; Manser, T.; Wysocki, L. J.; Breitman, L.; Stollar, B. D.; Gefter, L. M.; Schwartz, R. S.: Evolution of anti-arsonate antibodies from germline encoded autoantibodies (submitted).

128 Hahn, B. H.: Characterization of pathogenic subpopulations of antibodies to DNA. Arthritis Rheum. *25:* 747–752 (1982).

129 Dang, H.; Harbeck, R. J.: The in vivo and in vitro glomerular deposition of isolated anti-double stranded-DNA antibodies in NZB/W mice. Clin. Immunol. Immunopathol. *30:* 265–278 (1984).

130 Germuth, F. G.: A comparative histologic and immunologic study in rabbits of induced hypersensitivity of the serum sickness type. J. exp. Med. *97:* 257–282 (1983).

131 Dixon, F. J.; Feldman, J. D.; Vazquez, J. J.: Experimental glomerulonephritis. The pathogenesis of a laboratory model resembling the spectrum of human glomerulonephritis. J. exp. Med. *113:* 899–920 (1961).

132 Anderson, J.; Coutinho, A.; Melchers, F.: Frequencies of mitogen reactive B cells in the mouse. II. Frequencies of B cells producing antibodies which lyse sheep or horse erythrocyte and trinitrophenylated or nitroiodophenylated sheep erythrocytes. J. exp. Med. *145:* 1520–1529 (1977).

133 Levy, M.: Frequencies of phosphorylcholine-specific and T15-associated 10/13 idiotype-positive B cells within lipopolysaccharide-reactive B cells of adult BALB/c mice. Eur. J. Immunol. *14:* 864–868 (1984).

134 Holmberg, D.; Wennerstrom, G.; Andrade, L.; Coutinho, A.: The high idiotypic connectivity of 'natural' newborn antibodies is not found in adult mitogenic reactive B cell repertories. Eur. J. Immunol. *16:* 82–87 (1986).

135 Holmberg, D.; Coutinho, A.: Natural antibodies and autoimmunity. Immunol. Today *6:* 356 –357 (1985).

136 Morgan, A.; Isenberg, D. A.; Naparstek, Y.; Rauch, J.; Duggan, D.; Khiroija, R.; Staines, N. A.: Schattner, A.: Shared idiotypes are expressed on mouse and human anti-DNA autoantibodies. Immunology *56:* 393–399 (1985).

137 Lane, D.; Koprowski, H.: Molecular recognition and the future of monoclonal antibodies. Nature, Lond. *296:* 200–202 (1982).
138 Varga, J.M.; Konigsberg, W.H.; Richards, F.F.: Immunoglobulin with multiple binding functions. Induction of single immunoglobulin species with structurally dissimilar haptens. Proc. natn. Acad. Sci. USA *70:* 3268–3274 (1973).
139 Avrameas, S.; Dighiero, G.; Lymberi, P.; Guilbert, B.: Studies on natural antibodies and autoantibodies. Ann. Immunol., Paris *134D:* 103–113 (1983).
140 Ghearhart, P.J.; Bogenhagen, D.F.: Clusters of point mutations are found exclusively around rearranged antibody variable genes. Proc. natn. Acad. Sci. USA *80:* 3439–3445 (183).
141 Cohen, D.I.; Hedrick, S.M.; Nielsen, E.A.; D'Eustachio, P.; Ruddle, F.; Steinberg, A.D.; Paul, W.E.; Davis, M.M.: Isolation of cDNA clone corresponding to an X-linked gene family (XLR) closely linked to the murine immunodeficiency disorder Xid. Nature, Lond. *314:* 369–372 (1985).
142 Grabar, P.: Autoantibodies and immunological theories: an analytical review. Clin. Immunol. Immunopathol. *4:* 453–466 (1975).
143 Schrater, F.A.; Goidl, E.A.; Thorbecke, J.; Siskind, G.W.: Production of auto-anti-idiotypic antibody during the normal immune response to TNP-Ficoll. I. Occurence in AKR/J and BALB/C mice of hapten-augmentable anti-TNP plaque forming cells and their accelerated appearance in recipients of immune spleen cells. J. exp. Med. *250:* 138–153 (1979).
144 Goidl, E.A.; Schrater, A.F.; Siskind, G.W.; Thorbecke, G.J.: Production of auto-anti-idiotypic antibody during the normal immune response to TNP-Ficoll. II. Hapten reversible inhibition of anti-TNP plaque forming cells by immune serum as an assay for auto-anti-idiotypic antibody. J. exp. Med. *150:* 154–165 (1979).
145 Wieties, K.M.; Moticka, E.J.: Demonstration of hapten augmentable plaques in the bromelain treated anti-mouse red blood cell system: putative evidence for anti-idiotypic regulation of autoantibody secretion. Cell. Immunol. *98:* 68–77 (1986).
146 Hang, L.; Slack, J.H.; Amunolson, C.; Izui, S.; Theofilopoulos, A.N.; Dixon, F.J.: Induction of murine auto-immune disease by chronic polyclonal B cell activation. J. exp. Med. *157:* 974–986 (1983).

G. Dighiero, MD, Unité Immunohématologie et Immunopathologie,
Institut Pasteur, F-75724 Paris Cedex 15 (France)

Concepts Immunopathol., vol. 4, pp. 77–102 (Karger, Basel 1987)

Natural Cytotoxic (NC) Cell Activity in Murine and Human Systems

Effector Cells from Multiple Lineages with Antitumor Activity

Edmund C. Lattime

Immunology Program, Memorial Sloan-Kettering Cancer Center, New York, N. Y., USA

The term natural cell-mediated cytotoxicity (NCMC) has come to describe the lysis of a number of tumor cell lines in vitro by a family of related lymphoid cells which lack the characteristics of T cells, B cells and macrophages [1–5]. NCMC was first described as a unique activity as recently as the mid to late 1970s [6–8]. Initial studies into the presence of anti-tumor immunity both in humans [9, 10] and experimental animals [6, 7] had resulted in the finding that lymphoid cells from normal control subjects often exhibited significant in vitro lysis of a number of tumor cell lines without any evidence of overt exposure to the particular tumor. This cytotoxicity was initially considered 'background' and either subtracted from what was thought to be specific immunity, or else it was ignored. When the spontaneous lytic activity was first examined in its own right, studies were designed to examine its relationship to ongoing viral infection [11, 12] and in fact, the coining of the term natural killer (NK) cell was made in the study of such a possible relationship between target cell lysis and murine Moloney leukemia virus [6].

A number of characteristics have come to define the overall NCMC system. NCMC has been shown to be present in high levels without a need for specific priming [1, 2, 5, 13]; lack identifiable immunological memory [5, 13]; and lack major histocompatibility complex (MHC) restriction in killing [1–3, 5, 13]. Initially, a single effector, termed NK, was described [6], however studies in our laboratory exploring the cell-mediated cytotoxic response to non lymphoid tumors in mice revealed the presence of a second activity, which, while sharing the defining NCMC characteristics above, differed significantly enough from the NK cell to warrant the separate terminology natural cytotoxic (NC) cell [3, 4].

The purpose of this review is to summarize the findings which have been made regarding the effector cell(s) which mediate what we have termed NC activity [3], and discuss the evidence for an in vivo role for NC in tumor surveillance. In doing this, comparisons will be made to both NK and cytotoxic T lymphocytes (CTL). I should point out, however, that discussion of NK, etc. will only serve as a comparison, and references to non NC systems are not intended to be exhaustive [for recent comprehensive reviews of the NCMC area, see refs. 14, 15].

Before beginning a detailed discussion of the various facets of NC activity, a few words on nomenclature are in order. The principal defining characteristics of NCMC have been the lysis of tumor cells without priming and with a lack of MHC restriction. NK and NC cell activities were defined based on the cytotoxic activity of freshly harvested lymphoid populations against a series of tumor cell lines. Thus, the two effectors were defined not by a particular characteristic of the relevant population but by an *activity,* the lysis of tumor cells in vitro. While the initial definition of NC and NK were based on freshly harvested effectors, the term NCMC has been broadened in the literature to include any cellular mechanism which lyses tumor cells in vitro providing that the two tenets of lack of priming and MHC restriction are met. This broadened definition has come to encompass a variety of effectors generated in both short and long term culture systems as well as long term cell lines with only their non MHC restricted lytic activity required to term them NCMC. At a recent symposium on NCMC, held at Oakland University in Rochester, Mich., discussions by a committee of investigators resulted in subdividing the area into natural killer cells, which would include both NK and NC, and activated killers (AK) which would include both culture activated effectors as well as cloned long term lines.

For the purpose of this review, I will follow a similar approach i.e. examining NC, and where appropriate NK, characteristics as defined by freshly harvested populations, while addressing the question of activated killer cells and their relationship to NC in a separate section.

A Note on the Human Equivalent of Murine NC

The majority of the NC literature has been generated in the murine system, with only a small amount of data available on proposed human equivalents. Due to this limitation and in the interest of clarity, NC in the human will be discussed in a separate section of this review with reference to the similarities and differences from the murine system.

Assay Systems and Target Morphology

NK activity was first described in studies which utilized lymphoid tumor targets and short term ^{51}Cr release assays. In contrast, due to the adherent nature of the Meth-A and Meth-113 fibrosarcoma targets used in the early characterization of NC cell activity [3, 4], and adherence cell assay which measured the detachment of the tumor target following cell death was used [3]. These early studies found that NC activity required an extended (12–24 h) assay as opposed to the 4-hour assay for NK. Subsequently, studies using the BALB/c sarcoma WEHI-164 [16, 17] which grows nonadherently and was therefore assayed in the ^{51}Cr release system verified the requirement for an extended assay period characterized by a true 'lag' phase of 8–12 h before any target lysis was noted. It might be pointed out that when the original NC targets Meth-A and Meth-113 were assayed for susceptibility using the ^{51}Cr release assay, they were repeatedly found to be resistant to lysis [18], a finding which we have ascribed to the trypsinization required for preparing a suspension of the targets for the assay [18].

At least two mechanisms may be responsible for the lag period prior to measurable lysis in both the Meth-A, Meth-113 [3, 4] ^{3}H-proline and WEHI-164, ^{51}Cr release assay systems. Such a lag could be the function of a required activation of the effector population, the result of a target repair mechanism acting to counter lysis, or a combination of the above. In addressing the former, we began a series of studies in which murine spleen cells, as a source of NC, were pre-cultured with the Meth-A target for up to 18 h, washed and assayed for the kinetics of NC lysis with the premise in mind that if such a preactivation were required, then the 'activated' effectors would be capable of lysing the target in a short, 4-hour period. This was found not to be the case as precultured effector populations followed the same kinetics of lysis as did freshly harvested effector populations [19]. Elimination of both control and augmentable NK cells from the preactivation experiments also ruled out the generation of an activated NK population mediating the NC lysis [19]. A second possible mechanism for the requirement of a prolonged assay period is the presence of a target repair mechanism which may act to counter the lytic process and therefore result in delayed lysis. Such a mechanism has been described in both murine [20, 21] and human [22] NCMC systems. The evidence for such a repair mechanism will be described more fully in the section on target recognition and lytic mechanism to follow.

The question of target cell morphology and NC vs. NK susceptibility has led to a significant degree of confusion in the literature. The initial characterization of NK activity utilizing lymphoid tumor lines [1, 2, 6, 23], and NC using sarcoma lines [3, 4, 16, 17], resulted in the development of an NK-lymphoid, NC-nonlymphoid association. Using this reasoning, studies from a number of laboratories examining NCMC activity using nonlymphoid tumor targets were based on the assumption that the active effector cell was NC by the morphology of the target cell being examined. The question of target morphology alone identifying the class of effector cell involved was also studied in the rat system with findings that depending on the type of assay utilized, a number of nonlymphoid target cells were susceptible to lysis by effector cells with NK rather than NC characteristics [24]. I would point out that limiting our original studies to a very few prototype tumor cell lines was in part responsible for this premature association of target cell morphology and effector type.

In order to address the relationship between target cell morphology and NC/NK susceptibility, we examined a number of murine non-lymphoid tumor lines for relative sensitivity to NK and NC activities. We found that such tumors can be divided into three categories: NC susceptible, with all lysis the function of resting or activated Qa-5$^-$ effector cells; NK susceptible, with all lysis due to resting or activated Qa-5$^+$ effectors; and NK and NC susceptible with target cells lysed by a combination of NK and NC cells usually demonstrating susceptibility to NC with an activated NK component to lysis [25]. It should be pointed out that the prototype NC target WEHI-164 cell line was found to be the least NK susceptible with only occasional susceptibility to highly activated NK cells found [25] and thus may represent the preferred NC target. The finding that susceptibility to NC and NK lysis was independent of target morphology, contrary to the assumptions which followed the original NC/NK experiments demonstrates the danger in studying a restricted number of prototype target cell lines and extrapolating such data to describe the wider NCMC system.

Effector Cell Phenotype and Lineage

Following the advent of antisera and monoclonal antibodies directed towards lineage associated cell surface antigens, studies from a number of laboratories were carried out to characterize murine NCMC effector populations with the aim of both defining the specific cells involved as well as ascribing or associating the various NCMC activities to cells of a particular lineage. Negative selection experiments using C mediated elimination demonstrated that the cells manifesting murine NK cell activity expressed the T cell associated Qa-5 and Thy-1 antigens [16, 17, 26–28], as well as the more specific NK-1.1 [27, 29], NK-1.2 or 2.1 [16, 17, 30] and asialo-GMl [31] markers. Studies from both our [32] and other [16] laboratories demonstrated that while murine NK cells expressed the above antigens, NC activity was not eliminated when similar reagents were used in C mediated elimination protocols. In addition, negative selection with anti-class I MHC reagents which eliminated as many as 95% of spleen cells failed to eliminate NC activity [16, 17, 33]. Taken together, these findings led to the conclusion that NC activity was the function of a null cell population, and although no positive association between NC and lineage was possible, it was clearly shown that elimination of NK and T cells from the effector cell population did not eliminate NC activity.

In order to further characterize the effector cells manifesting NC, positive selection experiments using the fluorescence activated cell sorter (FACS) and a number of the monoclonal antibodies which were used for the negative selection studies above were carried out. In contrast to the conclusion reached above that NC activity was the function of a null cell population, it was found that spleen cells positive and negative for Qa-5 [34–36], NK-1.1 [34, 37], Thy-1 [35, 36] and IgG [36] all lysed the prototype NC target WEHI-164 as did cells sorted for high or low expression of MHC Class-I antigens [35, 36]. In order to confirm that the cells responsible for the lysis of WEHI-164 in the positively selected NK-1.1$^+$ spleen population were NK, it was also shown that treatment of the NK-1.1$^+$ spleen cells with anti-asialo GM1+C significantly reduced both NK and NC activities, while similar treatment of whole spleen cells failed to have measurable effects on NC [37].

In addition to confirming the above finding that freshly harvested Ig$^+$ as well as Ig$^-$ populations lyse WEHI-164, unpublished data kindly provided by Dr. R. Welsh, University of Massachusetts also demonstrates that spleen cells positive and negative for the macrophage antigen

MAC-1, MHC class-II antigens, and the B-220 B cell differentiation antigen all manifest significant NC activity as measured by the lysis of WEHI-164. It should be pointed out that while all of the populations tested for NC activity were capable of lysing WEHI-164, in three cases NC activity was clearly enriched. Cells having the highest NC activity were found to be Ig^-, $Qa\text{-}5^+$ and $Ly\text{-}2^-$ [36]. Therefore, whereas negative selection experiments resulted in the conclusion that NC was the function of a small null cell population, positive selection resulted in the demonstration that cells from both T and B cell lineages are capable of mediating NC activity, as are cells bearing the NK associated Qa-5 and NK 1.1 antigens.

While negative selection experiments in which NK cells were removed leaving NC intact were used to demonstrate that NK cells did not mediate NC activity, recent evidence would suggest to the contrary that NK cells are capable of NC activity, i.e. the lysis of NC susceptible targets, although they make up a small proportion of the total NC in spleen. The positive selection experiments cited above which use monoclonal antibody to the NK associated antigen NK 1.1 antigen (5% of spleen) or antisera to asialo GM-1 (11% of spleen) resulted in the isolation of cells which lysed the NC target WEHI-164 although NC activity was not reduced in the negative fractions [37]. Furthermore, it was shown that the majority of the NC activity in the $NK\text{-}1.1^+$ population was removed by treatment with antiasialo GM1+C which also eliminated NK [37]. Additional studies [Dr. C. Biron, personal commun.; 38] have also shown that enrichment for cells with NK activity (blast NK cells) from LCM virus infected or poly-IC injected mice resulted in a lytic population with significant NC activity.

In summarizing the phenotypic analysis of NC, it is clear from studies from a number of laboratories that positively selected cell populations from a number of defined lineages, as well as cells enriched for NK cell activity are all capable of mediating NC activity as measured by the lysis of WEHI-164. In addressing the apparent opposite results derived from negative selection experiments in which no treatment eliminated NC, it is assumed that with a number of distinct effector cells mediating NC activity, that the elimination of a small NC^+ population using antibody plus C was not detected because of the larger numbers of cells with NC activity which were not affected.

A second approach towards addressing the question of lineage of NC, and in particular the relationship of NC with NK and CTL, has involved the use of genetically mutant mice with defined immunologic deficiencies. In using these mutants, it was hoped that an association of decreased NC with decreases in other lymphoid or myeloid populations would yield further information on NC lineage. Towards this end, mice with the nude (nu/nu) mutation deficient in T cell function [3, 35]; motheaten (me) deficient in T and NK activity [35]; beige (bg/bg) deficient in NK [35, 39]; and the anemic WWv mouse deficient in myeloid and mast cell progenitors [35, 40] were all found to express significant levels of NC activity as assayed in the WEHI-164 or Meth-A tumor systems. Supporting the presence of NC in the absence of NK activity was the finding that mice treated from birth with anti-NK 1.1 which failed to express any NK activity had normal NC [35].

It should be pointed out that the myeloid and mast-cell-deficient WWv mutant, while having significant NC activity was the 1 mouse with consistently lower levels of NC than the control [35, 40, our unpubl. results] suggesting that a significant fraction of NC may lie within the myeloid compartment. Also in support of this conclusion are studies which show that bone marrow chimeras made with WWv marrow in normal recipients have lower NC as a function of total spleen cell numbers [37], although on a per cell basis demonstrate significant NC activity.

In summary, therefore, data derived from both positive selection as well as mutant mouse studies support the conclusion that NC activity is present in cells from more than one lineage. In describing this finding, we have previously coined the term 'horizontal lineage' by which we mean that rather than be the function of a single lineage, NC activity may be mediated by cells of multiple lineages, perhaps at different stages of differentiation [41]. These findings draw further attention to the caution raised at the beginning of this review, i.e. that by defining NK and NC by the 'activity' of lysing a particular prototype tumor cell line in vitro may falsely suggest that they are discreet cell populations, whereas the data presented above clearly demonstrates that, at least in the NC system, the defining activity is indeed the function of multiple cell types.

Regulation of NC Activity by Lymphokines

Following the early demonstration that NK cell activity was augmented by interferon [42] and subsequently that IL-2 also served to increase the activity of NK [43], studies from our and other laboratories examined the relative augmenting activity of a number of characterized lymphokines on NK and NC activities. These studies were begun for two reasons. The first was to better characterize the regulation of NCMC lysis. In addition, it was felt that by determining which in a series of lymphokines were active in augmenting NC, that this evidence would perhaps contribute to a better understanding of lineage, i.e. if NC activity was preferentially regulated by IL-2, an association might be made with the T cell lineage. In this second vein, it was felt that the relationship between NC and NK might be better established by determining if the two effectors shared similar regulatory mechanisms.

Short-term activation protocols, i.e. 12–18 h preincubation of murine spleen cells with graded doses of IL-2 (semipurified lectin free supernatant from Con-A stimulated murine and rat spleen cells) and IL-3 (produced by WEHI-3 cells and purified by Ihle et al. [44]) were found to augment NC activity at relatively low doses [45] while neither alpha/beta nor gamma interferon [our unpubl. results] nor the interferon inducing agent poly-IC [45, 46] increased NC activity. Therefore, while both NK and NC activities were augmented by IL-2, NK but not NC was augmented by IFN, while NC, but not NK, activity was increased by IL-3. In support of the IL-3 activation of NC, and reported independently at the same time were studies in which IL-3 dependent murine spleen cell lines manifested significant NC, but not NK activity [47].

Studies in the NK system have examined the interrelationship between IL-2 and IFN augmentation of activity with mixed results. The culture of spleen cells with IL-2 was shown to result in the induction of gamma-IFN [48] and studies from one laboratory showed that anti-IFN antibody inhibited the IL-2 augmentation of NK [49]. These two findings taken together suggested that IL-2 was not the activating moiety, but rather that IL-2 acted via secondary IFN production [48–50]. More recent studies in the human system have shown that gamma-IFN augments NK in only a minority of individuals [51] and likewise, we have found that recombinant murine gamma-IFN augments murine NK only weakly, if at all, following the same protocols which result in major augmentation by IL-2 [our unpubl. results].

The mechanism of IL-2 activation in NC, and whether it acts via IFN production was answered early on by the demonstration that in vitro culture neither alpha/beta nor gamma-IFN resulted in augmentation of NC, nor did the IFN inducing poly-IC molecule have any augmenting activity [45, 46; our unpubl. results]. Therefore, although it has not been elucidated whether IL-2 manifests its NC augmenting activity directly or via the induction of a second factor, it is clear that it does not act via IFN.

The second question addressed by the lymphokine studies was whether it was possible to associate NC activity with a particular cell type or lineage based on its activation by IL-2 and/or IL-3. IL-3 has been shown to cause the expansion of both early stem cell as well as committed precursors and end stage populations of a number of lineages [52], and thus the demonstration of its activating properties on NC would not help elucidate a particular lineage or lineages of NC active cells.

IL-2, on the other hand, has been principally associated with activities in the T cell lineage [53] and NK populations bearing Thy-1 [28], although it has been shown that the IL-2 receptor TAC is present on some human B cells [54]. It was therefore felt that this association of NC with IL-2 suggested a link between NC and the T cell lineage [45, 55]. Recent studies described in the lineage section above, however, in which a series of mutant mice strains, deficient in cells of one or more lineages, were examined resulted in the demonstration of an association of IL-2 augmentation with NC, in mice with major T cell deficiencies [35]. In these studies, mutant mice deficient in T cell activity (nude nu/nu as well as motheaten me/me); NK activity (beige bg/bg, me/me, and mice depleted of NK by administration of anti-NK 1.1 antibody); and mice with deficient myeloid and mast cell function (WWv) all manifested NC activity and in every case NC was augmented by IL-2.

In summary, therefore, studies into the regulation of NCMC by lymphokines have resulted in the finding that NC and NK activities are augmented by an overlapping group of lymphokines with NK augmented by IFN and IL-2, but not IL-3, while NC activity is augmented by IL-2 and IL-3, but not IFN. In addition, studies aimed at elucidating the lineage of NC and its relationship to NK by the relative augmenting effects of the various lymphokines have resulted in an apparent association of IL-2 augmentation and NC which crosses lineage lines.

Mechanism of NC Target Recognition and Antitumor Activity

While not characterized as thoroughly as the NK effector-target interaction [56], studies from a number of laboratories have examined NC target recognition and lytic mechanism against both tumor and transformed fibroblast cell lines. Taken together to form a consensus model, these studies have demonstrated a requirement for effector cell target cell contact, having a specificity for certain target cell lines, which results in the generation or release of a soluble cytotoxic factor which is responsible for target cell lysis.

With the above described finding that tumor cell targets can be divided into NK susceptible, NC susceptible and those susceptible to both, a number of studies have addressed the question of NC target recognition and its relationship to that of NK and CTL effector populations. In light of the findings that NC may be the property of several cell types, discussed more fully in the section on lineage above, it was decided that studies into target recognition and lytic mechanism might identify common characteristics of effectors with NC activity and thus help to better define the NC system. To this end, we will divide NC lysis into three phases.

Target Recognition

While lacking MHC restriction for lysis, the NC effector-target interaction has been shown to have specificity. Two lines of data have been presented which demonstrate specificity at the recognition phase of the effector target interaction, both of which supporting shared recognition determinants between the NC and NK systems.

In studies designed to examine the role of the extracellular matrix glycoprotein laminin on NK activity, it was found that the addition of laminin to NC or NK assays inhibited target cell lysis by inhibiting the effector target binding step in the reaction [57]. It was additionally found that target cells preincubated with laminin failed to cold compete with labeled NC targets, and effector populations treated with antilaminin antibodies exhibited decreased lytic activity [57]. This led to the conclusion that the laminin molecule was present on the effector cell with its corresponding receptor on the target [57, 58].

Similar evidence that cells which mediate NC and NK cell activities share common target recognition determinant(s) has been provided through the use of cold target inhibition experiments. Studies from our [18, 32, 33] and other [20, 59, 60] laboratories have demonstrated by the use of a number of NK and NC susceptible target cell lines that NK activity is competitively inhibited by NC targets and vice versa while NK and NC resistant lines fail to compete for the two activities.

An additional similarity between NC and NK, but not CTL activity was found in studies designed to determine the role of sugar moieties in NC target recognition and lysis. NC and NK, but not CTL mediated target lysis were shown to be inhibited by the addition of low levels of monosaccharides to the assay [61] leading to the conclusion that NC target recognition might involve a lectin like interaction shared by NK but not CTL effector populations. While both NK and NC activities were inhibited by monosaccharides, NK activity was susceptible to inhibition by a range of sugars whereas NC was particularly sensitive to inhibition by *D*-mannose [61]. While it has not been determined whether the sugar inhibition of NC acts at a pre- or post-binding event, this finding added further evidence for a similar mechanism of NC and NK activities. It is of interest to note that while the activity of CTL generated in five day mixed lymphocyte culture was not blocked by the addition of monosaccharide [61], target lysis by long-term CTL clones propagated in IL-2 was blocked by a similar panel of sugars as was found for NK [62], suggesting that the propagation of CTL lines in IL-2 may result in an altered recognition system similar to an NK/NC-like mechanism. A further discussion of the relationship between NK/NC and CTL lines can be found in a later section of this review.

Programming for Lysis

Preliminary studies into the cellular requirements for NC target lysis resulted in the finding that intact and viable effector cells were required for lysis, while dead cells and membrane fragments were incapable of lysing the target [16]. More recently, studies which describe tumor necrosis factor (TNF) as the putative lytic molecule have shown that the interaction between murine spleen cells and the NC target WEHI-164 are required for the release of significant levels of TNF, not found in supernatant from spleen cells cultured alone [63]. The conclusion that TNF is the active factor in NC lysis was made on the basis that (1) the NC susceptible WEHI-164 triggered the release of TNF from spleen cells; (2) WEHI-164 is particularly sensitive to the lytic activity of both naturally produced as well as recombinant murine TNF, and (3) that the spleen cell mediated lysis of the WEHI-164 target cell was inhibited by the addition of antisera produced against murine TNF [63, 64]. Further studies have demonstrated that the TNF-NC association is distinct from the mechanism involved in murine NK cell lysis. In this regard, it was found that in contrast to the NC target WEHI-164, the prototype NK target YAC-1 was resistant to the cytotoxic effects of TNF, did not induce TNF production upon coculture with spleen cells, and that splenic NK activity was not reduced by the addition of anti-TNF antisera [63].

Target Mechanisms in NC Lysis

In addition to the effector phase of NC lysis, studies have described the involvement of a target cell repair mechanism which may act to counter the NC lytic activity of the effector cell [21, 59]. Rather than act as an inert partner in the effector-target interaction, it has been found that the requirement for an extended assay period for NC lysis could be substantially shortened by the pretreatment of the target cell with protein synthesis inhibiting compounds [21, 59]. This finding has been used as support for the presence of a protein synthesis dependent target cell repair mechanism which acts to counter the lytic activity of the NC cell [21, 59]. These studies further contrast the mechanism of NC lysis with that for CTL an NK cell activities in that similar target cell treatment failed to alter the rapid kinetics of the two [21]. It should be pointed out that a similar acceleration has been reported in the lysis of certain human target cells requiring a long term assay [22] which may represent a human equivalent of that described in the murine system [21, 59].

Therefore, while NC and NK share the defining characteristics of NCMC populations, both similarities and differences exist in their interaction with targets. Studies into target recognition and binding of NC and NK effectors have demonstrated significant similarities and shared recognition structures. In contrast, both at the level of mechanism of lysis and the role of the target in the lytic interaction, significant differences have been identified between NC and NK activities.

In vivo Antitumor Activity of NC

As discussed in the introduction, both NC and NK have been defined by their in vitro lysis of a series of prototype tumor cell lines. While this has led to a great deal of mechanistic data, it is their ability to manifest antitumor activity in vivo which is required to demonstrate that the in vitro lytic activity is modeling a similar in vivo activity.

If NC and/or NK are to act as a true surveillance system as has been described by Burnet [65], then it should be possible to show that animals deficient in the relevant effector population(s) would manifest increased spontaneous tumor incidence over those with normally functioning NCMC systems. In order to prove a role for NCMC against spontaneous tumors in vivo requires the long-term observation of large numbers of animals for the development of spontaneous tumors. The few of such studies which have used NK deficient animals have not shown statistically significant increases in spontaneous tumor incidence [reviewed in refs. 39, 66]. As we have described obove, as yet no murine mutant or inbred strain has been identified which has a deficiency in populations which mediate NC. Therefore, such experiments have not been possible in the NC system.

On the other hand, two experimental tumor transplantation models have been used which support a role for NC and NK in in vivo elimination of tumor cells. In the first system, series of tumor cell lines have been studied for their susceptibility to NC- or NK-mediated lysis in the relevant in vitro assay, and these results correlated with the number of cells required to induce the in vivo growth of the tumor. When both NK [67]- and NC [18]-susceptible targets were examined in this fashion, statistically significant correlations were found between the susceptibility of the target to NC/NK and resistance to tumor growth in vivo. More recently, studies which extended the previous findings demonstrated that when NC-susceptible, NK-resistant cell lines were selected for NC-resistant variants either by in vivo passage or in vitro culture with normal spleen cells that the NC-resistant clones were more efficient at inducing tumors in vivo [68] thus supporting a role for NC in the in vivo elimination of transplanted tumors.

The second model system which has been used was designed to study the role of NK in surveillance against metastasis [69]. In these studies, single cell suspensions of NK susceptible tumor cell lines were injected i.v. and following a period of up to 30 days, the mice were sacrificed and the number of tumor foci in the lungs counted. Studies such as these have resulted in the most significant results to date supporting an in vivo role for NCMC. In the NK system, it was shown that mice deficient in NK such as young mice [70], or the bg/bg mutant mouse [71] were less efficient at clearing circulating tumor emboli than normal adult controls. Conversely, in vivo NK augmentation using such agents as the interferon inducing compound poly-IC or *Corynebacterium parvum* [69] resulted in increased clearance of circulating NK susceptible tumor cells. Similar lung clearance experiments have not been reported in the NC system due to the lack in NC-deficient animals, however, experiments using NC-susceptible, NK-resistant tumors have demonstrated increases in lung colonies in mice treated with antiasialo GM1 (shown to eliminate NK, but not NC). Such a finding would seem to be inconsistent with studies which have shown that in vitro elimination of asialo $GM\text{-}1^+$ cells failed to effect NC activity. Recent studies have, however, shown that such in vivo treatment results in the reduction of as much as 95% in the antiviral CTL response [72], and, therefore, until the cells responsible for the clearance of the NC susceptible target in this system are characterized, any conclusions as to the mechanism of increased tumor foci noted would be premature.

In summary, while a convincing role for NC and/or NK activity in the in vivo surveillance against spontaneously arising tumors has not been proven, significant evidence has been reported which links NK, and perhaps NC with elimination of circulating tumor emboli. In addition, although by correlation, studies in both the NK and the NC system would seem to demonstrate that NC- and NK-susceptible tumor cell lines are less efficient at inducing tumors than NC/NK-resistant lines.

Nontumor-Related Activities of NC

A number of studies in both human and murine systems have given rise to evidence supporting a role for NK in nontumor-related activities. While it has not been suggested that NK cells are the only population involved, NK activity has been associated with the regulation of normal hematopoiesis. Studies have shown that the preculture of bone marrow cells with NK-enriched populations results in decreased CFUc and BFUe colony formation [73]. Likewise, studies have shown the presence of an NK-sensitive 'target' cell in newborn thymus [74] and normal bone marrow [75] and NK activity has also been associated with the rejection of bone marrow engraftment [76].

Studies have also linked NK with the early surveillance of a number of infections and parasitic organisms. NK activity has been linked to the response to viruses such as herpes, cytomegalovirus and hepatitis; parasites such as Trypanosoma and microbial pathogens such as Shigella and malaria [for a series of articles on these subjects see the relevant sections in ref. 77].

While the above reports have linked the activity of NK cells with a number of nontumor-associated functions ranging from the regulation of hematopoiesis to surveillance against a number of infectious agents, a similar analysis of NC activities has not progressed to such an extent. The characterization of nontumor-related NK activities was made possible by the ability to enrich and/or deplete lymphoid populations of NK using either in vivo or in vitro techniques or through the use of NK-deficient mutant mouse strains. As an example, the demonstration that NK acted to down regulate CFUc und BFUe activities [73] was made possible by antibody + C elimination of NK activity from the accessory cell population. As we have discussed above in the sections on lineage and phenotype, the antitumor activity of NC is a function of cells from more than one lineage, and it has not been possible to eliminate NC through standard depletion techniques [35, 36]. Therefore, similar studies as those noted for NK have not been possible in the NC system.

NC activity has, in a recent report, however, been associated with the response to herpes virus (HSV-1) [78]. In this study, it was shown that HSV-1 infected WEHI-164 target cells were lysed more efficiently than uninfected targets, in a similar fashion as these investigators had previously shown in the NK system [79], and it was concluded that the effector mechanism responsible was NC based on the NK insensitivity of the WEHI-164 target, and the demonstration that the accelerated killing of the virus infected cell was not effected by the elimination of NK activity using anti-Qa-5 + C [78].

The recent finding that the antitumor activity of NC may be mediated via TNF production [63, 64] and the extension of these findings to conclude that the common factor of the multilineage populations with NC activity may be their ability to produce TNF [63] would suggest that lymphoid and myeloid populations which mediate NC, most likely are also involved in a number of nontumor-associated functions. Studies published this year alone have shown that TNF, and by extension the cells which produce TNF are involved in the regulation of hematopoiesis [80], the growth and factor production by vascular endothelial cells [81–83], neutrophil activation [84–86], the production and regulation of IL-1 and PGE2 [87], eosinophil toxicity to Schistosoma [88], and bone metabolism [89].

In summary, with the exception of the herpes virus study [78], there has not been a direct association of NC activity and nontumor-related activities as has been previously made for NK. As discussed above, however, it is likely that this lack of a link between NC and nontumor systems is based on technical problems in dealing with NC, most notably the inability to eliminate the cells mediating NC activity through conventional means. If, however, the recent association of NC and TNF proves to be the case and the ability to produce TNF upon stimulation is found to be the common characteristic of NC, then, cells which mediate NC may also prove to have significant nontumor activities.

Human Equivalent of Murine NC

The original demonstration of NC in the murine system, and its characterization as a distinct NCMC effector population was dependent on the identification of the prototype Meth-A, Meth-113 and WEHI-164 targets [3, 17]. A similar finding in the human system has resulted in the initial characterization of what would appear to be a human correlate of the murine NC [90, 91]. It should be noted that, as became the case in the murine system, there has been the tendency to identify a human NCMC effector cell as NC, based predominantly on the morphology of the target. As discussed above, this is insufficient evidence as the majority of murine nonlymphoid tumors were found to be sensitive to both NK and NC activities [25]. Therefore, given the current characterization of murine NC, four properties would be expected of a human equivalent which would differentiate it from NK and CTL: (1) the presence of lytic activity in freshly harvested lymphoid cells; (2) a requirement for a long term (greater than 8 h) assay period; (3) augmentation by IL-2, but not alpha/beta-interferon, and (4) presence of activity in the absence of NK. Given the demonstration that cells of a number of lineages are capable of manifesting NC activity, including those which express NK-associated antigens, determining an NC phenotype has not been possible in the murine system. With this in mind, however, studies from a number of laboratories have shown that NC activity is present in the absence of NK. This has been shown by eliminating NK activity with antibodies + C [17, 32]; positive selection experiments using the FACS (see earlier section on phenotype of NC); and in studies using NK-deficient mutant mice (see section on lineage of NC). Therefore, although NK cells may manifest NC activity, in all murine systems tested, removing cells with NK activity did not eliminate NC.

Our initial attempts at elucidating a human equivalent of the murine NC (unpubl. results with C. Platsoucas] involved the screening of a number of human nonlymphoid tumors including breast and colon carcinomas, lung adenomas and melanomas. While we found that a number of these lines were sensitive to NCMC in an 18-hour ^{51}Cr release assay, negative selection using monoclonal antibodies to the NK-associated Leu-7

(HNK-1), Leu-11 and OKM-1 +C resulted in depleting both the lysis of K-562 (NK activity) as well as the lysis of the nonlymphoid targets. Therefore, while these tumors were found to be NCMC sensitive, lysis was apparently due to NK cell activity which would be consistent with our findings in the murine system that most NCMC sensitive nonlymphoid tumors were NK sensitive [25]. Supporting our findings are unpublished results [provided by Drs. S. Golub and J.D. Gray, UCLA, Los Angeles] which show that the NCMC activity against human melanoma targets was reduced or eliminated by negative selection using the monoclonal antibody B73.1 which recognizes the Fc-gamma-receptor associated with human NK [73]. Therefore, in these earlier attempts, target cell lysis which might have been expected to be NC based solely on target morphology was shown to be due to the activity of NK cells.

More recent studies, however, using the human carcinoma cell line MA-160, have demonstrated that, similar to the murine NC system, target lysis requires a prolonged assay time, is augmented by IL-2 but not gamma-interferon, and is distinct serologically from human NK [90, 91]. The effector cells mediating this activity share the NK- and T cell-associated Leu-11 and OKM1 markers, but fail to express the NK marker Leu-7 and T cell antigen OKT-8 [91]. In addition, the description of a new monoclonal antibody (HNC-1), present on NC, but not NK, has allowed for the separation of the two effectors [90, 91]. While these results have been derived for the most part through the use of a single target cell line, based on cell surface phenotype, target cell repertoire, and lymphokine regulation, the putative human NC effector cell has similar characteristics to those shown in the murine system.

Culture-Generated Cytotoxic Populations, Cloned Cell Lines and Their Relationship to NC

While the topics discussed in this review were intended to center on the NCMC activity of freshly harvested cell populations, a defining characteristic of the system, a note is in order regarding the range of culture generated effector cells which have been shown to lyse NK and NC susceptible target cell lines, and by this activity have been associated with NK and NC.

As discussed above with regard to assigning an effector population based solely on the morphology of the target cell, in a number of cases the description of NK and NC as activities based on their lysis of prototype target cells resulted in the assumption that cells which lysed YAC-1 or WEHI-164 were NK and/or NC, respectively. This tendency to define a cytotoxic system based solely on the in vitro lysis of a prototype target in some cases resulted in the effector(s) inheriting other characteristics of the respective freshly harvested cytotoxic cell without their having been satisfactorily studied.

Cytotoxic cell populations which lyse a number of overlapping targets have been described following culture of spleen cells alone with fetal calf serum [16, 92–97, 107] or with a number of stimuli such as allogeneic cells [98–101], poly I [102], conditioned medium containing IL-2 [103, 104) and a number of tumor cell lines [95]. These culture systems have, for the most part, resulted in the generation of cells which preferentially lyse tumor targets over normal cells, and NK sensitive cells over NK resistant ones.

More specifically, in the case of culture generated cells which lyse the NC target WEHI-164, a recent report from our laboratory [101] highlighted the danger of calling any cell which lyses WEHI-164 NC. Using an allo-MLC system, it was found that a number of distinct anti-WEHI-164 effector cells were generated. Effector cells which lysed WEHI-164 were found to be both positive and negative for Ly 2, Thy 1, and L3T4 [101]. These studies identified the respective populations by C mediated elimination of lytic activity, which has not been possible using freshly harvested populations [32]. Whether these distinct populations share a similar mechanism of lysis or are the equivalent of the multilineage anti-WEHI-164 effectors which we have reported in freshly harvested populations [35, 36] has yet to be established. These studies, however, further point out the fact that the lysis of one or more prototype target is not sufficient to identify an effector cell type.

In addition to the studies described above which have characterized cytotoxic populations generated in short-term in vitro systems, studies from two laboratories have specifically examined cloned cell lines with NC anti-WEHI-164 but not NK activity. These studies have identified cell lines with lymphoid [47], as well as mast cell and basophil [40, 105] characteristics which share the ability to lyse WEHI-164, but not NK-sensitive targets. These findings would be consistent with the studies described in the lineage section above which show that freshly harvested cells from more than one lineage have NC activity. However, until it has been shown that these lines share more than just the ability to lyse

WEHI-164 with the freshly harvested effectors, it may be premature to equate their activity with NC.

The risk in characterizing or identifying a cell based on the lysis of one or more targets is probably best pointed out in studies by Brooks et al. [106] which demonstrated that the target cell repertoire as well as MHC restriction of lysis by cloned CTL lines with allo specificities varied based on the concentration of IL-2 used for their propagation. These cloned lines, as IL-2 concentration was increased, passed through a stage in which they were cytotoxic for the specific allo target and also NK-sensitive, but not NK-resistant targets, followed with higher IL-2 by a stage where they were capable of lysing a broad range of NK-sensitive and NK-resistant target cell lines [106]. Therefore, these studies in which the target repertoire of a monoclonal cell population is directly affected by the culture conditions used for its propogation raises a further caution in identifying a cytotoxic cell strictly based on its target spectrum.

Conclusions

As outlined at the beginning of this review, it was my intention to discuss the underlying experimental basis and conclusions which have been reached regarding the cells responsible for what we have termed NC activity. Until quite recently, it was the working hypothesis of the major investigators in the NC area, based particularly on serological data, that NC activity was the function of a small null cell population distinct from T cells, B cells or macrophages. More recently, however, it has become clear that cells from a number of defined lineages have the ability to express NC which raises new questions as to their shared characteristics and/or mechanisms of antitumor activity. The identification of TNF as a proposed mediator of NC target lysis, taken with its other activities, may shed light on the multiplicity of functions mediated by cells with NC activity.

Acknowledgements

I would like to thank Dr. Osias Stutman and Dr. Stuart Macphail for helpful discussions; and Drs. Christine Biron, Sidney Golub, John Hiserodt and Raymond Welsh for sharing unpublished results and preprints. The experimental work described in this text was supported by NIH grants CA-08748 and CA-15988 and American Cancer Society IM-188. Dr. Lattime is a scholar of the Leukemia Society of America. This text was completed August 25, 1986.

References

1 Herberman, R.B.; Holden, H.T.: Natural cell-mediated immunity. Adv. Cancer Res. *27:* 305–377 (1978).

2 Kiessling, R.; Haller, O.: Natural killer cells in the mouse: An alternative immune surveillance mechanism? Contemp. Top. Immunobiol. *8:* 171–201 (1978).

3 Stutman, O.; Paige, C.; Feo Figarella, E.: Natural cytotoxic cells against solid tumors in mice. I. Strain and age distribution and target cell susceptibility. J. Immun. *121:* 1819–1826 (1978).

4 Paige, C.J.; Feo Figarella, E.; Cuttito, M.J.; Cahan, A.; Stutman, O.: Natural cytotoxic cells against solid tumors in mice. II. Some characteristics of the effector cells. J. Immun. *121:* 1827–1835 (1978).

5 Herberman, R.B.; Djeu, J.D.; Kay, D.; Ortaldo, J.R.; Riccardi, C; Bonnard, G.D.; Holden, H.T.; Fagnani, R.; Santoni, A.; Puccetti, P.: Natural killer cells. Characteristics and regulation of activity. Immunol. Rev. *44:* 43 (1979).

6 Kiessling, R.; Klein, E.; Wigzell, H.: 'Natural killer' cells in the mouse. I. Cytotoxic cells with specificity for mouse Moloney leukemia cells. Specificity and distribution according to genotype. Eur. J. Immunol. *5:* 112–117 (1975).

7 Herberman, R.B.; Nunn, M.E.; Lavrin, D.H.: Natural cytotoxic reactivity of mouse lymphoid cells against syngeneic and allogeneic tumors. I. Distribution of reactivity and specificity. Int. J. Cancer *16:* 216–229 (1975).

8 Pross, H.F.; Jondal, M.: Cytotoxic lymphocytes from normal donors. A functional marker of human non-T lymphocytes. Clin. exp. Immunol. *21:* 226–232 (1975).

9 Rosenberg, E.B.; Herberman, R.B.; Levine, P.H.; Halterman, R.H.; McCoy, J.L.; Wunderlich, J.R.: Lymphocyte cytotoxicity reactions to leukemia-associated antigens in identical twins. Int. J. Cancer *9:* 648–658 (1972).

10 McCoy, J.L.; Herberman, R.B.; Rosenberg, E.B.; Donnelly, F.C.; Levine, P.H.; Alford, C.: 51 Chromium-release assy for cell-mediated cytotoxicity of human leukemia and lymphoid tissue-culture cells. Natn. Cancer Inst. Monogr. *37:* 59–67 (1973).

11 Herberman, R.B.; Nunn, M.E.; Lavrin, D.H.; Asofsky, R.: Effect of antibody to theta antigen on cell-mediated immunity induced in syngeneic mice by murine sarcoma virus. J. natn. Cancer Inst. *51:* 1509 (1973).

12 Gomard, E.; Leclerc, J.C.; Levy, J.P.: Spontaneous antylymphoma reaction of pre-leukemia AKR mice is a non-T killing. Nature, Lond. *150:* 671–673 (1974).

13 Kiessling, R.; Wigzell, H.: An analysis of murine NK cells as to structure/function and biological relevance. Immunol. Rev. *44:* 165–208 (1979).

14 Herberman, R.: Multiple functions of natural killer cells, including immunoregulation as well as resistance to tumor growth. Concepts Immunopathol. *1:* 96–132 (1985).

15 Stutman, O.; Lattime, E.: Lymphokines and natural cell-mediated cytotoxicity; in Landy, Lymphokines, vol. 12 pp. 107–159 (Academic Press, New York 1985).

16 Burton, R.: Alloantisera selectively reactive with NK cells: characterization and use in defining NK cell classes; in Herberman, Natural cell-mediated immunity against tumors, pp. 19–35, (Academic Press, New York 1980).

17 Burton, R.C.; Bartlett, S.P.; Kumar, V.; Winn, H.J.: Studies on natural killer (NK) cells. II. Serologic evidence for heterogeneity of murine NK cells. J. Immun. *127:* 1864–1868 (1981).

18 Stutman, O.; Feo Figarella, E.; Paige, C.; Lattime, E.: Natural cytotoxic (NC) cells against solid tumors in mice: General characteristics and comparison to natural killer (NK) cells, in Herberman, Natural cell-mediated immunity against tumors, pp.187–229 (Academic Press, New York 1980).

19 Lattime, E.C.; Pecoraro, G.A.; Stutman, O.: Natural cytotoxic cells against solid tumors in mice: IV. Natural cytotoxic (NC) cells are not culture activated natural killer (NK) cells. Int. J. Cancer *30:* 471–477 (1982).

20 Collins, J.L.; Patek, P.Q.; Cohn, M.: Tumorigenicity and lysis by natural killers. J. exp. Med. *153:* 89–106 (1981).

21 Patek, P.A.; Collins, J.L.; Cohn, M.: Evidence that cytotoxic T cells and natural cytotoxic cells use different lytic mechanisms to lyse the same targets. Eur. J. Immunol. *13:* 433–436 (1983).

22 Hudig, D.; Djobadze, M.; Redelman, D.; Mendelsohn, J.: Active tumor cell resistance to human natural killer lymphocyte attack. Cancer Res. *41:* 2803–2808 (1981).

23 Sendo, F.; Aoki, T.; Boyse, E.A.; Buafo, C.K.: Natural occurrence of lymphocytes showing cytotoxic activity to BALB/c radiation-induced leukemia RLol cells. J. natn. Cancer Inst. *55:* 603–609 (1975).

24 Brooks, C.; Flannery, G.; Webb, P.; Baldwin, R.: Quantitative studies of natural immunity to solid tumours in rats. The nature of the killer cell depends on the type of assay. Immunology *41:* 673–680 (1980).

25 Lattime, E.C.; Pecoraro, G.A.; Cuttito, M.J.; Stutman, O.: Murine nonlymphoid tumors are lysed by a combination of NK and NC cells. Int. J. Cancer *32:* 523–528 (1983).

26. Kumar, V.; Luevano, E.; Bennett M.: Hybrid resistance to EL-4 lymphoma cells. I. Characterization of natural killer cells that lyse EL-4 cells and their distinction from marrow dependent natural killer cells. J. exp. Med. *150:* 531–547 (1979).

27 Koo, G.; Jacobson, J.; Hammerling, G.; Hammerling, U.: Antigenic profile of murine natural killer cells. J. Immun. *125:* 1003–1006 (1980).

28 Minato, N.; Reid, L.; Bloom, B.R.: On the heterogeneity of murine natural killer cells. J. exp. Med. *154:* 750–762 (1981).

29 Jondal, M.; Targan, S.: In vitro induction of cytotoxic effector cells with spontaneous killer cell specificity. J. exp. Med. *147:* 1621–1636 (1978).

30 Pollack, S.; Emmons, S.: Anti-NK 2.1. An activity of NZB anti-BALB/c serum; in Herberman, NK cells and other natural effector cells, pp. 113–118 (Academic Press, New York 1980).

31 Kasai, M.; Iwamori, M.; Nagai, Y.; Ilumura, K.; Tada, T.: A glycolipid on the surface of mouse natural killer cells. Eur. J. Immunol. *10:* 175–180 (1980).

32 Lattime, E.C.; Pecoraro, G.A.; Stutman, O.: Natural cytotoxic cells against solid

tumors in mice. III. A comparison of effector cell antigenic phenotype and target cell recognition structures with those of NK cells. J. Immun. *126:* 2011–2014 (1981).

33 Lattime, E.; Ishizaka, S.; Pecoraro, G.; Koo, G.; Stutman, O.: NC cells do not express NK-associated cell surface antigens and are not culture activated NK cells; in Herberman, NK cells and other natural effector cells, pp. 187–192 (Academic Press, New York 1982).

34 Kumar, V.; Hackett, J.; Lipscomb, M.; Bennett, M.; Koo, G.: Studies of purified NK-1.1$^+$ natural killer (NK) cells. (Abstract). Fed. Proc. *44:* 1525 (1985).

35 Lattime, E.; Bykowsky, M.; Stutman, O.: Natural cytotoxic (NC) activity. A multi-lineage system regulated by IL-2. Immunol. Res. *5:* 5–15 (1986).

36 Bykowsky, M.J.; Stutman, O.: The cells responsible for natural cytotoxic (NC) activity: A multilineage system. J. Immun. *137:* 1120–1126 (1986).

37 Hackett, J.; Bennett, M.; Koo, G.; Kumar, V.: Origin and differentiation of natural killer cells. III. Relationship between the precursors and effectors of natural killer and natural cytotoxic activity. Immunol. Res. *5:* 16–24 (1986).

38 Biron, C.; Pedersen, K.; Welsh, R.: Purification and target cell range of in vivo elicited blast natural killer cells. J. Immun. *137:* 463–471 (1986).

39 Stutman, O.; Cuttito, M.J.: Normal levels of natural cytotoxic cells against solid tumors in NK-deficient beige mice. Nature, Lond. *290:* 254–257 (1981).

40 Ghiara, P.; Boraschi, D.; Villa, L.; Scapigliati, G.; Taddei, C.; Tagliabue, A.: In vitro generated mast cells express natural cytotoxicity against tumor cells. Immunology *55:* 317–324 (1985).

41 Stutman, O.; Lattime, E.: Natural killer and other effector cells; in Kripke, Frost, Immunology and cancer, pp. 221–258 (University of Texas Press, Houston, TX, 1986).

42 Senik, A.; Gresser, I.; Maury, C.; Gidlund, M.; Orn, A.; Wigzell, H.: Enhancement by interferon of natural killer cell activity in mice. Cell. Immunol. *44:* 186–200 (1979).

43 Henney, C.S.; Kuribayashi, K.; Kern, D.E.; Gillis, S.: IL-2 augments natural killer cell activity. Nature, Lond. *291:* 335–338 (1981).

44 Ihle, J.N.; Rebar, L.; Keller, J.; Lee, J.C.; Hapel, A.: Interleukin-3. Possible roles in the regulation of lymphocyte differentiation and growth. Immunol. Rev. *63:* 5–32 (1982).

45 Lattime, E.C.; Pecoraro, G.A.; Stutman, O.: The activity of natural cytotoxic (NC) cells is augmented by interleukin 2 and interleukin 3. J. exp. Med. *157:* 1070–1075 (1983).

46 Lattime, E.; Pecoraro, G.; Cuttito, M.; Stutman, O.: Solid tumors are killed by NK and NC cell populations. Interferon inducing agents do not augment NC cell activity under NK activating conditions; in Herberman, NK cells and other natural effector cells, pp. 179–186, Academic Press, New York 1982).

47 Djeu, J.Y.; Lanza, E.; Pastore, S.; Hapel, A.J.: Selective growth of natural cytotoxic but not natural killer effector cells in interleukin-3 Nature, Lond. *306:* 788–791 (1983).

48 Kawase, I.; Brooks, C.; Kuribayashi, K.; Olabuenaga, S.; Newman, W.; Gillis, S.; Henney, C.: Interleukin 2 induced-interferon production. Participation of macrophages and NK like cells. J. Immun. *131:* 288–292 (1983).

49 Weigent, D.; Stanton, G.; Johnson, H.: Interleukin 2 enhances natural killer cell activity through induction of gamma interferon. Infect. Immunity *41:* 992–997 (1983).

50 Ortaldo, J.; Mason, A.; Gerard, J.; Henderson, L.: Farrar, W.; Hopkin, R.; Herberman, R.; Rabin, H.: Effects of natural and recombinant IL 2 on regulation of IFN production and natural killer activity. Lack of involvement of the TAC antigen for these immunoregulatory effects. J. Immun. *133:* 779–783 (1984).

51 Sayers, T.; Mason, A.; Ortaldo, J.: Regulation of human natural killer cell activity by interferon-gamma. Lack of a role in interleukin-2 mediated augmentation. J. Immun. *136:* 2176–2180 (1986).

52 Ihle, J.; Keller, J.; Orszolan, S.; Henderson, L.; Copeland, T.; Prystowsky, M.; Goldwasser, E.; Schrader, J.; Palaszynski, E.; Dy, M.; Lebel, B.: Biological properties of homogeneous interleukin 3. I. Demonstration of WEHI-3 growth factor activity, mast cell growth factor activity, P cell stimulating factor activity, colony stimulating factor activity and histamine-producing cell-stimulating factor activity. J. Immun. *131:* 282–287 (1983).

53 Smith, K.A.; Ruscetti, F.W.: T cell growth factor and the culture of cloned functional T cells. Adv. Immun. *31:* 137 (1981).

54 Tsudo, M.; Uchiyama, T.; Uchino, H.: Expression of TAC antigen on activated normal human B cells. J. exp. Med. *160:* 612–617 (1983).

55 Lattime, E.; Stutman, O.: Natural cell-mediated cytotoxicity against tumors in mice. Surv. Synth. Path. Res. *2:* 57–67 (1983).

56 Hiserodt, J.C.; Britvan, L.J.; Targan, S.R.: Characterization of the cytolytic reaction mechanism of the human natural killer (NK) lymphocyte: Resolution into binding, programming, and killer cell-independent steps. J. Immun. *129:* 1782–1787 (1982).

57 Hiserodt, J.; Laybourn, K.; Varani, J.: Laminan inhibits the recognition of tumor target cells by murine natural killer (NK) and natural cytotoxic (NC) lymphocytes. Am.J. Path. *121:* 148–155 (1985).

58 Hiserodt, J.; Laybourn, K.; Varani, J.: Expression of a laminin-like substance on the surface of murine natural killer (NK) lymphocytes and its role in NK recognition of tumor target cells. J. Immun. *135:* 1484–1487 (1985).

59 Lin, Y.; Collins, J.L.; Patek, P.Q.; Cohn, M.: An analysis of the sensitivity of somatic cell hybrids to natural killer cell and natural cytotoxic cell-mediated lysis. J. Immun. *131:* 1154–1159 (1983).

60 Laybourn, K.A.; Hiserodt, J.C.; Abruzzo, L.V.; Varani, J.: In vitro and in vivo interaction between murine fibrosarcoma cells and natural killer cells. Cancer Res. *46:* 3407–3412 (1986).

61 Stutman, O.; Dien, P.; Wisun, R.; Lattime, E.: Natural cytotoxic cells against solid tumors in mice. Blocking of cytotoxicity by *D*-mannose. Proc. natn. Acad. Sci. USA *77:* 2895–2898 (1980).

62 Palladino, M.A.; Lattime, E.C.; Pecoraro, G.A.; Stutman, O.; Oettgen, H.F.: Characterization of IL-2-dependent cytotoxic T-cell clones. III. Inhibition of killing activity by monosaccharides. Cell. Immunol. *76:* 286–294 (1983).

63 Ortaldo, J.; Mason. L.H.; Mathieson, B.; Liang, S.; Flick, D.; Herberman, R.: Mediation of mouse natural cytotoxic activity by tumor necrosis factor. Nature, Lond. *321:* 700–702 (1986).

64 Ortaldo, J.; Mason, L.; Herberman, R.: Relationship of mouse natural killer (NK) cells to mouse natural cytotoxic (NC) cells. Effector cells and possible mechanisms of action. Immunol. Res. *5:* 25–32 (1986).

65 Burnet, F.: The concept of immunological surveillance. Prog. exp. Tumor Res. *13:* 1 (1970).

66 Haliotis, T.; Ball, J.; Dexter, D.; Roder, J.: Spontaneous and induced primary oncogenesis in natural killer (NK)-cell-deficient beige mutant mice. Int. J. Cancer *35:* 505–513 (1985).

67 Riesenfeld, I.; Orn, A.; Gidlund, M.; Axberg, I.; Alm, G.; Wigzell, H.: Positive correlation between in vitro NK activity and in vivo resistance towards AKR lymphoma cells. Int. J. Cancer *25:* 399–403 (1980).

68 Patek, P.; Lin, Y.; Collins, J.; Cohn, M.: In vivo or in vitro selection for resistance to natural cytotoxic cell lysis selects for variants with increased tumorigenicity. J. Immun. *136:* 741–745 (1986).

69 Hanna, H.; Fidler, I.J.: Role of natural killer cells in the destruction of circulating tumor emboli. J. natn. Cancer Inst. *65:* 801–809 (1980).

70 Hanna, N.: Expression of metastatic potential of tumor cells in young nude mice is correlated with low levels of natural killer cell-mediated cytotoxicity. Int. J. Cancer *26:* 675–680 (1980).

71 Hanna, N.; Fidler, I.J.: Relationship between metastatic potential and resistance to natural killer cell-mediated cytotoxicity in three murine tumor systems. J. natn. Cancer Inst. *66:* 1183–1190 (1981).

72 Stitz, L.; Baenziger, J.; Pircher, H.; Hengartner, H.; Zinkernagel: Effect of rabbit anti-asialo GM1 treatment in vivo or with anti-asialo GM1 plus complement in vitro on cytotoxic T cell activities. J. Immun. *136:* 4674–4680 (1986).

73 Degliantoni, G.; Perussia, B.; Mangoni, L.; Trinchieri, G.: Inhibition of bone marrow colony formation by human natural killer cells and by natural killer cell-derived colony-inhibiting activity. J. exp. Med. *161:* 1152–1168 (1985).

74 Hannson, M.; Karre, K.; Kiessling, R.; Roder, J.; Andersson, B.; Hayry, P.: Natural NK-cell targets in the mouse thymus. Characteristics of the sensitive cell population. J. Immun. *123:* 765–771 (1979).

75 Hansson, M.; Kiessling, R.; Andersson, B.: Human fetal thymus and bone marrow contain target cells for natural killer cells. Eur. J. Immunol. *11:* 8–12 (1981).

76 Cudkowicz, G.; Hochman, P.: Do natural killer cells engage in regulated reactions against self to ensure homeostasis? Immunol. Rev. *44:* 13–41 (1979).

77 Herberman, R.B.: NK cells and other effector cells, pp. 1–1546 (Academic Press, New York 1982).

78 Colmenares, C.; Lopez, C.: Enhanced lysis of herpes simplex virus type 1-infected mouse cell lines by NC and NK effectors. J. Immun. *136:* 3473–3480 (1986).

79 Lopez, C.; Kirkpatrick, D.; Fitzgerald, P.A.; Ching, C.Y.; Pahwa, R.N.; Good, R.A.; Smithwick, E.M.: Studies of the cell lineage of the effector cells that spontaneously lyse HSV-1 infected fibroblasts (NK(HSV-1)). J. Immun. *129:* 824–828 (1982).

80 Broxmeyer, H.E.; Williams, D.E.; Lu, L.; Cooper, S.; Anderson, S.L.; Beyer, G.S.; Hoffman, R.; Rubin, B.Y.: The suppressive influences of human tumor necrosis factors on bone marrow hematopoietic progenitor cells from normal

donors and patients with leukemia. Synergism of tumor necrosis factor and interferon-gamma. J. Immun. *136:* 4487–4495 (1986).

81 Stolpen, A.; Guinan, E.; Fiers, W.; Pober, J.: Recombinant tumor necrosis factor and immune interferon act singly and in combination to reorganize human vascular endothelial cell monolayers. Am. J. Path. *123:* 16–24 (1986).

82 Sato, N.; Goto, T.; Haranaka, K.; Satomi, N.; Nariuchi, H.; Mano, H.Y.; Sawasaki, Y.: Actions of tumor necrosis factor on cultured vascular endothelial cells. Morphologic modulation, growth inhibition, and cytotoxicity. J. natn. Cancer Inst. *76:* 1113–1122 (1986).

83 Libby, P.; Ordovas, J.M.; Auger, K.R.; Robbins, A.H.; Birinyi, L.K.; Dinarello, C.A.: Rapid communication. Endotoxin and tumor necrosis factor induce interleukin-1 gene expression in adult human vascular endothelial cells. Am. J. Path. *124:* 179–186 (1986).

84 Pohlman, T.H.; Stanness, K.A.; Beatty, P.G.; Ochs, H.D.; Harlan, J.M.: An endothelial cell surface factor(s) induced in vitro by lipopolysaccharide interleukin 1, and tumor necrosis factor-alpha increases neutrophil adherence by a CDw18-dependent mechanism. J. Immun. *136:* 4548–4553 (1986).

85 Klebanoff, S.J.; Vadas, M.A.; Harlan, J.M.; Sparks, L.H.; Gamble, J.R.; Agosti, J.M.; Waltersdorph, A.M.: Stimulation of neutrophils by tumor necrosis factor. J. Immun. *136:* 4220–4225 (1986).

86 Ruddle, N.H.: Activation of human polymorphonuclear neutrophil functions by interferon-gamma and tumor necrosis factors (letter). J. Immun. *136:* 2335–2336 (1986).

87 Bachwich, P.R.; Chensue, S.W.; Larrick, J.W.; Kunkel, S.L.: Tumor necrosis factor stimulates interleukin-1 and prostaglandin E2 production in resting macrophages. Biochem. biophys. Res. Commun. *136:* 94–101 (1986).

88 Silberstein, D.S.; David, J.R.: Tumor necrosis factor enhances eosinophil toxicity to Schistosoma mansoni larvae. Proc. natn. Acad. Sci. USA. *83:* 1055–1059 (1986).

89 Bertolini, D.; Nedwin, G.; Bringman, T.; Smith, D.; Mundy, G.: Stimulation of bone resorption and inhibition of bone formation in vitro by tumour necrosis factors. Nature, Lond. *319:* 516–518 (1986).

90 Rola-Pleszczynski, M.; Lieu, H.: Human natural cytotoxic lymphocytes definition by a monoclonal antibody of a subset which kills an anchorage dependent target cell line but not the K-562 cell line. Cell. Immunol. *82:* 326–333 (1983).

91 Rola-Pleszczynski, M.; Lieu, H.; Sullivan, A.; Girard, M.: Membrane markers, target cell specificity, and sensitivity to biologic response modifiers distinguish human natural cytotoxic from human natural killer cells. J. clin. Invest. *76:* 1927–1931 (1985).

92 Oshimi, K.; Kano, S.; Sumiya, M.; Gonda, N.; Takaku, F.: Cytotoxicity of cultured mouse spleen cells against natural killer-sensitive target cells. Characterization of the effector cell. Int. Archs. Allergy appl. Immun. *64:* 395–409 (1981).

93 Claesson, M.H.; Olsson, L.: Autoreactive natural killer-like cells from agar-cloned murine bone marrow cells. Nature, Lond. *283:* 578–580 (1980).

94 Kiyohara, T.; Tanino, T.; Egawa, K.: T cell-dependent nonspecific cytotoxicity induced by culture of mouse spleen cells against natural killer insensitive tumor cells. Jap. J. exp. Med. *52:* 201–208 (1982).

95 Shain, B.; Holt, C.A.; Lilly, F.: Lack of specificity for viral and H-2 antigens by

anomalous T killer cells generated in murine leukocyte cultures. J. Immun. *129:* 722–729 (1982).

96 Lattime, E.; Stutman, O.: The generation of culture activated killer cells (AK) is interleukin-2-dependent and requires self-Ia recognition. Int. J. Cancer *35:* 535–542 (1985).

97 Seeley, J.K.; Golub, S.H.: Studies on cytotoxicity generated in human mixed lymphocyte cultures. I. Time course and target spectrum of several distinct concomitant cytotoxic activities. J. Immun. *120:* 1415–1422 (1978).

98 Karre, K.; Seely, J.K.: Cytotoxic Thy-1.2 positive blasts with NK-like target selectivity in murine mixed lymphocyte cultures. J. Immun. *123:* 1511–1518 (1979).

99 Paciucci, P.A.; Macphail, S.; Bach, F.H.; Zarling, J.M.: Requirements for T cells in alloantigen-induced generation of non-T cell-mediated cytotoxicity against syngeneic mouse sarcoma cells. J. Immun. *125:* 36–39 (1980).

100 Macphail, S.; Paciucci, P.A.; Stutman, O.: Phenotypic heterogeneity of antisyngeneic tumor killer cells (ASTK) generated in allogeneic mixed lymphocyte reactions. J. Immun. *123:* 3205–3210 (1984).

101 Macphail, S.; Stutman, O.: Heterogeneous cytotoxic cells that kill NC-sensitive WEHI-164 tumor cells are activated in allogeneic mixed lymphocyte reactions. Immunol. Res. *5:* 40–49 (1986).

102 Dorfman, N.; Winkler, D.; Burton, R.C.; Kossayda, N.; Sabia, P.; Wunderlich, J.: Broadly reactive murine cytotoxic cells induced in vitro under syngeneic conditions. J. Immun. *129:* 1762–1769 (1982).

103 Kedar, E.; Ikejiri, B.L.; Gorelik, E.; Herberman, R.B.: Natural cell-mediated cytotoxicity in vitro and inhibition of tumor growth in vivo by murine lymphoid cells cultured with T cell growth factor (TCGF). Cancer Immunol. Immunother. *13:* 14–23 (1982).

104 Grimm, E.A.; Mazumber, A.; Zhang, H.Z.; Rosenberg, S.A.: Lymphokine activated killer cell phenomenon. Lysis of natural killer-resistant fresh solid tumor cells by interleukin 2-activated autologous human peripheral blood lymphocytes. J. exp. Med. *155:* 1823–1841 (1982).

105 Okuno, T.; Takagaki, Y.; Pluznik, D.; Djeu, J.: Natural cytotoxic (NC) cell activity in basophilic cells: Release of NC-specific cytotoxic factor by IgE receptor triggering. J. Immun. *136:* 4652–4658 (1986).

106 Brooks, C.G.; Urdal, D.L.; Henney, C.S.: Lymphokine-driven 'differentiation' of cytotoxic T-cell clones into cells with NK-like specificity. Correlations with display of membrane macromolecules. Immunol. Rev. *72:* 43–72 (1983).

107 Shustik, C.; Cohen, I.R.; Schwartz, R.S.; Latham-Griffin, E.: T lymphocytes with promiscuous cytotoxicity. Nature *263:* 699–701 (1976).

Edmund C. Lattime, MD, Immunology Program, Memorial Sloan-Kettering Cancer Center, 1275 York Avenue, New York, NY 10021 (USA)

Concepts Immunopathol., vol. 4, pp. 103–128 (Karger, Basel 1987)

Role of the Third Component of Complement in Immunoregulation[1]

John M. Weiler[a], Monte V. Hobbs[b]

[a]Iowa City Veterans Administration Medical Center and Division of Allergy/Immunology, Department of Internal Medicine, University of Iowa, Iowa City, Iowa, USA; [b]Scripps Clinic and Research Foundation, La Jolla, Calif., USA

Introduction

Since the early 1970s many reports suggest that complement is important in regulation of the immune response [reviewed in 1–5]. Most early investigators used in vivo systems and showed that immune responses could be abrogated in animals treated with complement activators that depressed hemolytic complement levels [1, 6]. As in vitro systems became more well defined, later investigators examined an immunoregulatory role for specific complement proteins and degradation products [2, 3].

A large portion of these studies focused upon the role that C3 and its fragments play in immune regulation. C3 has been studied by many investigators because of the following observations: (1) C3 is part of both the classical and alternative activating pathways of complement and serves in the alternative-amplification loop; (2) C3 is present in serum in the highest concentration of any complement protein making its isolation relatively easy; (3) Early in vivo studies used CoVF treatment of animals, which greatly reduces levels of C3 and alters immune functions [1, 6]; (4) Complement receptors for C3 (CR) are present on lymphocytes and macrophages, cells that participate in humoral and cellular immune responses, and these receptors are reported to play a role in the regulation

[1] The authors acknowledge Steve Rinderknecht, Luke Sloan and Drs. Thomas Feldbush, Zuhair Ballas and Barbara Needleman for their contributions to these studies. This work was supported in part by Meril Review Awards from the Veteran Administration and by a grant from the Kroc foundation.

of the immune response [7–12]; (5) C3 is secreted by macrophages, cells which are known to play a role in immune regulation; therefore complement is present in tissues where immune responses occur [13, 14]; (6) C3 may regulate the production of lymphokines [15]; and (7) C3 and antibody may play a role in tissue localization of antigen [16, 17].

In this review, we will examine the early studies which suggest a role for C3 in immune regulation. Then we will examine each fragment of C3 which is reported to have immunoregulatory capacity. Finally, we will speculate on the biological significance of these observations. This review must be viewed as a status report because work in this area continues.

C3 Structure and Activation

The third component of complement exists in plasma at a concentration of about 1.5 mg/ml, making it the most abundant of the complement proteins. Native C3 (fig. 1) is about 195,000 daltons and consists of an alpha-chain of 992 amino acid residues and a beta-chain of 645 residues [18]. C3 has been purified to homogeneity and the primary amino acid sequence has been derived from the cDNA coding sequence [18].

Functionally, in the hemolytic complement pathways, C3 serves as the pivotal termination point of both the classical and the alternative activating pathways and as the initiating point for the terminal pathway (fig. 2). The classical pathway is activated by substances such as antigen-antibody complexes while the alternative pathway is activated by substances such as yeast wall or rabbit erythrocytes. Classical activation leads to the formation of a complex consisting of C4b,C2a, the classical C3 converting enzyme (C3 convertase). Alternative activation leads to the formation of C3b,Bb,P, the alternative-amplification pathway C3 convertase. The formation of both convertases is magnesium and temperature dependent and decay is time and temperature dependent.

Both convertases have the capacity to act on their natural substrate, C3, to cleave it to C3a and C3b (fig. 1–3). C3a is the 9,300-dalton anaphylatoxin which consists of 77 amino acids. C3a has the capacity to cause basophils and mast cells to degranulate, an increase in vascular permeability, smooth muscle to contract and lysosomal enzymes to be released from macrophages [19]. The effects of C3a are short-lived because an inactivator (anaphylatoxin inactivator), a carboxypeptidase, acts in

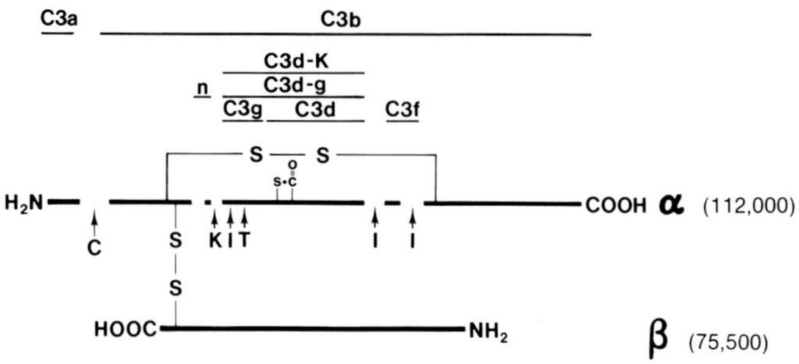

Fig. 1. C3 molecule [modified from ref. 18].

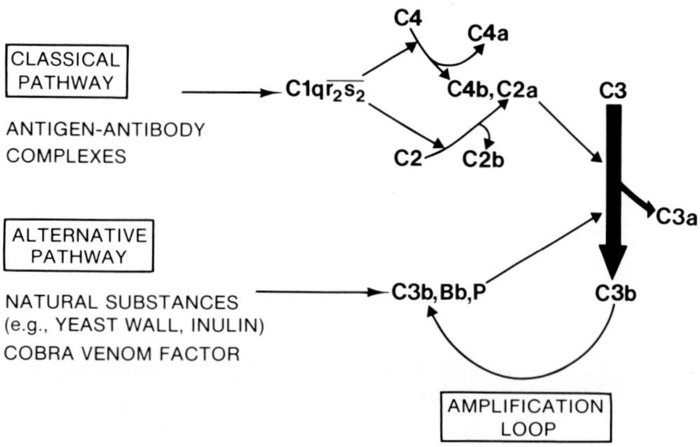

Fig. 2. Simplified schematic of events in classical and alternative activating pathways.

vivo on C3a within seconds to remove the carboxyterminal arginine and render the anaphylatoxin inactive.

The remaining portion of the molecule is C3b, a 185,000-dalton fragment, which in native C3 contains a thioester between cysteine (residue 1010) and glutamine (residue 1014) on the alpha-chain of the molecule [18]. Immediately upon cleavage of C3 by convertase, this internalized thioester bond is exposed allowing the C3b molecule to have momentary binding affinity for many membranes and surfaces or to react with water [20, 21]. A covalent bond is formed if the thioester reacts with R-OH groups on the surface of the membrane. If the C3b does not find a membrane rapidly, then the thioester binding site reacts with water and the C3b fragment remains in the fluid phase and loses ability to bind covalently to membranes.

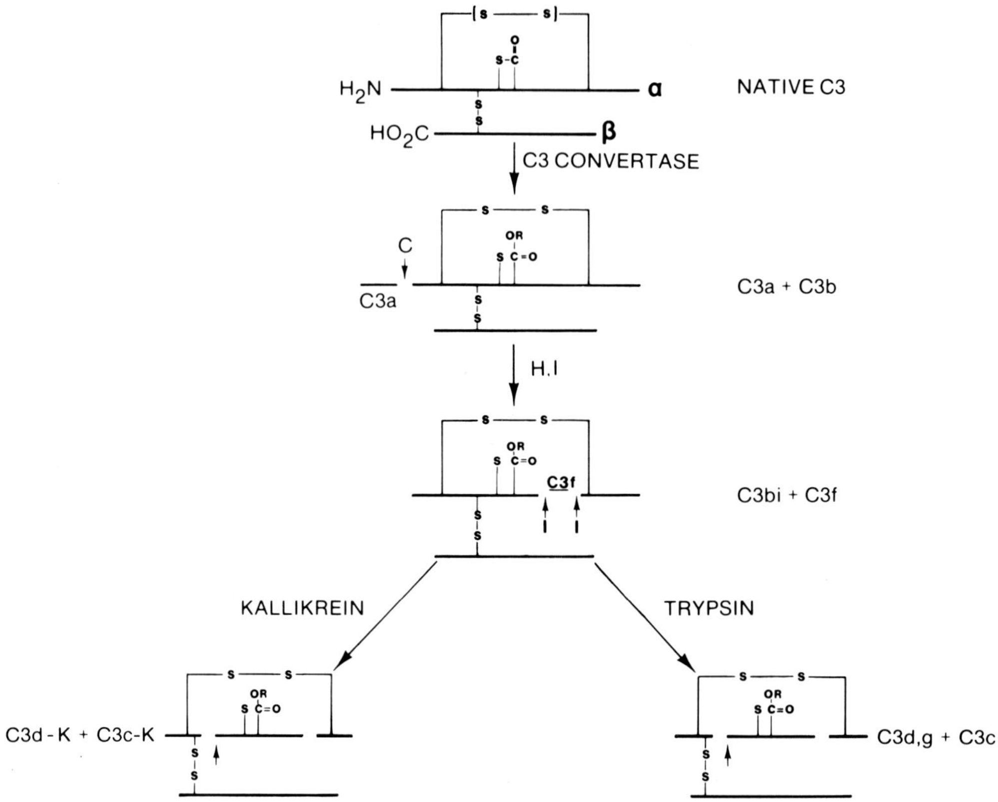

Fig. 3. Degradation of C3. Native C3 is acted upon by classical, alternative or amplification pathway convertase to produce C3a and C3b. C3b is acted upon by factors H and I to produce C3bi; C3f is the 2,000-dalton fragment cleaved by I. C3bi may be acted on by a variety of enzymes. Trypsin will produce C3d,g and C3c; C3d,g may decay to C3d and C3g. Kallikrein will produce C3d-K and C3c-K. C3d-K has nine amino acids on the amino terminal end that are not contained on C3d, g.

C3b which is bound to membrane may then lead to terminal pathway hemolytic events and lysis of the cell or membrane. In addition, membrane-bound C3b may stimulate a variety of immunological phenomena such as phagocytosis. Fluid phase C3b may compete with membrane bound C3b to inhibit hemolysis.

The degradation of C3b (fig. 3) has been studied extensively and involves the regulatory proteins, H and I (formerly known as β1H and C3b Inactivator) [22–28]. Reaction of C3b with H and I forms an intermediate molecule, C3bi, with the cleavage of a 2,000-dalton fragment known as C3f. C3bi may then react with a variety of enzymes such as trypsin, kallikrein, elastase, urokinase, plasmin, or cathepsin G to form C3c, C3c-K, C3d,g, C3d-K, C3d and C3g (fig. 1, 3) [23, 25, 28–31]. Trypsin treatment of C3bi causes formation of C3d,g and C3c [28]. Kallikrein treatment of C3bi leads to the formation of C3d-K and C3c-K [29]. C3d-K contains nine amino acids on its amino terminal end which are not contained by C3d,g. This nonapeptide is reported to be responsible for leukocyte mobilizing activity [32]. The natural enzyme responsible for the degradation of C3bi in vivo is not known, although breakdown products do form in vivo and are increased in some disease states [27]. Other fragments of C3 have also been described but their sequences have not been definitely mapped on the molecule and include fraction 2 protein [2], C3e [33], leukocyte mobilizing factor (LMF) [34] and C3-FP [35]. Many of these fragments have been studied for ability to regulate the immune response and will be discussed below.

Early Studies on the Immunoregulatory Role of C3

Many of the early studies to examine a role for complement in regulation of the immune response were in vivo and suggest that complement does have a role [1, 6]. Four main types of studies were employed early:

Often investigators used complement activators that were administered to animals and then attributed any effects to 'complement depletion' [1, 6]. Cobra venom factor (CoVF) was most frequently used for these studies because CoVF forms a very stable complex with factor B which then functions as a C3 convertase [36–39]. When CoVF is administered to animals there is rapid complement activation which leads to levels of total hemolytic complement (CH50) of less than 1% by day one; levels remain low for up to 6 days [37]. Investigators employed this tool to 'decomplement' animals for their studies and then reported that this treatment causes depression of the primary antibody response to T-dependent antigens, with IgG, IgA and IgE being more suppressed than IgM [1, 6, 40, 41]. In contrast, the antibody response to T-independent antigen is not generally suppressed by CoVF treatment [1, 6, 39]. CoVF treatment also was shown to impair the ability of mice to localize both T-dependent and T-independent antigens in splenic follicles, to form splenic antigen-binding cells and to form germinal centers [42–46]. These observations suggested to investigators that C3 is necessary for immune responses to occur [1]. However, this interpretation is confounded by the fact that complement activators, which deplete animals of hemolytic complement, also lead to greatly increased levels of complement activation fragments (e.g. C3a). Therefore, many of the effects that were observed in these early studies may have come from activation fragments [2]. Alternatively, the CoVF itself could have been immunoregulatory [47].

Some early studies used in vitro systems to examine a role for complement in the immune response [1, 15, 47–51]. In some cases serum was treated in some manner and then used in vitro in tissue culture as an indirect way to manipulate the complement system. For example, zymosan treatment of serum renders it incapable of supporting an antibody response to sheep red blood cells in mouse lymph node cultures [47]. In other cases, isolated protein preparations were examined in vitro in tissue culture but we now know that many of these preparations may have contained more than one protein or fragment. As an example, some studies suggested that C3 is mitogenic while other studies suggested that C3 is capable of inhibiting either mitogen and/or antigen stimulation of lymphocytes, but it has been reported that these C3 preparations may have contained factor H [51, 52]. In other reports anti-C3 antibody in vitro in mouse spleen cell cultures was shown to reduce primary and secondary responses to T-dependent antigens but not to T-independent antigens [1]. Almost all of these studies used serum in the tissue culture medium and serum contains complement components, activators and inhibitors which may confound interpretation of the data. In addition, activation of serum by CoVF or zymosan produces activation products in vitro and the same reservations that apply to the in vivo studies apply to these in vitro studies.

In other early studies investigators separated cells on the basis of surface receptors for complement [40, 41]. For example, Lewis et al. [40, 41] suggested that the in vitro T-dependent antibody response to sheep red blood cells from CR+ B cells can be suppressed when anti-C3 antibody is added to cultures; CR-negative B cells are not inhibited by the presence of anti-C3. However, we now know that there are at least three and perhaps four distinct receptors for C3 and there is no information which receptor(s) plays a role in this phenomenon [8–12]. It is possible that one receptor suppresses while another augments immune responses.

Finally, some investigators have examined genetic deficiency states to study a role for complement in the immune response [53–56]. Deficiency states offer a rare opportunity to examine the contribution of one specific complement component on the immune response and are the only true 'complement depletion' studies. In general, these studies suggest that complement deficiency is not associated with aberration in the immune response [53, 54]. In particular, deficiency of C3 in the human has been examined and, although the patients are susceptible to infection, they do not appear to have impaired immune responses [54]. Only C4 deficiency appears to predispose animals and humans to have impaired immune responses [57–59]. However, C4 has not been well enough studied in vitro to understand the role that it plays in the immune response. Although the genetic deficiency studies suggest then that C3 is not necessary for normal immune responses to occur, they do not exclude the possibility that C3 fragments may down-regulate immune responses. Therefore, there may be an alternative explanation for the observations reported in early studies in which animals were said to be 'decomplemented'. In those cases, when complement activators (e.g. CoVF) were used, the attenuated immune responses may have been due to the production of suppressive C3 fragments.

While these early studies suggest that complement may play a role in the immune response, they do not demonstrate which components and fragments regulate the immune response, under what circumstances these proteins play a role and what role each protein plays. It is difficult to make unified hypotheses about the role of complement in immune regulation on the basis of the early observations. Since 1980, there has been a resurgence of interest in the role of complement proteins and fragments in regulating the immune response [2–5]. These more recent studies have used proteins and fragments that often have high levels of purity. In addition, they have employed biological systems that now allow in vitro dissection of the immune response in ways that were not available in the 1970s. Even today, however, there are many studies that remain to be performed before we will have a full understanding of the mechanisms of complement regulation of the immune response. This review then is a status report on the role of C3 fragments on the immune response.

C3a

C3a has now been studied extensively for regulation of a variety of immune functions [60–70]. Early studies by Ferluga suggested that C3a is cytotoxic for lymphocytes but these observations were not confirmed by later studies [60, 61]. Others examined C3a for inherent mitogenicity and failed to demonstrate any effects [15, 51]. In one of these early studies, C3a appeared to cause inhibition of serum-induced proliferation of murine lymphocytes although the authors did not comment on this observation [51].

More recently, Charriaut et al. [62] suggested that C3a contaminating their C3 preparations is responsible for inhibition of in vitro natural killer (NK) cytotoxicity of mouse (YAC-1) and human (K562) target cells. C3 preparations at 35 μg/ml inhibit by 50% the response in a time- and dose-dependent manner. Effector cells can be preincubated with C3 and subsequently are able to inhibit lysis of target cells. However, preincubation of C3 with target cells does not inhibit lysis suggesting that the effect of C3 is on the NK cells and not on the target cell population. Charriaut et al. [62] examined C3a derived from trypsin-treated C3 and C3a des arg and reported that both are capable of inhibiting NK cell activity. This is an unusual observation since C3a des arg is inactive in virtually all other assays in which it has been examined [19].

In 1982, Payan et al. [63] reported that C3a and a single C3a synthetic peptide which included the 8 carboxy terminal amino acids, (C3a [70–77]), inhibit mitogen-(phytohemagglutinin [PHA] and concanavalin A [ConA]) and antigen-(streptokinase-streptodornase)-induced generation of leukocyte inhibitory factor at $10^{-7}\,M$ concentrations. In these studies, C3a and C3a(70–77) also inhibit mitogen-induced random migration of human T lymphocytes but not mitogen- or antigen-induced human lymphocyte blastogenesis in a serum-containing medium [63].

Morgan et al. [65–70] then reported that C3a inhibits polyclonal and antigen-specific antibody responses in vitro in a serum-containing medium supplemented with an inhibitor of anaphylatoxin inactivator (2-mercaptomethyl-5-guanidinopentanoic acid). They showed that C3a inhibits Fc fragment-induced and sheep red blood cell (SRBC)-induced immunoglobulin (Ig) synthesis by human peripheral blood leukocytes (PBL) and murine splenic lymphocytes [65, 70]. In contrast, C3a has no effect on mitogen- or antigen-induced T cell or B cell proliferative responses or on the proliferative response of a murine B cell tumor line. Furthermore, PHA-, pokeweed mitogen (PWM)- and Fc fragment-induced proliferative responses are unmodified by the presence of C3a at concentrations ten times greater than those at which C3a inhibits antibody responses. C3a must be present for only 30 min for significant inhibition to be seen. The earlier C3a is present, the more inhibition that is observed [70].

The effect of C3a may be through the generation of non-antigen-specific suppressor T cells [66]. Soluble T cell factor will override the effects of C3a on Fc fragment-induced polyclonal responses. Incubation of C3a with T cells makes them unable to provide help in Fc fragment-induced polyclonal response [67, 70]. C3a may act on a population of Lyt1+ suppressor T inducer cells or may act indirectly through macrophages [70]. Ultimately, C3a appears to induce Lyt2+ suppressor T cells. C3a probably does not induce a soluble factor when incubated with T cells and does not appear to regulate IL-2 production. However, IL-2 may abolish the suppressive effects of C3a [66]. As might be expected, C3a has no effect on T cell-independent antigens (TNP-LPS or TNP-Ficoll) [66].

These data suggest that macrophages with C3a receptors may be necessary for C3a to regulate T cells [69]. When indomethacin is present in the tissue culture medium, C3a suppression of immune responses is blocked suggesting a role for prostaglandins (PG). Furthermore, C3a is capable of stimulating adherent macrophages to release magnitudes more PG of the E series into tissue culture supernatant than in control cultures [69]. Taken together, these observations suggest that C3a augments macrophage production of prostaglandins which then leads to a decrease in T helper cell function and/or an increase in T suppressor cells.

Morgan et al. [65] examined a series of synthetic oligopeptides of C3a for ability to regulate polyclonal and antigen-specific antibody responses and found that all of the synthetic peptides are less active than is native C3a. Some activity is seen when the carboxyterminal five amino acids are present (leu-gly-leu-ala-arg) and this activity increases with an increase in the size of the oligopeptide; the carboxyterminal 5-mer is 0.03% as active as the native molecule while the carboxyterminal 21-mer is about 44% as active as native C3a. When the terminal arginine is deleted, there is absolutely no activity [65]. The species of the C3a may be important in these in vitro studies; 100-fold less human C3a is needed to inhibit the response of human lymphocytes than to suppress murine cells.

The levels of C3a that are immunosuppressive are in the range that may be generated by complement activation. One tenth to one microgram C3a/ml is immunoregulatory in vitro whereas 50–100 μg C3a/ml may be generated from the available C3; therefore only 0.2–2% of the C3 available in vivo must be activated to produce levels of C3a that are immunosuppressive in vitro.

Thus, C3a is capable of regulating immune responses in vitro. However, the biological significance of these observations with C3a is not clear. In most cases C3a is degraded rapidly in vivo to C3a des arg by anaphylatoxin inactivator and C3a des arg is totally inactive in regulating immune responses [70]. These studies require serum in the tissue culture medium and serum contains carboxypeptidase [70]. Consequently, there is also an absolute requirement for a carboxypeptidase inhibitor. Therefore, for these studies to be biologically relevant, C3a would have to act very rapidly, which has not been demonstrated in vivo or in vitro, or it would have to be present in tissue in which anaphylatoxin inactivator is absent, which has also not been demonstrated, or C3a would have to be present in high local concentrations.

C3b and C3b Degradation Products (C3d,g, C3d-K, Fraction 2 Protein, C3d)

A number of laboratories have reported that C3b and fragments derived from C3b have an immunoregulatory role [2, 5, 15, 29, 35, 50, 51, 71–81]. Pepys and Butterworth reported in 1974 that C3b, C3c and C3d inhibit the blastogenic response of human lymphocytes to antigen (purified protein derivative (PPD) and Candida) but not to mitogen (PHA) [50]. Hartmann and Bokisch [51] in 1975 reported that C3b is mitogenic in human lymphocyte cultures. Koopman et al. were unable to confirm that C3b is mitogenic [15] and recently it was suggested that early C3 preparations contained contaminating amounts of factor H which may also be mitogenic in tissue culture [52]. Koopman et al. [15] did show that C3b is able to induce lymphokine secretion in tissue culture medium.

In 1979, Schenkein and Genco [71] reported that C3c and C3d, produced by trypsin treatment of C3, inhibit antigen-induced but not mitogen-induced blastogenesis. The concentrations of C3c (30–120 μg/ml) and C3d (10–40 μg/ml) required in their study to inhibit were quite high. When excess adherent cells are added to the cultures, the effects of C3c and C3d can be overcome, suggesting to these authors that the effects of these C3 fragments might be on the macrophage [71].

In more recent studies, Erdei et al. [72] used purified native human C3, cross-linked C3 or Sepharose-bound C3 and found that none of these preparations have any effect on resting murine splenic lymphocytes in serum-free medium. However, they showed that cross-linked or immobilized C3 but not soluble C3 stimulate LPS-activated splenic B cells to proliferate and produce Ig. In addition, these studies suggest that soluble C3 or treatment with anti-C3 antibody can inhibit the ability of crosslinked or immobilized C3 to cause proliferation and maturation of the Ig-secreting cells [72].

In other studies, Tsokos et al. [73] reported that addition of soluble C3b early in tissue culture may inhibit PWM-induced human B lymphocyte synthesis of Ig. Similarly, zymosan coated with C3b is inhibitory. These authors postulated that C3b acts directly on B cells and not on helper T cells because C3b inhibits the plaque forming cell (PFC) response of mononuclear cells depleted of T cells and stimulated with the T cell-independent mitogen, Epstein-Barr virus. Suppressor cells were not generated in these studies by treatment with C3b [73]. Rather large amounts of C3b were required to cause significant effects in these studies (100 μg C3b/ml).

C3d-K, which overlaps with C3d,g on the alpha-chain of C3 (fig. 1, 3), has also been widely studied [29,66]. C3d-K contains 9 amino acids on the amino terminal end of the molecule which are not found in C3d,g. Meuth et al. [29] reported that C3d-K inhibits the mixed lymphocyte response of human spleen cells and the proliferative response of human spleen cells to tetanus toxoid and to PHA. There is 50% inhibition of this response in the presence of C3d-K at levels which would result from conversion of only 0.2% of the circulating C3. C3d-K is capable of inhibiting mitogen-induced proliferative responses by T cells and B cells and spontaneous proliferation of several murine tumor cell lines [74]. C3d-K inhibits IL-2-induced mitogenesis of T cells by blocking synthesis of IL-2; in contrast, Con A-induced IL-2 synthesis is not blocked by C3d-K [74]. Therefore, C3d-K suppresses immune responses probably through an effect on the lymphocyte directly. The concentrations of C3d-K required for these various effects are relatively high with 50% inhibition seen at a dose of 20–30 μg/ml [74].

Studies in our laboratory beginning in the late 1970s utilized serum-free conditions and purified proteins to study the effects of C3 on a variety of cellular immune phenomena [reviewed in 2]. These studies suggested that a C3 degradation product called fraction 2 is capable of inhibiting human and rat antigen- and mitogen-induced T and B cell proliferation, T-dependent and T-independent rat memory B cell responses, mixed lymphocyte responses in the human and mouse and the generation of cytotoxic T cells but not NK cells or augmented NK cells [2,75–79].

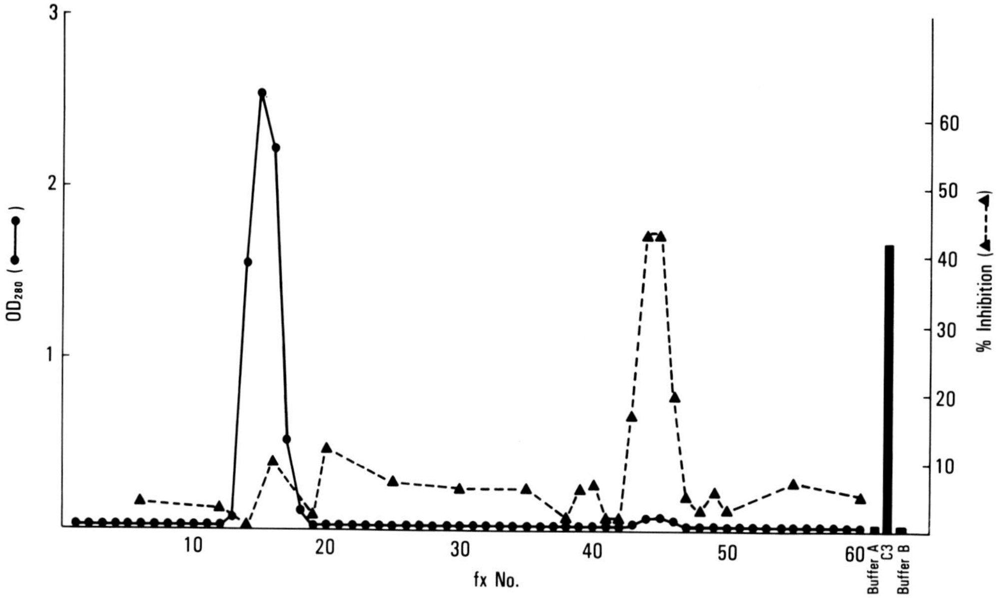

Fig. 4. Isolation of fraction 2 from C3 preparations. C3 [82] was passed over a column containing Sephadex G75 equilibrated with veronal-buffered 1.15 *M* saline, 2 m*M* ethylenediamine-tetraacetate, pH 7.4 and fractions screened at A_{280} (●) and for ability to inhibit 10 μg/well of PHA-induced human T cell proliferation (▲) [83]. Also shown here is inhibition caused by 25 μg/ml of C3 and by C3 buffers. PHA wells had 139,410 cpm and wells containing no mitogen had 3,699 cpm.

For our studies and for many of the other recent studies, C3 was isolated from human plasma by a modification of the method of Tack and Prahl [82]. This 'native C3' is capable of inhibiting the immune responses described above. In an effort to determine if the native C3 or a fragment contained therein is responsible for the inhibition that was observed, we passed the C3 over a column containing Sephadex G–200 (fig. 4). This procedure resolved a 10,000-dalton fragment (called fraction 2) which contains all of the inhibitory capacity and the remaining material which chromatographs at an apparent weight of 195,000 daltons and is totally inactive (fraction 1). Therefore, native C3 is not responsible for the inhibition that we had observed.

We showed initially that fraction 2 is capable of inhibiting antigen- and mitogen-induced proliferative responses in concentrations as low as 0.1μg/ml [75] in serum-free medium [83]. We found that fraction 2 is stable to heating and acid treatment, however its effects are reduced but

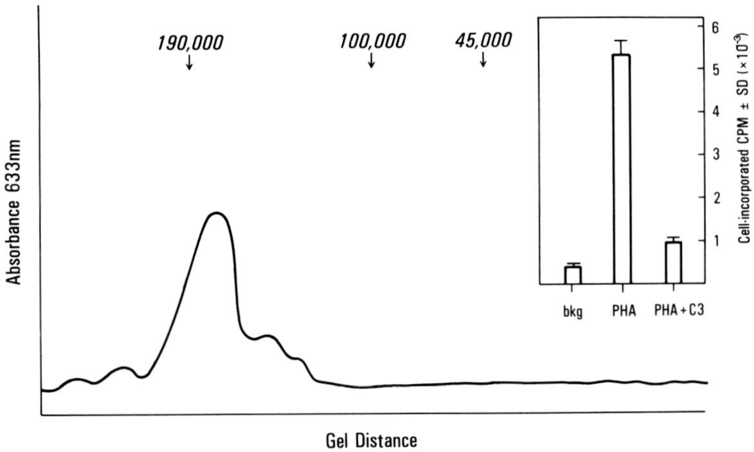

Fig. 5. C3 was examined by SDS-PAGE. 100 μg C3 [82] was in 0.1 % SDS in 5 % gels under nonreducing conditions. The gels were stained with Coomassie blue and scanned at A_{633} using a soft laser densitometer. In insert are results of human peripheral blood leukocyte cultures treated with medium (background), PHA, or PHA+C3.

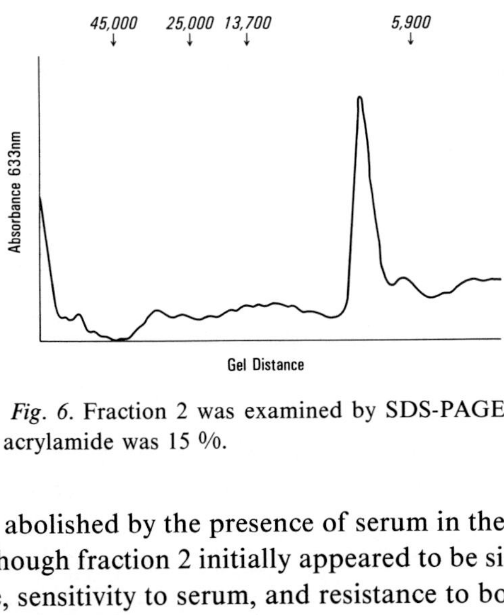

Fig. 6. Fraction 2 was examined by SDS-PAGE as described in figure 5 except that acrylamide was 15 %.

not abolished by the presence of serum in the tissue culture medium [76]. Although fraction 2 initially appeared to be similar to C3a on the basis of size, sensitivity to serum, and resistance to boiling and low pH, it clearly is not C3a [2,75,79].

C3, fraction 1 and fraction 2 were also examined using sodium dodecyl sulfate polyacrylamide gel electrophoresis (SDS-PAGE). Under non-

Table I. Effect of immunoadsorbent columns on the inhibitory capacity of fraction 2[a]

Immunoadsorbent	% Inhibition fraction 2 (μg/ml)[b]		
	0.4	0.2	0.1
Anti-fraction 1	12	1	9
Anti-C3-deficient human serum	65	48	30

[a] Rabbits were immunized with 100 μg of human C3-deficient serum or fraction 1 protein (fig. 4) in Freund's complete adjuvant, boosted 3 and 6 weeks later, then bled weekly. Anti-fraction 1 antiserum was monospecific against normal human serum and did not react with C3-deficient serum on IEP, whereas anti-C3 deficient serum did not react with C3 on IEP. The immunoglobulin fractions of each antiserum were precipitated by 33% ammonium sulfate, coupled to Sepharose 6B beads using activated cyanogen bromide, washed extensively with PBS and packed into 1 ml columns. Fraction 2 was then passed over these columns.

[b] Several doses of adsorbent-treated fraction 2 were added on day 0 to cultures of human PBL stimulated with Con A and proliferation was measured on day 3. The cpm (mitogen-stimulated)/cpm (nonstimulated) from control cultures was 135. Percent inhibition was determined as:

$$1-\frac{\text{cpm (mitogen and fraction 2)} - \text{cpm (nonstimulated)}}{\text{cpm (mitogen)} - \text{cpm (nonstimulated)}} \times 100.$$

reducing conditions, inhibitory C3 preparations contain a major 195,000-dalton protein corresponding to the known molecular weight for human C3 and minor contamination with possible C3 breakdown products (fig. 5). Analysis of fraction 2 by SDS-PAGE reveals the presence of a single protein of about 10,000 daltons (fig. 6).

To determine whether fraction 2 originated from C3 or merely copurified as a contaminant, we performed immunosorbent experiments. We used antisera raised in rabbits against human C3-deficient serum or against noninhibitory fraction 1 material. The anti-fraction 1 antiserum was monospecific against normal human serum and did not react with C3-deficient serum on immunoelectrophoresis (IEP) gels while the anti-C3-deficient serum produced several precipitin lines against normal human serum but did not react with purified human C3 on IEP gels. Fraction 2 protein was then passed through columns containing either the anti-fraction 1 adsorbent or the anti-C3-deficient serum adsorbent and

Table II. Effect of fraction 2 on rat B cell proliferation[a]

Mitogen[b]	Fraction 2 μg/ml[c]	cpm/well ± SD (% inhibition[d]) experiment 1	experiment 2
–	–	1,861 ± 180	7,085 ± 2,841
LPS	–	50,216 ± 3,768	59,800 ± 4,479
LPS	0.38	48,421 ± 273 (5)	50,516 ± 8,349 (15)
LPS	0.75	48,246 ± 4,140 (4)	45,522 ± 679 (21)
LPS + DxS	–	127,072 ± 12,827	73,723 ± 6,229
LPS + DxS	0.38	91,770 ± 3,575 (29)	44,240 ± 8,619 (43)
LPS + DxS	0.75	49,867 ± 12,429 (62)	23,180 ± 1,196 (71)
Anti-Ig	–	64,510 ± 3,900	38,260 ± 3,679
Anti-Ig	0.38	62,515 ± 9,934 (0)	43,633 ± 4,784 (0)
Anti-Ig	0.75	64,845 ± 5,795 (0)	47,715 ± 7,928 (0)

[a] Female F1 hybrid Lewis × Brown Norway rats were sacrificed and lymph node suspensions prepared from mesenteric and cervical lymph nodes. B cell-enriched lymph node cells were obtained by panning with affinity-purified goat antirat $F(ab')_2$ fragments. B cells were at least 95% surface Ig positive and were cultured in triplicate at 2.5×10^5 in 100 μl medium (RPMI 1640 containing 5×10^{-5} 2-mercaptoethanol and 10% fetal calf serum) for 3 days at 37 °C in 10% CO_2. Mitogens were: 50 μg lipopolysaccharide (LPS 055;B5 Sigma Chemical Co.), 10 μg/LPS ml + 10 μg dextran sulfate/ml (DxS; MW 500,000, 17% sulfur, Sigma Chemical Co.) or 5% v/v anti-Ig conjugated beads (prepared by coupling IgG goat antirat $F(ab')_2$ to Sepharose 4B).

[b] Two experiments are shown in which cultures of purified rat B cells were stimulated with medium (–), 50 μg LPS/ml, 10 μg LPS/ml plus 10 μg DxS/ml, or 5% (v/v) anti-Ig beads on day 0 and proliferation was measured on day 3.

[c] Fraction 2 was added on day 0 at the doses shown.

[d] % inhibition was calculated as in table I.

the two effluents were tested at various concentrations for ability to regulate Con A-induced blastogenesis. As shown in table I, the anti-fraction 1 adsorbent removed most of the proliferation-inhibiting activity in fraction 2. In contrast, no activity was removed by passing the fraction 2 protein over the anti-C3-deficient serum adsorbent column. Since the anti-fraction 1 antiserum was raised against a purified human C3 preparation that was *not* inhibitory (fig. 4), it seems likely that fraction 2 is a breakdown product of C3. An additional observation suggests that fraction 2 is derived from the native C3 molecule. A monoclonal antibody (called

Table III. Effect of fraction 1 and LMF on rat B cell proliferation

Mitogen	Inhibitor (µg/ml)	cpm/well±SD	(% inhibition)
–	–	20,720±1,711	
LPS+D×S	–	67,981±7,500	
LPS+D×S	fraction 1 (75)	104,113±1,538	(0)
LPS+D×S	fraction 2 (0.1)	61,198±3,587	(14)
LPS+D×S	fraction 2 (0.5)	7,655±1,153	(100)
LPS+D×S	LMF (0.4)	44,256±4,075	(50)
LPS+D×S	LMF (0.8)	18,632±1,449	(100)

This experiment was performed as in table II.

'clone 9') recognizing C3g [25] also showed reactivity with fraction 2 [Lachmann, personal commun.]. Taken together, these data strongly suggest that fraction 2 is a product of the low level C3 degradation which occurs during the purification procedure and handling of the C3 preparations. Alternatively, it is possible to conclude that fraction 2 is an in vivo C3 breakdown product and merely copurifies with C3.

Previous studies revealed that fraction 2 inhibits in vitro antibody responses and, based on its ability to inhibit mitogen- or antigen-induced T cell proliferation, one mechanism of action may be inhibition of T helper cell function [2,75,77]. Alternatively, fraction 2 may act directly on B cells, inhibiting triggering, cell proliferation or differentiation. To assess the effect of fraction 2 on B cell activation, we utilized cultures of purified rat B cells stimulated with the B cell mitogens lipopolysaccharide (LPS), LPS plus dextran sulfate (DxS), or anti-Ig beads. As shown in table II, all three mitogens are able to induce marked cell proliferation. Fraction 2 is a potent inhibitor of LPS plus DxS-induced proliferation, however, anti-Ig-induced proliferation is not suppressed and LPS-induced proliferation is suppressed only marginally. Fraction 1 is noninhibitory in LPS plus DxS-treated cultures even at a 100-fold greater dose than the inhibitory fraction 2 dose (table III). The present studies suggest that in addition to its effects on T cell proliferation, fraction 2 is able to inhibit mitogen-induced rat B cell proliferation, although the level of inhibition is dependent on the mitogen used in culture. Two possibilities for this observed mitogen-dependency are: (1) that each mitogen stimulates a separate subset of B cells and that only certain subsets are sensitive to inhibition by fraction 2, or (2) that the stage at which each mitogen

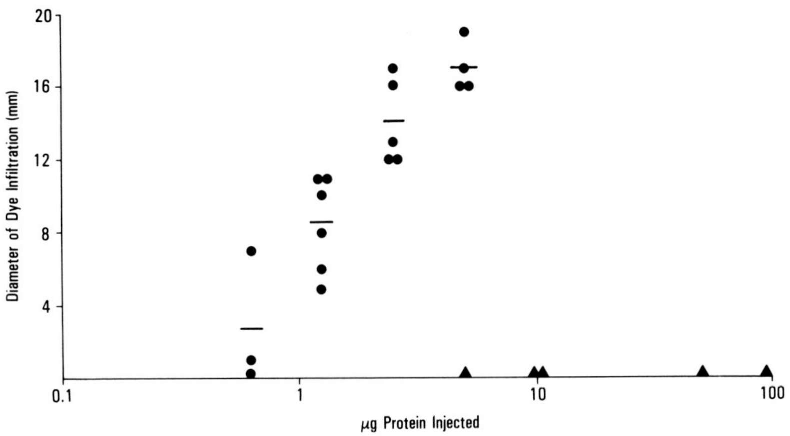

Fig. 7. Vascular permeability of fraction 1 and fraction 2. Abdominal skin of rats was shaved and challenged intradermally with 0.1 ml of concentrations of fraction 1 (▲), fraction 2 (●) or PBS control buffer. After 3 min, 0.5 ml of Evans blue dye in PBS (4 % v/v) was injected into the tail vein. After an additional 10 min the rats were sacrificed and the skin was bluntly dissected and measured for dye infiltration. Each point represents dye diameter from a single injection minus the control buffer diameter (approximately 1 mm).

stimulates B cells is differentially sensitive to fraction 2. We are currently examining these two possibilities.

Fraction 2 was then examined for ability to increase vascular permeability. Rats were challenged with fraction 1, fraction 2, or a buffer control. As shown in figure 7, various doses of fraction 2 were able to increase dye infiltration in the skin in a dose-dependent manner. Fraction 1 was inactive at all doses tested. Therefore, fraction 2 has the capacity to increase vascular permeability.

Fraction 2 was also examined for ability to cause leukocyte mobilizing factor activity (kindly performed by Drs. Rother [34]). The assay for leukocyte release from isolated, perfused rat femurs has been described in detail [34]. As shown in figure 8, fraction 2 or LMF (positive control) when added to the perfusion medium resulted in transient, significant increases in the number of cells released into the perfusate. In contrast, neither the perfusion medium alone nor phosphate-buffered saline (PBS) was active.

Because of the similarities of fraction 2 and leukocyte mobilizing factor (LMF) in causing this leukocyte mobilization [34], LMF was also

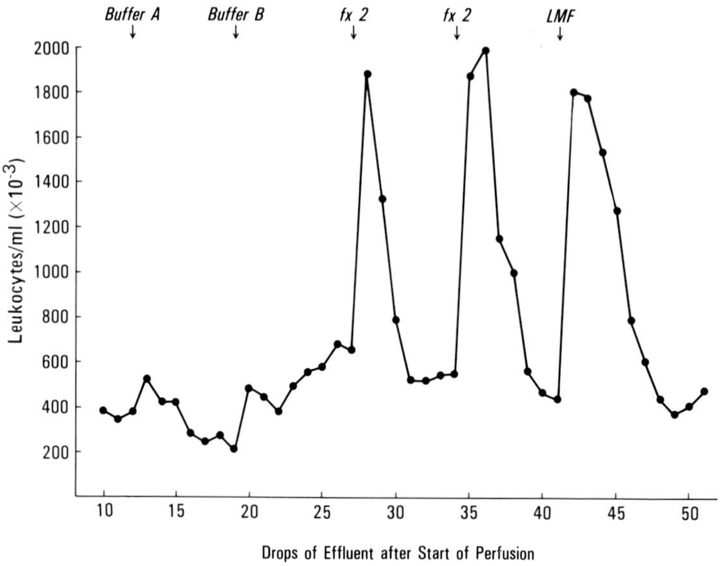

Fig. 8. Leukocyte mobilizing factor activity of fraction 2. Isolated, perfused rat femurs were perfused with 0.2-ml aliquots of medium (buffer A; medium 199, 1 % bovine serum albumin, 1 % heparin), fraction 2 (80 and 120 μg/ml) and LMF (50 μg/ml) as described [34]; this experiment was performed by Drs. Rother and colleagues.

tested in LPS plus DxS-treated cultures. LMF was graciously provided by K. and U. Rother of Heidelberg, FRG, for these studies and had been isolated from antigen-antibody complex-activated human serum, as described previously [34]. We found that LMF, like fraction 2, inhibits in this system (table III). Moreover, LMF, like fraction 2, is unable to suppress anti-Ig-induced B cell proliferation (data not shown).

Our observations suggest that a small molecular weight fragment derived from C3 breakdown is capable of immunosuppression. This fragment acts in very low concentration. Inhibition by this fragment is reduced but not abolished by the presence of serum in tissue culture medium [76]. Although the fragment has not been mapped on the C3 molecule, it does appear to be an important down-regulator of the immune response produced when C3 undergoes degradation.

Melchers et al. [80] have subsequently observed a similar phenomenon and have reported that a fragment of the alpha chain of C3, which they called 'soluble C3d' is capable of regulating B cell activation.

In contrast, they reported that 'cross-linked C3d' stimulates cells presumably through the CR2 receptor. Unfortunately, their fragment was not fully mapped on the alpha-chain of C3 [80].

Recently, Walker et al. [35] reported that CoVF-convertase treated C3 contains a low molecular fragment, termed C3-FP, which is capable of blocking the IL-2 dependent transition of cells from the Gla to the Glb portion of the cell cycle. C3-FP also inhibits proliferation of cell lines but only if they are IL-2 dependent. However, addition of IL-2 does not reverse the effects of C3-FP and cause the cells to progress beyond the Gla phase. In addition, C3-FP does not inhibit IL-2 production or IL-2 receptor formation [35]. Unfortunately, this C3 fragment has also not been fully characterized but does confirm that a small molecular weight C3 fragment has immunoregulatory capacity.

Therefore, at least four laboratories have now described fragments derived from the breakdown of C3b which have immunoregulatory capacity [5,29,35,80]. Only one of these fragments, C3d-K, has been fully mapped on the alpha chain of C3. The remaining fragments-fraction 2, C3d described by Melchers et al., C3-FP described by Walker et al., and LMF-may all be derived from a similar area of the alpha-chain of C3 so that a single peptide sequence could be responsible for the inhibition of T cell and B cell responses.

It is clear that C3 and its cleavage products may be important regulators of the immune response. LMF, C3d-K, C3d, C3-FP and fraction 2 all inhibit mitogen-induced proliferation [5,29,35,80]. LMF shares with fraction 2 and C3d-K both the lymphocyte-inhibiting and leukocytosis-inducing functions. The nine amino acids on the amino terminal end of C3d-K (TLDPERLGR) have been reported to be responsible for the leukocytosis seen with C3d-K [32]; this could explain why C3d,g, which does not contain these nine amino acids but which is otherwise identical with C3d-K, does not have leukocytosis-inducing activity.

However, we still do not know the enzyme responsible in vivo for the release of these active fragments from C3. Furthermore, we do not know the sequence of amino acids responsible for these activities. It will be important to determine if a single sequence is responsible for inhibition of B cell responses, inhibition of T cell responses, leukocytosis and leukocyte mobilization from bone marrow. Finally, it is difficult at the present time to assess the in vivo significance of these observations. Evidence for a physiological role awaits the identification of the biologically-active fragment(s) in tissues or body fluids.

Biological Significance of Complement Regulation of the Immune Response

The in vivo studies performed to date examining the role of C3, or indeed any of the complement components, on the immune response are inconclusive and provide neither the mechanism of action nor the precise amino acid sequence responsible for the effects that have been observed. Nevertheless, it will be important in the future to employ in vivo studies to demonstrate a biological role for complement in the regulation of the immune response [81].

In this review we must speculate on the biological significance of complement in the regulation of the immune response based upon clinical observation, early in vivo studies and more recent in vitro observations. It is clear from clinical observation that deficiency of C3 does not predispose a patient to aberrant immune responses. How then can complement play an important role in immunoregulation? The answer is that complement must play an ancillary role. Complement serves with other systems to control immune response. In general, C3 fragments, C3a and the C3b degradation products, appear to attenuate immune responses. This explains why a deficiency of C3 would not be manifested by *lack* of a response but rather as inability to *down regulate* an immune response. The absence of C3 would only be clinically apparent when other systems that also down regulate antibody responses are missing and this probably only occurs rarely. C3a, is short lived in vivo, with a half life of seconds, and inhibits lymphocyte responses until it is degraded to inactive C3a des arg. C3b degradation products probably have a much longer immunoregulatory life because they remain in circulation much longer in an active form.

We propose that in normal individuals, C3 is fixed in areas in which there is increased antibody production. C3 then serves to down regulate lymphocyte responses. C3a has short-term effects and C3b degradation products act much longer. In immune complex disease in which there is active complement consumption, one would predict the degradation products of C3 would serve to prevent even more activation of the lymphocytes in the areas of consumption. However, patients with such autoimmune diseases as rheumatoid arthritis and systemic lupus erythematosus exhibit a hyperactive immune system [84]. It will be interesting to test whether C3a and the inhibitory C3b degradation products are able to regulate in vitro lymphocyte responses in these patients, or, alternatively, whether the signal that causes this hyperactivity simply overcomes the suppressive effects of these fragments.

Early studies suggested a role for native C3 in immunoregulation, however the more recent observations suggest that all of the phenomena might be explained by C3 degradation products contained in native C3 preparations. Therefore, we cannot at present ascribe any immunoregulatory role to native C3. This is fortunate because otherwise we would have to explain why a component which circulates at a concentration of about 1.5 mg/ml regulates immune responses.

Postscript

Studies on the role of complement proteins on the immune response have been advanced greatly by recent elucidation of the primary amino acid sequences of these proteins. In addition, we now have available purified receptor preparations and monoclonal antibodies directed against these receptors and against specific regions of the complement molecules. Synthetic peptide analogues are also readily available for these studies.

Future studies will examine specific regions of these complement molecules for immunoregulatory activity. Immunoregulatory sequences will be examined in structure-function studies using synthetic peptides with an ultimate goal to produce important immunopharmacological agents. It might be possible with synthetic analogues to attenuate hyperactive immune responses that occur in immune complex diseases. Alternatively, it might be possible to generate leukocyte mobilizing factor activity in patients deficient in this activity. Finally, the studies with C3d-K suggest that immunoregulatory peptides might be used to inhibit the growth of tumor cells. The future holds the promise that the basic observations reviewed here will lead to significant therapeutic advances.

References

1 Pepys, M.B.: Role of complement in the induction of immunological responses. Transplant. Rev. *32:* 93–120 (1976).

2 Weiler, J.M.; Ballas, Z.K.; Needleman, B.W.; Hobbs, M.V.; Feldbush, T.L.: Complement fragments suppress lymphocyte immune responses. Immunol. Today *3:* 238–243 (1982).

3 Weigle, W.O.; Goodman, M.G.; Morgan, E.L.; Hugli, T.E.: Regulation of immune response by components of the complement cascade and their activated fragments. Springer Semin. Immunopathol. *6:* 173–194 (1983).

4 Egwang, T.G.; Befus, A.D.: The role of complement in the induction and regulation of immune responses. Immunology *51:* 207–224 (1984).

5 Weiler, J.M.: Complement and the Immune Response; in Whaley, Complement in health and disease (MTP Press, Lancaster 1986).

6 Pepys, M.B.: Role of complement in induction of antibody production in vivo: Effect of cobra factor and other C3-reactive agents on thymus-dependent and thymus-independent antibody responses. J. exp. Med. *140:* 126–145 (1974).

7 Bianco, C.; Patrick, R.; Nussenzweig, V.: A population of lymphocytes bearing a membrane receptor for antigen-antibody-complement complexes. I. Separation and characterization. J. exp. Med. *132:* 702–720 (1970).

8 Berger, M.; Gaither, T.A.; Frank, M.M.: Complement receptors. Clin. Immunol. Rev. *1:* 471–545 (1981–1982).

9 Ross, G.D.: Structure and function of membrane complement receptors. Fed. proc. *41:* 3089–3093 (1982).

10 Fearon, D.T.; Wong, W.W.: Complement ligand-receptor interactions that mediate biological responses. A. Rev. Immunol. *1:* 243–271 (1983).

11 Schreiber, R.D.: The chemistry and biology of complement receptors. Springer Semin. Immunopathol. *7:* 221–249 (1984).

12 Ross, G.D.; Medof, M.E.: Membrane complement receptors specific for bound fragments of C3. Adv. Immunol. *37:* 217–267 (1985).

13 Colten, H.R.; Ooi, Y.M.; Edelson, P.J.: Synthesis and secretion of complement proteins by macrophages. Ann. N.Y. Acad. Sci. *332:* 482–490 (1979).

14 Zimmer, B.; Hartung, H.-P.; Scharfenberger, G.; Bitter-Suermann, D.; Hadding, U.: Quantitative studies of the secretion of complement component C3 by resident, elicited and activated macrophages. Comparison with C2, C4 and lysosomal enzyme release. Eur. J. Immunol. *12:* 426–430 (1982).

15 Koopman, W.J.; Sandberg, A.L.; Wahl, S.M.; Mergenhagen, S.E.: Interaction of soluble C3 fragments with guinea pig lymphocytes. Comparison of effects of C3a, C3b, C3c, and C3d on lymphokine production and lymphocyte proliferation. J. Immun. *117:* 331–336 (1976).

16 McConnell, I.; Hurd, C.M.: Lymphocyte receptors. I. Receptors for Fc of IgG and complement (C3b) on immunoglobulin-bearing, antigen-binding and antibody-secreting cells. Immunology *30:* 825–833 (1976).

17 Gjal-Peczalska, K.J.; Fish, A.J.; Meuwissen, H.J.; Frommel, D.; Good, R.A.: Localization of immunological complexes fixing B_{1C} (C3) in germinal centers of lymph nodes. J. exp. Med. *130:* 1367–1393 (1969).

18 de Bruijn, M.H.L.; Fey, G.H.: Human complement component C3: cDNA coding sequence and derived primary structure. Proc. natn. Acad. Sci. USA *82:* 708–712 (1985).

19 Hugli, T.E.: Structure and function of the anaphylatoxins. Springer Semin. Immunopathol. *7:* 193–219 (1984).

20 Law, S.K.; Levine, R.P.: Interaction between the third complement protein and cell surface macromolecules. Proc. natn. Acad. Sci. USA *74:* 2701–2705 (1977).

21 Tack, B.F.; Harrison, R.A.; Janatova, J.; Thomas, M.L.; Prahl, J.W.: Evidence

for presence of an internal thioester bond in third component of human complement. Proc. natn. Acad. Sci. USA *77:* 5764–5768 (1980).

22 Weiler, J.M.; Daha, M.R.; Austen, K.F.; Fearon, D.T.: Control of the amplification convertase of complement by the plasma protein β1H Proc. natn. Acad. Sci. USA *73:* 3268–3272 (1976).

23 Nilsson, U.R.; Mandle, R.J.; McConnell-Mapes, J.A.: Human C3 and C5. Subunit structure and modifications by trypsin and C_{42}–C_{423}. J. Immun. *114:* 815–822 (1975).

24 Harrison, R.A.; Lachmann, P.J.: Novel cleavage products of the third component of human complement. Molec. Immunol. *17:* 219–228 (1980).

25 Lachmann, P.J.; Pangburn, M.K.; Oldroyd, R.G.: Breakdown of C3 after complement activation. Identification of a new fragment, C3g, using monoclonal antibodies, J. exp. Med. *156:* 205–216 (1982).

26 Davis, A.E.; Harrison, R.A.: Structural characterization of factor I mediated cleavage of the third component of complement. Biochemistry *21:* 5745–5749 (1982).

27 Chaplin, H.; Monroe, M.C.; Lachmann, P.J.: Further studies of the C3g component of the α2D fragment of human C3. Clin. exp. Immunol. *51:* 639–646 (1982).

28 Davis, A.E.; Harrison, R.A.; and Lachmann, P.J.: Physiologic inactivation of fluid phase C3b: Isolation and structural analysis of C3c, C3d,g (α2D), and C3g. J. Immun. *132:* 1960–1966 (1984).

29 Meuth, J.L.; Morgan, E.L.; DiScipio, R.G.; Hugli, T.E.: Suppression of T lymphocyte functions by human C3 fragments. I. Inhibition of human T cell proliferative responses by a kallikrein cleavage fragment of human iC3b. J. Immun. *130:* 2605–2611 (1983).

30 Matsuda, T.; Nagasawa, S.; Koide, T.; Koyama, J.: Limited proteolysis of a chemically modified third component of human complement, C3, by cathepsin G of human leukocytes. J. Biochem. *98:* 229–236 (1985).

31 Seya, T.; Nagasawa, S.; Matsukura, M.; Hasegawa, H.; Atkinson, J.P.: Generation of C3d,g and C3d by urokinase-treated plasma in association with fibrinolysis. Complement *2:* 165–174 (1985).

32 Hoeprich, P.D.; Dahinden, C.A.; Lachmann, P.J.; Davis, A.E.; Hugli, T.E.: A synthetic nonapeptide corresponding to the NH_2-terminal sequence of C3d-K causes leukocytosis in rabbits. J. biol. Chem. *260:* 2597–2600 (1985).

33 Ghebrehiwet, B.; Müller-Eberhard, H.J.: C3e: An acidic fragment of human C3 with leukocytosis inducing activity. J. Immun. *123:* 616–621 (1979).

34 Rother, K.: Leukocyte mobilizing factor: a new biological activity derived from the third component of complement. Eur. J. Immunol. *2:* 550–558 (1972).

35 Walker, C.; Kristensen, F.; Bitter-Suermann, D.; Stadler, B.M.; de Weck, A.L.: Interference of a C3-fragment preparation with IL 2-dependent proliferation. J. Immun. *136:* 3396–3401 (1986).

36 Vogel, C.-W.; Smith, C.A.; Müller-Eberhard, H.J.: Cobra venom factor: Structural homology with the third component of human complement. J. Immun. *133:* 3235–3241 (1984).

37 Cochrane, C.G.; Müller-Eberhard, H.J.; Aiken, B.S.: Deletion of plasma complement in vivo by a protein of cobra venom: Its effects on various immunologic reactions. J. Immun. *105:* 55–69 (1970).

38 Pepys, M.B.: Studies in vivo of cobra factor and murine C3. Immunology *28:* 369–377 (1975).

39 Pryjma, J.; Humphrey, J.H.: Prolonged C3 depletion by cobra venom factor in thymus-deprived mice and its implication for the role of C3 as an essential second signal for B-cell triggering. Immunology *28:* 569–576 (1975).

40 Lewis, G.K.; Ranken, R.; Nitecki, D.E.; Goodman, J.W.: Murine B-cell subpopulations responsive to T-dependent and T-independent antigens. J. exp. Med. *144:* 382–397 (1976).

41 Lewis, G.K.; Ranken, R.; Goodman, J.W.: Complement-dependent and -independent pathways of T cell–B cell cooperation. J. Immun. *118:* 1744–1747 (1977).

42 Klaus, G.G.B.; Humphrey, J.H.: The generation of memory cells: I. The role of C3 in the generation of B memory cells. Immunology *33:* 31–40 (1977).

43 Romball, C.G.; Ulevitch, R.J.; Weigle, W.O.: Role of C3 in the regulation of a splenic PFC response in rabbits. J. Immun. *124:* 151–155 (1980).

44 Spry, C.J.F.; Lane, J.T.; Vyakaranam, A.: The effects of complement activation by cobra venom factor on the migration of T and B lymphocytes into rat thoracic duct lymph. Immunology *32:* 947–954 (1977).

45 McConnell, I.; Hopkins, J.: Lymphocyte traffic through antigen-stimulated lymph nodes. I. Complement activation within lymph nodes initiates cell shutdown. Immunology *42:* 217–223 (1981).

46 Humphrey, J.H.: The still unsolved germinal centre mystery. Adv. exp. Med. Biol. *66:* 711–723 (1976).

47 Dukor, P.; Schumann, G.; Gisler, R.H.; Dierich, M.; König, W.; Hadding, U.; Bitter-Suermann, D.: Complement-dependent B-cell activation by cobra venom factor and other mitogens? J. exp. Med. *139:* 337–354 (1974).

48 Waldmann, H.; Lachmann, P.J.: The failure to show a necessary role for C3 in the in vitro antibody response. Eur. J. Immunol. *5:* 185–193 (1975).

49 Feldmann, M.; Pepys, M.B.: Role of C3 in vitro lymphocyte cooperation. Nature, Lond. *249:* 159–160 (1974).

50 Pepys, M.B.; Butterworth, A.E.: Inhibition by C3 fragments of C3-dependent rosette formation and antigen-induced lymphocyte transformation. Clin. exp. Immunol. *18:* 273–282 (1974).

51 Hartmann, K.-U.; Bokisch, V.A.: Stimulation of murine B lymphocytes by isolated C3b. J. exp. Med. *142:* 600–610 (1975).

52 Hammann, K.P.; Raile, A.; Schmitt, M.; Mussel, H.H.; Peters, H.; Scheiner, O.; Dierich, M.P.: β1H stimulates mouse-spleen B lymphocytes as demonstrated by increased thymidine incorporation and formation of B cell blasts. Immunobiology *160:* 289–301 (1981).

53 Ross, S.C.; Densen, P.: Complement deficiency states and infection: Epidemiology, pathogenesis and consequences of neisserial and other infections in an immune deficiency. Medicine *63:* 243–273 (1984).

54 Alper, C.A.; Colten, H.R.; Gear, J.S.S.; Rabson, A.R.; Rosen, F.S.: Homozygous human C3 deficiency. The role of C3 in antibody production, C_{1s}-induced vasopermeability, and cobra venom-induced passive hemolysis. J. clin. Invest. *57:* 222–229 (1976).

55 Blum, J.R.; Cork, L.C.; Morris, J.M.; Olson, J.L.; Winkelstein, J.A.: The clinical

manifestations of a genetically determined deficiency of the third component of complement in the dog. Clin. Immunol. Immunopathol. *34:* 304–315 (1985).
56 Böttger, E.C.; Hoffmann, T.; Hadding, U.; Bitter-Suermann, D.: Influence of genetically inherited complement deficiencies on humoral immune response in guinea pigs. J. Immun. *135:* 4100–4107 (1985).
57 Jackson, C.G.; Ochs, H.D.; Wedgwood, R.J.: Immune response of a patient with deficiency of the fourth component of complement and systemic lupus erythematosus. New Engl. J. Med. *300:* 1124–1129 (1979).
58 Sjöholm, A.G.; Hammarström, L.; Smith, C.I.E.; Kjellman, N.-I.M.: Immunoglobulin synthesis in a patient with C4 deficiency: Functional immaturity of peripheral blood lymphocytes. Acta pathol. microbiol. immunol. scand., C. *93:* 169–173 (1985).
59 Ochs, H.D.; Wedgwood, R.J.; Frank, M.M.; Heller, S.R.; Hosea, S.W.: The role of complement in the induction of antibody responses. Clin. exp. Immunol. *53:* 208–216 (1983).
60 Ferluga, J.; Schorlemmer, H.U.; Baptista, L.C.; Allison, A.C.: Cytolytic effects of the complement cleavage product, C3a. Br. J. Cancer *34:* 626–634 (1976).
61 Goodman, M.G.; Weigle, W.O.; Hugli, T.E.: Inability of the C3a anaphylatoxin to promote cellular lysis. Nature Lond. *283:* 78–80 (1980).
62 Charriaut, C.; Senik, A.; Kolb, J.-P.; Barel, M.; Frade, R.: Inhibition of in vitro natural killer activity by the third component of complement: Role for the C3a fragment. Proc. natn. Acad. Sci. USA *79:* 6003–6007 (1982).
63 Payan, D.G.; Trentham, D.E.; Goetzl, E.J.: Modulation of human lymphocyte function by C3a and C3a(70–77). J. exp. Med. *156:* 756–765 (1982).
64 Glovsky, M.M.; Hugli, T.E.; Ishizaka, T.; Lichtenstein, L.M.; Erickson, B.W.: Anaphylatoxin-induced histamine release with human leukocytes. Studies of C3a leukocyte binding and histamine release. J. clin. Invest. *64:* 804–811 (1979).
65 Morgan, E.L.; Weigle, W.O.; Erickson, B.W.; Fok, K.-F.; Hugli, T.E.: Suppression of humoral immune responses by synthetic C32a peptides. J. Immun. *131:* 2258–2261 (1983).
66 Morgan, E.L.; Thoman, M.L.; Hoeprich, P.D.; Hugli, T.E.: Bioactive complement fragments in immunoregulation. Immunol. Lett. *9:* 207–213 (1985).
67 Morgan, E.L.; Thoman, M.L.; Hobbs, M.V.; Weigle, W.O.; Hugli, T.E.: Human C3a-mediated suppression of the immune response. II. Suppression of human in vitro polyclonal antibody responses occurs through the generation of nonspecific OKT8+ suppressor T cells. Clin. Immunol. Immunopathol. *37:* 114–123 (1985).
68 Morgan, E.L.: Modulation of the immune response by anaphylatoxins. Complement (in press, 1986).
69 Morgan, E.L.: Immunoregulatory properties of human complement fragments C3a and C5a; in Goldstein, Bach, Wigzell, Immune regulation by defined polypeptides (Liss., New York 1986).
70 Morgan, E.L.; Weigle, W.O.; Hugli, T.E.: Anaphylatoxin-mediated regulation of the immune response. I. C3a-mediated suppression of human and murine humoral immune responses. J. exp. Med. *155:* 1412–1426 (1982).
71 Schenkein, H.A.; Genco, R.J.: Inhibition of lymphocyte blastogenesis by C3c and C3d. J. Immun. *122:* 1126–1133 (1979).
72 Erdei, A.; Melchers, F.; Schulz, T.; Dierich, M.: The action of human C3 in solu-

ble or cross-linked form with resting and activated murine B lymphocytes. Eur. J. Immunol. *15:* 184–188 (1985).

73 Tsokos, G.C.; Berger, M.; Balow, J.E.: Modulation of human B cell immunoglobulin secretion by the C3b component of complement. J. Immun. *132:* 622–626 (1984).

74 Thoman, M.L.; Meuth, J.L.; Morgan, E.L.; Weigle, W.O.; Hugli, T.E.: C3d-K, a kallikrein cleavage fragment of iC3b is a potent inhibitor of cellular proliferation. J. Immun. *133:* 2629–2633 (1984).

75 Needleman, B.W.; Weiler, J.M.; Feldbush, T.L.: The third component of complement inhibits human lymphocyte blastogenesis. J. Immun. *126:* 1586–1591 (1981).

76 Weiler, J.M.; Ballas, Z.K.; Feldbush, T.L.; Needleman, B.W.: Inhibition of human lymphocyte blastogenesis by C3: The role of serum in the tissue culture medium. Immunology *45:* 247–252 (1982).

77 Hobbs, M.V.; Feldbush, T.L.; Needleman, B.W.; Weiler, J.M.: Inhibition of secondary in vitro antibody responses by the third component of complement. J. Immun. *128:* 1470–1475 (1982)

78 Ballas, Z.K.; Feldbush, T.L.; Needleman, B.W.; Weiler, J.M.: Complement inhibits immune responses: C3 preparations inhibit the generation of human cytotoxic T lymphocytes. Eur. J. Immunol. *13:* 279–284 (1983).

79 Feldbush, T.L.; Hobbs, M.V.; Severson, C.D.; Ballas, Z.K.; Weiler, J.M.: Role of complement in the immune response. Fed. Proc. *43:* 2548–2552 (1984)

80 Melchers, F.; Erdei, A.; Schulz, T.; Dierich, M.P.: Growth control of activated synchronized murine B cells by the C3d fragment of human complement. Nature, Lond. *317:* 264–267 (1985).

81 Klaus, G.G.B.; Humphrey, J.H.: A re-evaluation of the role of C3 in B-cell activation. Immunol. today *7:* 163–165 (1986).

82 Tack, B.F.; Prahl, J.W.: The third component of human complement. Purification from plasma and physicochemical characterization. Biochemistry *15:* 4513–4521 (1976).

83 Needleman, B.W.; Weiler, J.M.: Human lymphocyte transformation induced by mitogens and antigens in a serum-free tissue culture system. J. immunol. Methods *44:* 3–14 (1981).

84 Möller, E.; Ström, H.; Al-Balaghi, S.: Role of polyclonal activation in specific immune responses. Scand. J. Immunol. *12:* 177–182 (1980).

John M. Weiler, MD, SW34E University Hospital,
University of Iowa, Iowa City, IA 52242 (USA)

Concepts Immunopathol., vol. 4, pp. 129–143 (Karger, Basel 1987)

Multigenic Basis of Autoimmune Disease in New Zealand Mice

Thomas M. Chused, Kathleen L. McCoy, Renu B. Lal, Elinor M. Brown, Phillip J. Baker

Laboratories of Immunology and Microbial Immunity, National Institute of Allergy and Infectious Diseases, National Institutes of Health, Bethesda, Md., USA

Introduction

The occurrence of a high incidence of spontaneous autoimmune disease in several strains of inbred mice indicates that this process has a genetic basis. Similarly, studies of human families [1–5] provide convincing evidence of a very strong genetic component underlying the several human autoimmune diseases examined. The much higher concordance for systemic lupus erythematosus in twins than in nontwin siblings [6, 7] indicates that the genetic influence is much stronger than any possible infectious or other environmental agents. Because the pathogenetic mechanisms of spontaneous autoimmune diseases in human patients have not been elucidated, animal models have been investigated with the expectation that their experimental accessibility, genetic homogeneity and controlled environment would facilitate understanding of the autoimmune process. These efforts have focused on several lines of inbred mice that spontaneously develop genetically conditioned autoimmune disease. Our work has emphasized the development of autoimmune disease in New Zealand mice because their clinical disorders and genetic complexity most closely resemble human disease. The New Zealand strains of mice originated at the University of Otago in Dunedin, New Zealand, during the 1950s where they were inbred, selecting for coat color, by Dr. Marianne Beilschowsky. In the eleventh inbred generation, it was noted that the mice of the New Zealand Black (NZB) strain developed autoimmune hemolytic anemia – the first animal model of autoimmune disease [8, 9]. Subsequent crosses with other strains revealed that the F_1 hybrid of NZB with New Zealand White (NZW) mice develops lupus erythematosus in which anti-DNA and anti-gp70 autoantibodies cause immune complex glomerulonephritis [10]. Interestingly, the NZW strain itself is immunologically normal, at least until very late in life. Like most human autoimmune disorders, female (NZB × NZW) F_1 mice are more severely affected than males. The results of castration and sex hormone replacement experiments have shown that this is a hormonal effect [11–13].

A number of pertinent observations on the immunologic disorder of New Zealand mice have been reported. These include the fact that B cells in NZB mice are polyclonally activated to IgM (but not IgG) production at the beginning of life [14–16]. Splenic B cells from all F_1 hybrids derived from crosses between NZB mice and other inbred strains produce one third to one half the amount of IgM produced by the NZB parent, indicating that this trait is semidominant. This abnormality is independent of T lymphocytes because it occurs in nu/nu and T cell deprived thymectomized, irradiated, fetal liver reconstituted NZB mice [17]. It is accompanied by increased expression of surface IgM receptors and decreased levels of surface IgD on the B cells of NZB mice [18, 19]. In addition, NZB mice are resistant to the experimental induction of immunologic tolerance prior to the onset of autoimmune disease [20–22]. Investigators using different methods and a variety of test antigens have attributed the difficulty in inducing tolerance to both T and B cell dysfunction; thus, the nature of this defect has not been clarified [23–28].

The genetic basis of autoimmune disease in New Zealand mice is extremely complex. Abnormalities such as B cell hyperactivity, tolerance resistance, as well as the formation of antithymocyte and antierythrocyte autoantibodies appear to be controlled by different genes or groups of genes as determined by conventional backcross analysis [29–35] or by the use of recombinant-inbred (RI) lines [36–39]. It is clear, however, that NZW immune response genes within the major histocompatibility complex of the H-2^z haplotype facilitate the immunologic recognition of DNA [40, 41]. Replacement of the H-2^z haplotype of NZW mice with the H-2^d haplotype from NZB mice (to generate the NZW strain congenic for H-2^d, named ZWD) greatly reduces the level of anti-DNA antibodies, but not of serum immunoglobulin, in the (NZB × ZWD) F_1 hybrid; this prolongs the survival of (NZB × ZWD) F_1 hybrids in comparison with the unmanipulated (NZB × NZW) F_1 mice [42].

An important feature of New Zealand mouse disease is that B cell hyperactivity and resistance to tolerance are fully established by 6–8 weeks of age, but overt autoimmune disease (formation of antierythrocyte and anti-DNA autoantibodies, and the development of hemolytic anemia and/or immune complex glomerulonephritis) does not appear until 6–12 months of age. This review will summarize our recent studies on enlargement of Lyt-2^+ T cells, tolerance resistance and the genetic analysis of NZB recombinant inbred lines.

Results

Changes in NZB Lymphocytes with Age

Longitudinal analysis of splenic T, B and null cell populations in NZB mice during the first year of life by flow cytometry revealed several important changes: (1) a progressive shift in the B cell population from surface IgD bright, IgM dull to IgD dull, IgM bright and the appearance of IL-2 receptors on some B cells, but not on T cells; (2) progressive elevation of IgG containing plasma cells after 6 months of age; (3) the sudden onset of splenomegaly, due to proliferation of null cells, beginning about 10 months of age, and (4) an increase in cell size (determined by narrow angle forward light scatter) of the Lyt-2^+, but not the Lyt-2^-, T cells after 10 months of age [43]. Although larger in size, two-color flow cytometry with the DNA stain Hoechst 33342 and anti-Lyt-2 showed that the Lyt-2^+ cells were blocked in G_1 and did not enter the S phase of the cell cycle. Consistent with the lack of proliferation, the total number of splenic Lyt-2^+ T cells did not change as NZB mice age.

The unusual enlargement of the Lyt-2^+ T cells in aging NZB mice prompted us to ask whether enlargement is correlated with the onset of disease. We examined individual NZB mice for Lyt-2^+ T cell size, anti-erythrocyte autoantibodies, anemia, proteinuria and splenomegaly. Lyt-2^+ T cell size was found to correlate with the level of antierythrocyte autoantibodies ($p < 0.002$) and the severity of hemolytic anemia ($p < 0.04$), but not with proteinuria or splenomegaly [44]. NZB mice congenic for *xid,* the gene causing X-linked immunodeficiency, which inhibits B cell hyperactivity and prevents the development of autoimmune disease [45], failed to develop enlarged Lyt-2^+ T cells. Similarly, the phenomenon was not observed in (NZB×NZW) F_1 or (NZB×NFS) F_1 hybrids. Thus, the enlargement of the Lyt-2^+ T cells appears to depend on both the NZB B cell hyperactivity and recessive genetic factors.

The functional status of the enlarged Lyt-2^+ T cells in old NZB mice was examined by exposure of such cells to concanavalin A in vitro and in vivo. Proliferative responses of both L3T4$^+$ and Lyt-2$^+$ T cells from old mice cultured with the mitogen were reduced by 75%; the induction of IL-2 receptor was reduced by 50%. After in vivo treatment, however, IL-2 receptors were induced on the L3T4 T cells from old mice at 35% of the level observed in young mice, but not at all on Lyt-2$^+$ cells. Thus in vivo activation of Lyt-2$^+$, but not L3T4$^+$, T cells is completely blocked in old NZB mice. That this block is partially relieved upon culture of these cells suggests that in vivo it depends either on a short-lived factor or intact lymphoid architecture.

Flow cytometric examination indicated that in old NZB and (NZB×NZW) F_1 mice splenic L3T4$^+$ and Lyt-2$^+$ T cells had similar amounts of autoantibody on their cell surfaces. Since Lyt-2$^+$ T cells enlarge in NZB, but not (NZB×NZW) F, mice it is unlikely that anti-T cell autoantibodies play a role in this process.

Loss of T Suppressor Function in Aging NZB Mice

To assess the functional capacity of enlarged Lyt-2$^+$ T cells in NZB mice, old and young animals were given concanavalin A to nonspecifically activate T suppressor cells involved in the antibody response to type III pneumococcal polysaccharide (SSS-III); the degree of suppression induced was then determined [46]. As in normal strains, the anti-SSS-III antibody response of young NZB mice was suppressed substantially by concanavalin A, whereas the response of old NZB mice, having enlarged Lyt-2$^+$ T cells, was paradoxically enhanced [44].

The expression of regulatory T cell activity for the antibody response to SSS-III also was used to further analyze the state of T suppressor cells in aging NZB mice. Treatment (priming) with a subimmunogenic dose of SSS-III prior to immunization induces an antigen-specific state of unresponsiveness mediated by T suppressor cells [47]. Although low-dose paralysis can be induced in nonautoimmune BALB/c mice at all ages tested, it is significantly diminished in NZB mice at 36 weeks of age, and nearly absent in NZB mice at 52 weeks of age.

Adoptive transfer of Lyt-2$^+$ T cells from low-dose SSS-III primed BALB/c mice to naive animals of the same strain resulted in antigen-specific suppression of the antibody response to SSS-III upon subsequent immunization of recipients. Suppression also could be transferred by primed Lyt-2$^+$ T cells from young to old animals and vice versa in this nonautoimmune strain. By contrast, normal-sized Lyt-2$^+$ T cells from low-dose primed old NZB mice were able to transfer suppression to young NZB mice; however, enlarged Lyt-2^+ T cells from old NZB mice were without effect [48]. Studies in which cells were transferred from young into old NZB mice demonstrated still another immunologic defect: the antibody response of old NZB mice to SSS-III was not reduced by Lyt-2^+ T cells, even though the same cells were effective upon transfer to young mice. These results suggest that two defects are involved in the decline of low-dose paralysis to SSS-III in aging NZB mice: (1) enlarged Lyt-2^+ T cells appear to lose their ability to function as mediators of suppression, and (2) B cells become resistant to T cell mediated suppression. B cell resistance to suppression may be related to alteration in cell surface antigen phenotype and activation as suggested by the expression of IL-2 receptors.

Amplifier T Cell Activity

The observation of decreased suppressor activity associated with enlargement of Lyt-2^+ T cells in old NZB mice prompted an examination of amplifier T cell function in this strain. Spleen cells from NZB mice given a subimmunogenic dose of SSS-III 72 h before sacrifice were treated with anti-Lyt-2 and complement to remove suppressor T cells and adoptively transferred to young recipients that had received an immunogenic dose of SSS-III 48 h previously [49]. Amplifier activity – a fourfold enhancement of response – was observed in old, but not in young, mice. Further experiments indicated a biphasic expression of amplifier activity: present in young mice and in mice older than 40 weeks but absent at 24 and 35 weeks. T helper activity, which differs from amplifier function in acting within 24 h after immunization and being sensitive to thymectomy and hydrocortisone, was absent in 48-week-old mice. Thus, T suppressor activity decreases and T amplifier activity increases at the onset of overt autoimmune disease in NZB mice.

Tolerance Defects in New Zealand Mice

The loss of tolerance to particular self antigens is associated with the development of autoimmune disease in NZB and (NZB × NZW) F_1 mice. Experimental induction of tolerance to foreign antigens has been examined to better understand the failure to maintain self-tolerance in autoimmune mice. Abnormalities of both B and T cells have been implicated in the resistance to tolerance induction of New Zealand mice [23–27]. To resolve this question, we developed a system that allows separate assessment of tolerance in the T and B cell compartments in vivo

Table I Resistance of NZB mice to induction of tolerance

Mouse strain	Monomeric BSA, μg	Percent reduction of response to: BSA	DNP
NFS	10	99	99
	100	99	99
	1000	99	99
NZW	10	98	99
	100	98	99
	1000	99	99
NZB	10	–28	26
	100	11	82
	1000	–45	99
NZB×B10.D2 F_1	1000	–23	79
NZB×NFS F_1	1000	33	96
NZB×NZW F_1	1000	–35	20
NZB.*xid* ♀	1000	99	99
NZB.*xid*×NZW F_1 ♀	1000	55	–56
NZB.*xid*×NZW F_1 ♂	1000	16	2

[50]. Unresponsiveness was induced with monomeric bovine serum albumin (BSA). The effectiveness of tolerance induction was determined by challenging with dinitrophenyl (DNP)-conjugated BSA and measuring the serum antihapten and anticarrier antibody levels of individual mice. Treatment with monomeric BSA induced tolerance in the T helper population, whereas B cells specific for DNP remain capable of responding to hapten. Obviously, a defect affecting T helper tolerance would prevent the development of tolerance to both hapten and carrier; by contrast, a defect affecting only B cells would impair tolerance only to the carrier.

Application of this system to normal NFS and NZW mice showed that doses of 10–1,000 μg of monomeric BSA induced tolerance to both BSA and DNP (table I). In NZB mice, tolerance to BSA was not induced by any dose. Unlike the anticarrier response, the anti-DNP response of NZB mice decreased with increasing doses of BSA, so that 1,000 μg BSA induced the same reduction of antihapten antibodies as in control mice.

The mode of inheritance of this abnormality in the induction of tolerance was determined by testing NZB F_1 hybrids. NZB, (NZB×B10.D2) F_1 and (NZB×NFS) F_1 mice express the same phenotype for the induction of tolerance, i.e., monomeric BSA induced a lack of response to

DNP – but not to BSA – when presented as a conjugate. This suggests that BSA-specific B cells were primed by the monomeric BSA but the naive DNP-specific B cells did not receive sufficient T cell help to respond. Surprisingly, (NZB × NZW) F_1 mice generated an antibody response to both DNP and BSA after receiving the same treatment. These results suggest that (NZB × NZW) F_1 mice express a major defect in T helper cell tolerance, whereas the parental NZB exhibits a less profound abnormality. The severe (NZB × NZW) F_1 defect presumably results from the combined effects of genes from both strains.

To further characterize the lymphocyte subsets responsible for the NZB and (NZB × NZW) F_1 tolerance defects, we examined the effect of the *xid* gene on the abnormal antibody responses. The presence of this gene, which suppresses the spontaneous polyclonal B cell activation of NZB mice [45], but does not affect T cells, causes NZB mice to become susceptible to tolerance induction. NZB.*xid* mice treated with monomeric BSA do not produce anti-BSA after challenge; this suggests that the anti-BSA response of similarly treated NZB mice may be associated with B cell hyperactivity. By contrast, (NZB.*xid* × NZW) ♂ (which are phenotypically *xid*) and (NZB.*xid* × NZW) ♀ (which are phenotypically normal) both manifest resistance to tolerance induction to BSA and DNP. The failure of the *xid* gene to correct the tolerance defect of (NZB × NZW) F_1 mice provides further evidence that this hybrid manifests substantial tolerance resistance in the T helper population.

Genetic Features of NZB Recombinant Inbred Lines

We have studied 16 NZB × NFS (a nonautoimmune inbred Swiss line) recombinant inbred lines. Lymphocyte phenotype distribution, B cell activation, Ly-1 expression by B lymphocytes, susceptibility to tolerance induction, null cell levels, and leukemia virus antigen expression were examined at 2–3 months of age. The animals were observed as they aged for the development of antierythrocyte autoantibodies, anemia, enlargement of Lyt-2^+ T cells, and proteinuria.

(NZB × NFS) F_1 mice and 9 of 14 lines examined were resistant to tolerance induction, indicating that two genes, at least one of which is semidominant, determine this phenotype. Murine leukemia virus antigen was expressed by 7 of 16 RI lines, consistent with control by a single dominant gene as concluded by other investigators. Null cells were normal in (NZB × NFS) F_1 mice but elevated in half the RI lines, suggesting that this trait is regulated by a single recessive gene. One or more B cell abnormalities (increased δ dull B cells, elevated plasma cells, or increased Ly-1$^+$μ$^+$ cells) were detected in 13 of the 16 RI lines. (NZB×NFS) F_1 mice were intermediate for all three traits indicating the involvement of semidominant genes. Only 2 of the 16 RI lines expressed the NZB level of plasma cells, suggesting the involvement of three genes. Twelve of the 16 lines manifested increased Ly-1 μ$^+$ cells, implying that either of two genes could produce the phenotype.

Most of the traits analyzed in the young RI lines did not segregate independently. All lines with elevated δ dull B cells also had increased Ly-1$^+$μ$^+$ cells. Increased δ dull B cells was also associated with increased plasma cells. Elevated plasma cells was associated with increased null cells. In addition, all RI lines with supranormal null cells were resistant to tolerance induction. Only the expression of leukemia virus antigen was unrelated to any of the other early NZB anormalities examined.

NFS and (NZB×NFS) F_1 mice did not produce antierythrocyte autoantibodies or develop anemia, indicating a critical role for either disease-inducing recessive NZB gene(s) or disease-suppressing dominant NFS genes. Five of the RI lines developed antierythrocyte autoantibodies but only three of these became anemic despite repeated testing, suggesting that a second gene is required for the development of anemia. Four of the five Coombs-positive lines had B cell abnormalities, including elevated plasma cells. All five had elevated null cells and were resistant to tolerance induction. The three that became anemic were H-2^d.

Seven of the RI lines developed significant proteinuria, four with a high incidence rate (>80%) and three with incomplete penetrance (30–40%). It appears that one gene could condition the development of renal disease and a second determine the incidence rate. There was no relationship between the development of proteinuria and any of the abnormal B cell traits expressed early in life. However, the four strains with high incidence renal disease were all H-2^q.

Enlargement of Lyt-2$^+$ T cells occurred in the (NZB×NFS) F_1 animals, indicating semidominant inheritance. This feature was observed in five of the RI lines, all of which had B cell abnormalities. In contrast to the parental NZB strain, there was no relationship between Lyt-2$^+$ T cell enlargement and anemia in the RI lines. Thus, Lyt-2$^+$ T cell enlargement may require an additional gene in the presence of B cell activation.

A scheme for the genetic basis of hemolytic anemia consistent with these observations is presented in table II. Development of the disease appears to require three sequential genetic steps. In the first, the com-

Table II. Genetic requirements for development of hemolytic anemia in NZB mice

Stage I			Stage II			Stage III		
trait	inheritance		trait	inheritance		trait	inheritance	
↑Ly^{-1+} μ^{+} ↑Plasma cells	Dom		Inducer of anti-RBC Ab ↓	Rec		Inducer of hemolytic anemia ↓	?	
↑Ly^{-1+} μ^{+} ↑Plasma cells ↑δ dull	Dom	Abnormal B cells	— or →		Anti-RBC	→		Hemolytic anemia
↑Null cells ↓Tolerance ↑Plasma cells	Rec		Suppressor of anti-RBC Ab ↑	Dom				
↓Tolerance	Dom							

bined effects of three dominant and one recessive genes determine the extent and type of B cell abnormalities. If sufficiently severe, a second stage gene can allow the production of antierythrocyte autoantibody. The data does not distinguish between two possible modes of inheritance for this gene: either the presence of a recessive enhancing gene or the absence of a dominant suppressing gene [51]. Finally, a third stage gene is required for the development of hemolytic anemia. This gene could, for example, condition a switch in antierythrocyte antibody isotype from IgM to IgG [52, 53].

Conclusions

These studies indicate that complex genetic and functional interactions, unfolding over the life of the animals, cause the development of autoimmune disease in New Zealand mice. Although each strain of autoimmune mice follows a unique path, our results suggest that the factors playing a role in New Zealand mice include: (1) Polyclonal B cell activation, which appears necessary, but not sufficient for the development of hemolytic anemia. Only IgM production is elevated in young animals, and this abnormality is intrinsic to B cells. (2) There are age-related changes in the distribution of NZB B cell subsets. The expression of IL-2 receptors by B cells late in life when disease develops indicates a type of B cell activation distinct from that occurring in young animals. Either or both of these changes could be related to the age-dependent loss in B cell susceptibility to regulatory T cell signals. (3) NZB mice lose T suppressor function as they age. T amplifier activity is not only present but may even be elevated whereas T helper activity is virtually absent. (4) New Zealand mice exhibit two types of tolerance defect. B cells in NZB and NZB F_1 mice manifest resistance to tolerance induction. The (NZB × NZW) F_1 hybrid is unique in also demonstrating a major block to the induction of tolerance in T helper cells. (5) Finally, the analysis of NZB × NFS RI lines indicates that a sequence of genetic 'gates' determines the development of autoimmune hemolytic anemia.

Our results suggest a difference between the pathogenesis of hemolytic anemia and renal disease in New Zealand mice and their hybrids. Hemolytic anemia is highly correlated with B cell hyperactivity and resistance to tolerance in the B cell compartment, which appears to be controlled by four interacting genes. In the presence of B cell abnormalities, an additional gene permits the production of antierythrocyte autoantibodies. If such antibodies are present, a final gene in the pathway, which may induce an isotype switch, causes hemolytic anemia. The complexity of this genetic pathway provides an explanation for the absence of hemolytic anemia in all NZB crosses except with the related NZC strain [30].

In the NZB×NFS RI lines, there is no correlation between renal disease and either hemolytic anemia or the degree of underlying B cell hyperactivity. Similarly, there is not a strong relationship between B cell activation and glomerulonephritis in F_1 and F_2 progeny of the NZB×SWR cross [54, 55]. It is likely that a group of genes that only partially intersects those related to hemolytic anemia is responsible for renal disease. This group probably includes immune response genes linked to $H\text{-}2^z$ in the (NZB×NZW) F_1 hybrid and possibly, because of the association we observed, to $H\text{-}2^q$ in the NZB×NFS RI lines. The uniquely impaired susceptibility of T cells in (NZB×NZW) F_1 mice to tolerance induction, which is apparent at immunologic maturity in contrast to the late-life T suppressor defect of the parental NZB strain, may well contribute to the early development of anti-DNA antibodies and immune-complex glomerulonephritis in this hybrid.

The complexity of the hereditary mechanism responsible for autoimmune disease in NZB mice, their F_1 hybrids and RI lines derived from them limits the precision of understanding attainable by genetic analysis of the type we and others have performed. Nevertheless, sufficient information is available to conclude that the number of genes necessary for the development of overt autoimmune disease is surprisingly large. Our estimate that five or six separate genes are required for hemolytic anemia must be considered a minimal value, in part because any gene common to both NZB and NFS would not be detected. Further, these genes may not be deleterious except in the presence of the others. Spontaneous autoimmune disease in humans almost certainly has a genetic mechanism similar to, but much more complex and varied than that of New Zealand mice. It is likely that a limited number of the genes involved may enhance individual survival and thus confer benefits to the species that outweigh the adverse effect of the rare occurrence of excessive numbers or unusual combinations of these genes. Such genes could, in fact, improve reproductive performance in an outbred population, e.g., by enhancing immunologic responsiveness, while causing autoimmune disease in a limited number of individuals. The multigenic basis of spontaneous autoimmune disease in mammalian species clearly poses obstacles to identification of the relevant genes and their mechanisms. Further analysis of New Zealand mice, however, and isolation of the responsible genes may provide gene probes that will prove useful in the investigation of human subjects.

References

1 Winchester, R.J.: Genetic aspects of rheumatoid arthritis. Springer Semin. Immunopathol. *4:* 89 (1981).

2 Lippman, S.M.; Arnett, F.C.; Conley, C.L.; Ness, P.M.; Meyers, D.A.; Bias, W.B.: Genetic factors predisposing to autoimmune diseases. Autoimmune hemolytic anemia, chronic thrombocytopenic purpura, and systemic lupus erythematosus. Am. J. Med. *73:* 827 (1982).

3 Reveille, J.D.; Wilson, R.W.; Provost, T.T.; Bias, W.B.; Arnett, F.C.: Primary Sjögren's syndrome and other autoimmune diseases in families. Prevalence and immunogenetic studies in six kindreds. Ann. intern. Med. *101:* 748 (1984).

4 Jabs, D.A.; Arnett, F.C.; Bias, W.B.; Beale, M.G.: Familial abnormalities of lymphocyte function in a large Sjögren's syndrome kindred. J. Rheimatol. *13:* 320 (1986).

5 Torfs, C.P.; King, M.C.; Huey, B.; Malmgren, J.; Grumet, F.C.: Genetic interrelationship between insulin-dependent diabetes mellitus, the autoimmune thyroid diseases, and rheumatoid arthritis. Am J. hum. Genet. *38:* 170 (1986).

6 Block, S.R.; Winfield, J.B.; Lockshin, M.D.; D'Angelo, W.A.; Christian, C.L.: Studies of twins with systemic lupus erythematosus. A review of the literature and presentation of 12 additional sets. Am. J. Med. *59:* 533 (1975).

7 Block, S.R.; Lockshin, M.D.; Winfield, J.B.; Weksler, M.E.; Imamura, M.; Winchester, R.J.; Mellors, R.C.; Christian, C.L.: Immunologic observations on 9 sets of twins either concordant or discordant for SLE. Arthritis Rheum. *19:* 545 (1976).

8 Bielschowsky, M.; Heyler, B.J.; Howie, J.B.: Spontaneous haemolytic anemia in mice of the NZB/Bl strain. Proc. Univ. Otago Med. Sch. *39:* 9 (1959).

9 Helyer, B.J.; Howie, J.B.: Spontaneous auto-immune disease in NZB/Bl mice. Br. J. Haemat. *9:* 119 (1963).

10 Lambert, P.H.; Dixon, F.J.: Pathogenesis of the glomerulonephritis of NZB/W mice. J. exp. Med. *127:* 507 (1968).

11 Roubinian, J.R.; Papoian, R.; Talal, N.: Androgenic hormones modulate autoantibody responses and improve survival in murine lupus. J. clin. Invest. *59:* 1066 (1977).

12 Roubinian, J.R.; Talal, N.; Greenspan, J.S.; Goodman, J.R.; Siiteri, P.K.: Effect of castration and sex hormone treatment on survival, anti-nucleic acid antibodies, and glomerulonephritis in NZB/NZW F_1 mice. J. exp. Med. *147:* 1568 (1978).

13 Roubinian, J.R.; Talal, N.; Greenspan, J.S.; Goodman, J.R.; Siiteri, P.K.: Effect of castration and sex hormone treatment on survival, anti-nucleic acid antibodies, and glomerulonephritis in NZB/NZW F_1 mice. J. exp. Med. *147:* 1568 (1978).

14 Moutsopoulos, H.M.; Boehm-Truitt, M.; Kassan, S.S.; Chused, T.M.: Demonstration of activation of B lymphocytes in New Zealand black mice at birth by an immunoradiometric assay for murine IgM. J. Immun. *119:* 1639 (1977).

15 DeHeer, D.H.; Edgington, T.S.: Evidence for a B lymphocyte defect underlying the anti-X anti-erythrocyte autoantibody response of NZB mice. J. Immun. *118:* 1858 (1977).

16 Izui, S.; McConahey, P.J.; Dixon, F.J.: Increased spontaneous polyclonal activation of B lymphocytes in mice with spontaneous autoimmune disease. J. Immun. *121:* 2213 (1978).

17 Chused, T.M.; Moutsopoulos, H.M.; Sharrow, S.O.; Hansen, C.T.: Evidence of a primary B lymphocyte abnormality of NZB mice; in Cooper, Mosier, Scher, Vitetta, B lymphocytes in the immune response, p. 363 (Elsevier/North-Holland, New York 1979).

18 Cohen, P.; Ziff, M.; Vitetta, E.S.: Characterization of a B cell defect in the NZB mouse manifested by an increased ratio of surface IgM to IgD. J. Immun. *121:* 973 (1978).

19 Manohar, V.; Brown, E.; Leiserson, W.M.; Chused, T.M.: Expression of Lyt-l by a subset of B lymphocytes. J. Immun. *129:* 532 (1982).

20 Weir, D.M.; McBride, W.; Naysmith, J.D.: Immune response to a soluble protein antigen in NZB mice. Nature, Lond. *219:* 1276 (1968).

21 Staples, P.J.; Talal, N.: Rapid loss of tolerance induced in weanling NZB and B-W F_1 mice. Science *163:* 1215 (1969).

22 Staples, P.J.; Talal, N.: Relative inability to induce tolerance in adult NZB and NZB-NZW F_1 mice. J. exp. Med. *129:* 123 (1969).

23 Taurog, J.D.; Smathers, P.A.; Steinberg, A.D.: Evidence for abnormalities in separate lymphocyte populations in NZB mice. J. Immun. *125:* 485 (1980).

24 Laskin, C.A.; Taurog, J.D.; Smathers, P.A.; Steinberg, A.D.: Studies of defective tolerance in murine lupus. J. Immun. *127:* 1743 (1981).

25 Goldings, E.A.; Cohen, P.L.; McFadden, S.F.; Ziff, M.; Vitetta, E.S.: Defective B cell tolerance in adult (NZB X NZW) F_1 mice. J. exp. Med. *152:* 730 (1980).

26 Laskin, C.A.; Smathers, P.A.; Reeves, J.P.; Steinberg, A.D.: Studies of defective tolerance induction in NZB mice. Evidence for a marrow pre-T cell defect. J. exp. Med. *155:* 1025 (1982).

27 Goldings, E.A.: Defective B cell tolerance induction in New Zealand black mice. I. Macrophage independence and comparison with other autoimmune strains. J. Immun. *131:* 2630 (1983).

28 Laskin, C.A.; Smathers, P.A.; Lieberman, R.; Steinberg, A.D.: NZB cells actively interfere with the establishment of tolerance to BGG in radiation chimeras. J. Immun. *131:* 1121 (1983).

29 Ghaffar, A.; Playfair, J.H.: The genetic basis of autoimmunity in NZB mice studied by progeny-testing. Clin. ecx. Immunol. *8:* 479 (1971).

30 Warner, N.L.: Genetic control of spontaneous and induced antierythrocyte autoantibody production in mice. Clin. Immunol. Immunopathol. *1:* 353 (1973).

31 Knight, J.G.; Adams, D.D.: Three genes for lupus nephritis in NZB×NZW mice. J. exp. Med. *147:* 1653 (1978).

32 Davidson, W.F.; Chused, T.M.; Morse, H.C. III: Genetic control of B- and T-lymphocyte abnormalities of NZB mice in crosses with Bl0.D2 mice. Immunogenetics *13:* 421 (1981).

33 Yoshida, H.; Kohno, A.; Ohta, K.; Hirose, S.; Maruyama, N.; Shirai, T.: Genetic studies of autoimmunity in New Zealand mice. III. Associations among antiDNA

antibodies, NTA, and renal disease in (NZB×NZW) F_1×NZW backcross mice. J. Immun. *127:* 433 (1981).

34 Maruyama, N.; Furukawa, F.; Nakai, Y.; Sasaki, Y.; Ohta, K.; Ozaki, S.; Hirose, S.; Shirai, T.: Genetic studies of autoimmunity in New Zealand mice. IV. Contribution of NZB and NZW genes to the spontaneous occurrence of retroviral gp70 immune complexes in (NZB×NZW) F_1 hybrid and the correlation to renal disease. J. Immun. *130:* 740 (1983).

35 Hirose, S.; Sekigawa, I.; Ozaki, S.; Sato, H.; Shirai, T.: Genetic regulation of hypergammaglobulinaemia and the correlation to autoimmune traits in (NZB×NZW) F_1 hybrid. Clin. exp. Immunol. *58:* 694 (1984).

36 Raveche, E.S.; Novotny, E.A.; Hansen, C.T.; Tjio, J.H.; Steinberg, A.D.: Genetic studies in NZB mice. V. Recombinant inbred lines demonstrate that separate genes control autoimmune phenotype. J. exp. Med. *153:* 1187 (1981).

37 Miller, M.L.; Raveche, E.S.; Laskin, C.A.; Klinman, D.M.; Steinberg, A.D.: Genetic studies in NZB mice. VI. Association of autoimmune traits in recombinant inbred lines. J. Immun. *133:* 1325 (1984).

38 Bocchieri, M.H.; Cooke, A.; Smith, J.B.; Weigert, M.; Riblet, R.J.: Independent segregation of NZB immune abnormalities in NZB×C58 recombinant inbred mice. Eur. J. Immunol. *12:* 349 (1982).

39 Datta, S.K.; Owen, F.L.; Womack, J.E.; Riblet, R.J.: Analysis of recombinant inbred lines derived from 'autoimmune' (NZB) and 'high leukemia' (C58) strains: independent multigenic systems control B cell hyperactivity, retrovirus expression, and autoimmunity. J. Immun. *129:* 1539 (1982).

40 Papoian, R.; Talal, N.: Ability of NZW but not NZB antigen-presenting cells to support T cell proliferative response to DNA methylated albumin. J. Immun. *124:* 515 (1980).

41 Hirose, S.; Nagasawa, R.; Sekikawa, I.; Hamaoki, M.; Ishida, Y.; Sato, H.; Shirai, T.: Enhancing effect of H-2-linked NZW gene(s) on the autoimmune traits of (NZB×NZW) F_1 mice. J. exp. Med. *158:* 228 (1983).

42 Hirose, S.; Nagasawa, R.; Sekikawa, I.; Hamaoki, M.; Ishida, Y.; Sato, H.; Shirai, T.: Enhancing effect of H-2-linked NZW gene(s) on the autoimmune traits of (NZB×NZW) F_1 mice. J. exp.Med. *158:* 228 (1983).

43 Manohar, V.; Brow E.M.; Leiserson, W.M.; Edison, L.J.; Chused, T.M.: Ly-2^+ T cell enlargement and null cell proliferation occur at the onset of splenomegaly and autoantibody production in New Zealand Black mice. J. Imm. *133:* 3020 (1984).

44 McCoy, K.L.; Baker, P.J.; Malek, T.R.; Chused, T.M.: Enlargement of Lyt-2-positive T cells is associated with functional impairment and autoimmune hemolytic anemia in New Zealand Black mice. J. Immun. *135:* 2432 (1985).

45 Taurog, J.D.; Moutsopoulos, H.M.; Rosenberg, Y.J.; Chused, T.M.; Steinberg, A.D.: CBA/N X-linked B-cell defect prevents NZB B-cell hyperactivity in F_1 mice. J. exp. Med. *150:* 31 (1979).

46 Markham, R.B.; Stashak, P.W.; Prescott, B.; Amsbaugh, D.F.; Baker, P.J.: Effect of concanavalin A on lymphocyte interactions involved in the antibody response to type III pneumococcal polysaccharide I. Comparison of the suppression induced by Con A and low dose paralysis. J. Immun. *118:* 952 (1977).

47 Baker, P.J.; Amsbaugh, D.F.; Stashak, P.W.; Caldes, G.; Prescott, B.: Direct evi-

dence for the involvement of T suppressor cells in the expression of low-dose paralysis to type III pneumococcal polysaccharide. J. Immun. *128:* 1059 (1982).
48 McCoy, K. L.; Baker, P. J.; Stashak, P. W.; Chused, T. M.: Two defects in old New Zealand Black mice are involved in the loss of low-dose paralysis to type III pneumococcal polysaccharide. J. Immun. *135:* 2438 (1985).
49 Baker, P. J.; Fauntleroy, M. B.; Stashak, P. W.; McCoy, K. L.; Chused, T. M.: Increased amplifier T cell activity in autoimmune NZB mice and its possible significance in the expression of autoimmune disease. Immunobiology *171:* 400 (1986).
50 McCoy, K. L.; Kendrick, L.; Chused, T. M.: Tolerance defects in New Zealand Black and New Zealand Black×New Zealand White F_1 mice. J. Immun. *136:* 1217 (1986).
51 Ozaki, S.; Honda, H.; Maruyama, N.; Hirose, S.; Hamaoki, M.; Sato, H.; Shirai, T.: Genetic regulation of erythrocyte autoantibody production in New Zealand black mice. Immunogenetics. *18:* 241 (1983).
52 Papoian, R.; Pillarisetty, R.; Talal, N.: Immunological regulation of spontaneous antibodies to DNA and RNA. II. Sequential switch from IgM to IgG in NZB/NZW F_1 mice. Immunology *32:* 75 (1977).
53 Kohno, A.; Yoshida, H.; Sekita, K.; Maruyama, N.; Ozaki, S.; Hirose, S.; Shirai, T.: Genetic regulation of the class conversion of dsDNA-specific antibodies in (NZB×NZW) F_1 hybrid. Immunogenetics *18:* 513 (1983).
54 Manny, N.; Datta, S. K.; Schwartz, R. S.: Synthesis of IgM by cells of NZB and SWR mice and their crosses. J. Immun. *122:* 1220 (1979).
55 Eastcott, J. W.; Schwartz, R. S.; Datta, S. K.: Genetic analysis of the inheritance of B cell hyperactivity in relation to the development of autoantibodies and glomerulonephritis in NZB×SWR crosses. J. Immun. *131:* 2232 (1983).

Thomas M. Chused, MD, Laboratory of Immunology, National Institute of Allergy and Infectious Diseases, National Institutes of Health, Bethesda, MD 20205 (USA)

Concepts Immunopathol., vol. 4, pp. 144–170 (Karger, Basel 1987)

Antigenic Mimicry Between Mycobacteria and Cartilage Proteoglycans:

The Model of Adjuvant Arthritis

Willem van Eden[a], *Joseph Holoshitz*[b], *Irun Cohen*[b]

[a]Department of Immunology, Faculty of Veterinary Medicine, University of Utrecht, The Netherlands; [b]Department of Cell-Biology, Weizmann Institute of Science, Rehovot, Israel

The discrimination between self and non-self is considered an essential and primary function of the immune system. It is therefore surprising to see how easily the discrimination between self and non-self seems to fail resulting in autoimmunity. As it is widely recognized at present, the potential for autoimmunity is present in virtually all individuals. Treatment of populations of normal lymphocytes with polyclonal activators can induce the secretion of autoantibodies to a variety of self antigens [1] and a multitude of autoimmune disorders in mice were seen to be evoked by stimulation of the immune system in graft-versus-host reactions [2]. Furthermore, autoreactive T cell clones have been isolated even from experimental animals, known to be resistant to induction of the relevant experimental autoimmune disease [3, 4]. The autoreactive potential is manifested in the frequent occurrence of autoimmune phenomena in infectious diseases. Infectious diseases are believed to have exerted the selective forces which shaped the structure and function of the immune system [5]. In infectious diseases we should expect to see the immune system functioning most adaptively. Therefore, autoimmunity arising as a result of infection could be seen to occur as a natural by-product of the physiologically normal immune response. And indeed, as we will discuss in this chapter, T cells with reactivity for self elements may arise as a consequence of the immune response directed against an exogenous microbial stimulus. In parallel, counter-autoimmune regulatory T cells may arise, activated by different epitopes present on the same exogenous stimulus. This places autoimmunity in the midst of immune regulation. It is this regulation, the tuning of the balance between counteracting functional elements in the immune response, which is, in our opinion, central to the actual function of the immune system. Especially, when this balance is disturbed by an exogenous stimulus bearing the potential of triggering pernicious self reactivity.

Microbial Infection and Rheumatic Disease

Although solid microbiological evidence for infective agents at sites of rheumatic inflammation has not been obtained, none of the diseases of supposed autoimmune origin has been seen in association with infective processes as often as inflammatory rheumatic diseases [6]. The best-known example is the association of acute rheumatic fever with streptococcal infection [7]. This association is strengthened by the observation that recurrence of rheumatic fever is accompanied by immunological evidence of intercurrent infection with Streptococci group A [8].

In addition, it has been shown to be possible to induce arthritis experimentally in rats, by inoculation with peptidoglycan-polysaccharide fragments of streptococcal bacterial cell wall [9]. Despite the availability of an experimental model of streptococcal induced arthritis, the effector mechanisms causing acute rheumatic fever, however, have yet to be elucidated.

Rheumatoid arthritis (RA) too has been associated with streptococcal infection. Elevated serum antibodies to streptococcal antigens have been observed in RA patients [6, 10], and the group B streptococcus, *Streptococcus agalactiae,* was reported to be isolated specifically from the nasopharynx and joints of RA patients. Furthermore, it was claimed that inoculation of such isolates into rats would lead to a seropositive chronic progressive polyarthritis [see ref. 6]. Although these studies are still awaiting independent confirmation, evidence implicating streptococci in the aetiology of RA has been obtained more than once, and therefore one has to accept the possibility that, at least in a number of cases, RA may be precipitated by streptococcal infection.

Besides acute rheumatic fever, which has become the classical example of so-called reactive arthritis, another group of sero-negative reactive arthritides has received much attention: Reiter's disease or arthritis triggered by microorganisms such as *Shigella, Salmonella, Campylobacters* and *Chlamydiae* [11]. Especially intriguing is their strong association with the B27 allele of the HLA system. Another bacterium to be mentioned in this context is *Klebsiella,* linked by some investigators to ankylosing spondylitis [12–15], which is also a B27 associated rheumatological disorder of autoimmune pathogenesis. In the latter case evidence has been collected for the existence of immunological cross-reactivity between the HLA-B27 molecule and antigens from *Klebsiella* and additional enteric microorganisms. Although a monoclonal anti-HLA-B27 antibody was found to detect a cross-reactive epitope present in both *Yersinia* and *Klebsiella* [16], it is an open question whether all these different bacteria share a common feature which enables them to cause reactive arthritis. At present no satisfactory etiological hypothesis for this group of reactive arthritides has been formulated. In Reiter's disease the infective hypothesis is still the most likely, especially since chlamydiae have been isolated from synovia, urethra or conjunctiva in a number of patients. Furthermore these chlamydial isolates were reported to cause chronic arthritis upon intra-articular injection in monkeys [17, 18]. The observation that acute viral diseases, such as influenza, hepatitis B, mumps and rubella, are frequently accompanied by transient inflammation of the joints, fostered the hypothesis that viruses may be etiological agents in rheumatological inflammatory disease. So far, however, most of the evidence is circumstantial and frequently disputed. In cases such as hepatitis B, polyarthritis may be explained by the presence of immune complexes [19]. Rubella virus has been considered as a potentially 'arthrotropic' virus, which was supposed to be etiologically related to RA [20–22]. Although interest in rubella virus as an infective agent causing RA has waned a recent report of isolation of rubella virus from lymphoreticular cells of children with chronic arthritis [23] may renew interest.

In table I microorganisms suspected of being able to induce arthritic disease are listed. As already mentioned, not all of them are held to cause true reactive arthritis. In some cases the causative microbe could be isolated from the joints. It is, however, possible that in such cases the presence of the microbe at the site of inflammation is required to maintain autoimmune reactivity directed to the self tissue elements. This for instance could be the case in Lyme arthritis [26]. While in Lyme arthritis the histological features of the synovium are very much like those in RA, the arthritis can be treated successfully with penicillin [32] and in some cases the etiological agent, the spirochete *Borrelia burgdorferi,* has been seen near arterioles in the synovium of patients [33]. Of obvious interest with respect to the model of adjuvant arthritis, to be discussed next, are the observations of arthritis in the presence of mycobacteria. Although

Table I. Microorganisms and arthritic disease in humans

Microorganism	Nature of arthritis	Clinical situation	Reference No.
Streptococcus group A	migratory polyarthritis	pharyngitis	7,8
Shigella	limited polyarthritis	antecedent diarrhea/B27	24
Salmonella	limited polyarthritis	antecedent diarrhea/B27	25
Yersinia	limited polyarthritis	antecedent diarrhea/B27	11
Klebsiella?	ankylosing spondylitis	?/B27	12, 13
Borrelia burgdorferi	intermittent, large joints	Lyme disease	26
Meningococcus	migratory polyarthritis	immune complexes	27
My. tuberculosis	migratory polyarthritis	erythema nodosum?	28
My. leprae	migratory polyarthritis	cutaneous vasculitis	29
My. bovis	polyarthritis small joints	cancer immunotherapy	30
Chlamidia	relapsing polyarthritis	Reiter's disease?/B27	17, 18
Rubella virus	transient/juvenile RA	vaccination/infection	20–23
Hepatitis-B virus	subacute migratory	infection, immune complexes	19
(Para) Myxovirus	subacute migratory	vaccination/infection	31

the arthritis seen in lepromatous leprosy is thought to be due to circulating immune complexes [29], the arthritis seen in association with tuberculosis could possibly be of a reactive nature [28]. In addition, arthritis has been observed to develop in a significant number of patients treated with BCG for cancer immunotherapy [30].

Adjuvant Arthritis is Mediated by T Cells

Indirect evidence that microorganisms could play a role in human autoimmune diseases, in arthritis, as discussed above, and also in diseases such as diabetes, multiple sclerosis and myasthenia gravis, has stimulated speculation that exogenous agents could trigger directly immune-reactivity to self structures. However, experimental models to test this hypothesis are scarce. Most models of experimental autoimmune diseases depend on immunization with the supposed self target antigen. Experimental autoimmune encephalomyelitis (EAE) in rats is induced by immunization with the basic protein antigen of myelin [34], experimental autoimmune thyroiditis (EAT) in mice by immunization with mouse thyroglobulin [35], autoimmune tubulointerstitial nephritis in guinea pigs with tubular basement membrane [36], collagen arthritis in rats with collagen type II [37], and so on. Adjuvant arthritis (AA) is therefore exceptional, since it is induced by immunization with an exogenous microbial agent, *Mycobacterium tuberculosis* (MT). For this reason AA provides rather unique possibilities to study the mechanism of how an exogenous trigger may lead to autoimmune reactivity. That AA is, indeed, an autoimmune disease has now been proven using T cell lines. AA may be induced in susceptible Lewis rats, by immunization intradermally with 1 mg of heat-killed ground MT suspended in mineral oil, i.e. Freund's complete adjuvant (CFA) [38]. Within 10–14 days all rats immunized this way develop inflammation with swelling, redness and tenderness manifested in the small joints of all four extremities. Macroscopically the acute inflammatory response subsides after 2–3 weeks. Microscopically, the process will continue for more than half a year and in most cases progress to ankylosis and crippling deformaties of the paws. Extraarticular lesions have also been noted [39]. Histologically, the arthritic process is remarkably similar to that seen in human RA, with a proliferative and inflammatory reaction in synovial membranes, pannus formation and eventually destruction of cartilage and erosion of bone [40]. That the arthritis is not due to mere entrapment of mycobacterial components into the joints causing local inflammation, was already made clear by the fact that disease could be succesfully transferred to normal recipients by lymphocytes obtained from diseased animals in the absence of bacterial antigens [41]. Formal proof that the relevant immunizing antigen is indeed of mycobacterial origin and not a self antigen present at the site of immunization with MT, was obtained when Holoshitz et al. [42] were able to transfer disease into irradiated syngeneic recipients by means of an MT-specific T cell line, called A2. Although this T cell line was originally obtained from a rat immunized with MT, the line was maintained by repeated restimulation in vitro with MT and was shown to proliferate specifically in the presence of MT or the mitogen Con A, and syngeneic irradiated thymocytes from naive rats as accessory cells. In order to induce this passive arthritis, the A2 line had to be activated by restimulating with either MT or Con A, prior to inoculation. The passive arthritis mediated by this A2 T cell line was similar to the arthritis seen of active, MT-induced AA in all respects [43]. Subsequent cloning in this A2 cell line revealed the heterogenous composition of A2. Subclones with varying functional phenotypes were obtained, amongst which was a clone, called

Table II. Comparison of arthritis mediated by the A2 line and its subclone A2b

Cells (2×10^7)	Recipient rats irradiated (750R)	Arthritis incidence %	mean day of onset	duration, days	Arthritis score
A2	no	0	–	–	–
	yes	100	8.0	18.0	4.5
A2b	no	0	–	–	–
	yes	100	5.0	31.0	6.8

A2b, with a more virulent arthritogenic capacity [44] (table II). This A2b clone too proliferated specifically in the presence of MT. Thus, the same T lymphocyte could be immunologically specific for a bacterial antigen and perniciously autoimmune at one and the same time. Was it possible that the T cell clone recognized an epitope present in mycobacteria and also in joints? That this question had to be answered positively was indicated by information collected from different models. In the model of EAE, disease was induced, in analogy to the A2-mediated arthritis, by the inoculation of a myelin basic protein (BP) specific T cell line [45]. Upon radioactively labelling the anti-BP line cells and injecting them into recipient rats, the onset of disease was accompanied by the accumulation of line cells in the brain and spinal cord, while the line cells reactive to other antigens were never found in the central nervous system [46]. So, the in vitro cultured line cells were, upon inoculation, capable of migrating to specific sites or organs where they induced disease. It is therefore reasonable to suppose that they were guided somehow in their migration by the local recognition of antigen. The latter supposition was supported by the observation that introduction of purified protein derivative (PPD) of MT into the brain following intravenous inoculation of a PPD specific T cell line led to influx of line cells into the brain and consequently to encephalomyelitis. Similary, introduction of PPD or BP into joints, following intravenous inoculation of PPD or BP specific cell lines, respectively, resulted in bystander arthritis [47]. From these observations it may be concluded that antigen can act as a specific signal for local accumulation of effector T lymphocytes. Therefore, we asked ourselves whether the arthritogenic A2b can recognize a component of normal joint tissues.

Structural Mimicry Underlying Adjuvant Arthritis

As already mentioned, autoimmune arthritis can be induced by immunization with collagen type II [37]. Because of this and in addition because it had been observed that rats with AA demonstrated some immunity to collagen type II [48], collagen type II was an obvious candidate for harboring the relevant target antigen of AA. However, although the original A2 cell line did show some weak reactivity to collagen type II, the A2b clone did not (table III). This finding clearly argued against collagen type II being the critical self antigen in AA [44]. Additional evidence against the same had already been derived from the finding that rats that had been rendered resistant to AA by pretreatment with low doses of CFA were still susceptible to induction of arthritis by collagen type II [49]. Furthermore, the observation that tolerance induced by cyclosporin A treatment during disease was found to be specific for each of the two model systems [50] and that the arthritogenic potential of CFA and collagen type II was seen to act synergistically [51], were also interpreted as showing the independent effector mechanisms involved in adjuvant and collagen type II-induced arthritis. In addition to collagen, the other main constituent of cartilage is a family of large molecules, called proteoglycans [52]. As represented schematically in figure 1, proteoglycans are composed of a long repeating disaccharide molecule hyaluronic acid, to which are anchored strands of protein, called core proteins. The interaction between the two molecules is stabilized by a distinct protein known as link protein. On each core protein three regions can be distinguished by differences among the polysaccharide chains attached to it. The first region has relatively few N-linked oligosaccharide chains. Then there is a region dominated by keratansulfate polysaccharide chains, and finally a region rich in chondroitin sulfate polysaccharide chains. Although the chemistry of the proteoglycan family of molecules has been worked out, it is hard to obtain pure preparations of the composing subunit molecules. The first evidence that the relevant target determinant of AA had to be located in the proteoglycan fraction of cartilage came from observations that the A2b and also the original cell line A2, did show a significant degree of in vitro proliferation in the presence of crude preparations of rat and pork proteoglycans (table III). Since A2b was a monoclonal population of lymphocytes, deploying antigen receptors of a uniform shape, the sensitivity of the A2b to both MT and proteoglycans argued for the existence of structural mimicry between their parts. That,

Table III. Arthritogenic T cell line A2 and its subclone A2b recognize both MT and crude proteoglycans

Cells	Proliferative responses in the presence of					
	MT	Coll. II	Coll. I	PG (rat)	PG (pork)	BP
A2	+	±	–	+	+	–
A2b	+	–	–	+	+	–
Z1a	–	–	–	–	–	+

Coll. = Collagen; PG = proteoglycan; BP = basic protein.

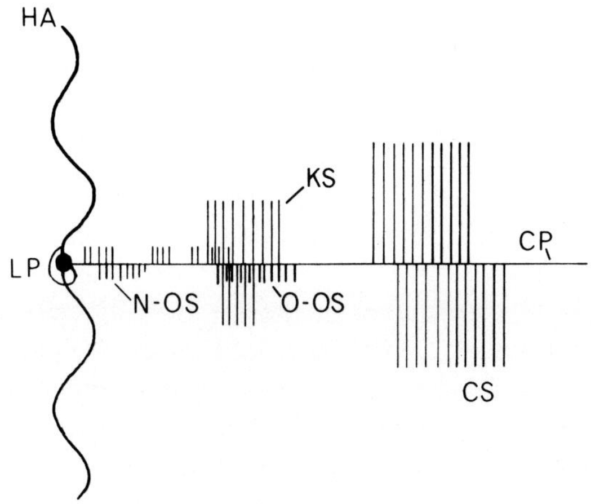

Fig. 1. Schematic representation of the proteoglycan macromolecule. HA = Hyaluronic acid; LP = link protein; N-OS = N-linked oligosaccharides; O-OS = O-linked oligo-saccharides; KS = keratan sulfate; CS = chondroitin sulfate; CP = core protein.

however, the magnitude of proliferation of clone A2b in response to proteoglycans was lower than that in response to MT suggested that this mimicry could be imperfect or alternatively that the relevant epitope might be only a minor component of the proteoglycan preparations tested. Be that as it may, subsequent testing of a preparation enriched for chondroitin sulfate did show responses of the A2b to the same order of magnitude as obtained with the crude rat and pork proteoglycans [54]. No responses were seen with preparations enriched for keratan sulfate or hyaluronic acid. In addition, synovial fluids, which are known to contain proteoglycans, aspirated from the knees of patients with RA or osteoarthrosis, were found to stimulate the A2b clone. The responses of A2b to the proteoglycan preparations and synovial fluids were specific since no responses to these preparations were seen using irrelevant control clones or cell lines.

Previously we had shown that T cell lines could transfer antigen-specific delayed type hypersensitivity (DTH) skin reactivity to naive recipients and that irradiation of recipient rats enhanced the magnitude of the reactivity transferred [47]. Therefore, we decided to test the ability of clone A2b, which bears the W3/25 marker of helper/DTH T lymphocytes [47], to transfer DTH for not only MT but also for the cross-reactive determinants as supposed to be present in proteoglycans. To this end, ear swelling was measured 24 and 48 h after injection of minute amounts of MT, preparations enriched for proteoglycan fractions or synovial fluids into ears of rats, some of which had been irradiated and/or had received clone A2b five days earlier. Remarkable DTH reactivity for MT was observed in both nonirradiated and irradiated A2b primed rats and not in the unprimed control rats. Moreover, reactivity to the chondroitin sulfate enriched preparation, to synovial fluids and in addition to a core-protein-enriched preparation was observed in A2b-primed animals that had been irradiated [53]. Histological examination of the ear-swelling confirmed that the response was caused by DTH. Thus, transfer of A2b with its double specificity for both MT and proteoglycans as observed by in vitro proliferation, appeared to sensitize naive recipients simultaneously for MT and proteoglycans. Since, the nonirradiated A2b inoculated recipients did not develop DTH to the proteoglycans and synovial fluids, it is conceivable that radiosensitive regulatory mechanisms control responsiveness to proteoglycan self determinants, a hypothesis supported by the finding that irradiation of the recipient is a prerequisite for induction of arthritis by line A2 or clone A2b [42, 44]. However, irradiation of the recipient was not required for other line-mediated autoimmune diseases such as EAE in rats [45] or EAT in mice [54].

Also in rats suffering from active, CFA-induced AA, DTH reactivity to proteoglycans could be shown to exist [53]. In this case the reactivity for chondroitin sulfate was clearly inferior to the reactivity for synovial fluid and especially the core protein. Taken together the responses to the core-protein-enriched preparations tended to be stronger than those to the chondroitin sulfate enriched preparations. Therefore the core protein, or maybe the oligosaccharides linked to it, are likely candidates for bear-

Table IV. Structural mimicry between MT and proteoglycan components as defined in various assays

Antigens	A2b proliferation	DTH after priming with		Binding in RIA of anti-MT monoclonal antibodies
		A2b	CFA	
MT	+	+	+	+
Chondroitin sulfate	+	+	±	–
Synovial fluid	+	+	+	±
Core protein		+	+	+
Keratan sulfate	–	–	–	–
Hyaluronic acid	–	–		–

ing the target determinant(s) in AA. It is clear, however, that a more precise identification of the relevant molecules was hampered thus far by the paucity of techniques suitable for isolation of undenaturated fragments of proteoglycans.

Additional, albeit indirect, evidence pointing to coreprotein, was obtained by screening a battery of 30 different monoclonal antibodies raised against mycobacteria for reactivity to proteoglycans [55]. In a radioimmunoassay 4 out of these thirty monoclonals were found to specifically recognize core protein [Lapidot, unpubl. results]. We are currently isolating the molecules recognized, both in mycobacteria and in the core protein preparation or synovial fluids. It should be stressed that we have, at this stage no proof that the determinants, recognized by those monoclonal antibodies are the same as those recognized by the A2b T cell clone. That antibodies do exist which recognize determinants shared between mycobacteria and cartilage constituents had been noted previously. Sera of rabbits immunized with a fraction of MT, that had been found to be particularly stimulatory to the A2b arthritogenic clone, were shown to contain antibodies, which gave a positive reaction in an immunofluorescence assay to snap-frozen human cartilage. This positive fluorescence could be specifically absorbed with crude proteoglycans of pork or rat origin [56].

In conclusion, one may say that both the cells and the sera do indicate the presence of epitopes shared between mycobacteria and cartilage proteoglycans (table IV). The demonstration of cross-reactivity by itself does not, however, prove its role in pathogenesis. But the fact that the arthritogenic clone A2b itself is the very agent that defines a structural mimicry between MT and joint cartilage argues strongly that this mimicry indeed may incite the immune attack on the joints characteristic of AA.

Antigenic Mimicry and Human Autoimmunity

In the human, a number of different crossreactivities between microorganisms and selfstructures have been detected, suggesting that structural mimicry between microbial and mammalian antigens is widespread and that this mimicry might be the germ of some autoimmune diseases [57] (table V). However, a direct role of the mimicry in the effector mechanisms leading to autoimmunity has in these cases not been shown, which makes the role of the mimicry in these diseases as yet hypothetical [60]. A most likely candidate of a bacterium inducing autoimmunity by structural mimicry with host tissues, is the group A Streptococcus [61]. Firstly, epitopes present in sarcolemmal membrane proteins of human myocardium, likely targets for the autoimmune attack causing carditis in acute rheumatic fever, have been found crossreactive with streptococcal M proteins [62]. Secondly, antibody reactivity for heparan sulfate proteoglycans isolated from the glomerular basement membranes, detected in sera of patients with poststreptococcal glomerulonephritis, could be inhibited specifically with streptococcal hyaluronic acid indicating structural mimicry between this bacterial product and proteoglycans present in the glomerulus [62].

Evidence that the constant parts of immunoglobulins contain epitopes cross-reactive with bacterial peptidoglycans stems from observations in experimental animals that rheumatoid factors arise following bacterial immunization [64]. The role of this cross-reactivity, and the role of rheumatoid factor in the pathogenesis of rheumatoid arthritis remains, however, to be established. The origin of anti-DNA antibodies in patients with SLE is unexplained. It is, however, conceivable that these antibodies arise in response to antigens introduced by microbial infection. A large proportion of monoclonal DNA antibodies obtained from SLE patients were found to react with both nucleic acid antigens and the phospholipid cardiolipin [65, 66]. Similar auto-antibodies were found in sera of patients with SLE [67]. This cross-reactivity is likely to explain the biologically false-positive test for syphilis that occurs frequently in patients with SLE [68]. Conversely, monoclonal antibodies obtained from

Table V. Structural mimicry and autoimmune disease

Microorganism	Exogenous inducer antigen	Endogenous target antigen	'Disease'	Reference No.
Streptococcus group A	M protein	cardiac glycoprotein	rheumatic fever	61
Streptococcus group A	hyaluronic acid	proteoglycan (heparansulf.)	poststreptoccal GN	63
Streptococcus group A	?	neurocytoplasm	Sydenham's chorea	58
Streptococcus/Staphylococcus	peptidoglycan	Fc of IgG	rheumatoid factor	64
Bacteria?/Myobacterium	cardiolipin/?	DNA/proteoglycan	SLE	65, 66, 70
E. coli (Proteus vulgaris, Klebsiella pneumoniae)	OmpC protein	α-Subunit of actylcholine receptor	myasthenia gravis	72
Klebsiella (Shigella, Yersinia)	?	B27, (M1, M2)	ankylosing spondylosis	73, 75, 15, 16
MT	?	proteoglycan (core protein?)	rheumatoid arthritis	53, 56
Trypanosoma cruzi	?	Purkinje neurons cardiac muscle	Chagas' disease	59
Yersinia	?	thyrotropin receptor	Grave's disease	78

mice immunized with cardiolipin from bacterial origin also reacted with double-stranded DNA [69]. That the double-stranded DNA itself is not immunogenic and the antibodies produced after immunization with exogenous single-stranded DNA are not cross-reactive, gives additional support to the hypothesis that immunization with a cross-reactive phospholipid, such as bacterial cardiolipin, may give rise to anti-DNA antibodies in human SLE. Recently the cross-reactivity of patient and also mouse monoclonal anti-DNA antibodies was extended to reactivity to proteoglycans. The presence of repeating negatively charged groups seemed to be essential for the binding of such cross-reactive antibodies [70]. Therefore, it may be of interest that anti-DNA antibodies were recently observed to react with MT [Shoenfeld, unpubl. results], suggesting that cross-reactivity similar to that seen in AA could be present in SLE. However that may be, the role of autoantibodies in the pathogenesis of SLE is still far from clear.

This is in contrast to the autoantibodies as seen in myasthenia gravis. The pernicious role played by antibodies specific for the acetylcholine receptor in this disease has been elegantly exploited in alleviating the disease in the experimental situation, by means of anti-idiotypic antibodies directed against the acetylcholine receptor antibodies [71]. It is therefore of interest that monoclonal antibodies directed against acetylcholine receptors have now been shown to recognize proteins present in *Proteus* and *Klebsiella* bacteria [72].

Mysterious but intriguing is the relationship between *Klebsiella* bacteria, ankylosing spondylitis (AS) and HLA-B27. Although the clinical association between *Klebsiella* infection and AS is unclear, *Klebsiella* seems to share antigenic specificity with antigens on lymphocytes of AS patients bearing the B27 allele [73]. This allele is furthermore present in over 95% of the individuals suffering from AS, while it occurs in 6–8% of the healthy population of European origin [74]. This sharing of antigenic specificity was convincingly shown by the fact that rabbit anti-*Klebsiella* sera were found to be cytotoxic for B27-positive patient lymphocytes and not for B27 positive lymphocytes of healthy individuals [73], a finding recently reproduced in a blind set-up [75]. The reason for this is not clear, and it appears that B27 lymphocytes might actually become modified by contact with bacterial antigens [76]. Similar cross-reactivity was concluded from the finding that monoclonal antibodies directed against variants of B27 were reactive with antigens present in *Klebsiella, Shigella* and *Yersinia* bacteria [16]. How this structural mimicry could lead to AS remains an open question. It is however possible that a partial tolerance for certain cross-reactive bacterial epitopes, may lead to immune recognition of other, usually silent, epitopes, with resultant autoimmune reactivity specifically occurring in B27 positive individuals in their confrontation with these bacteria.

A situation similar to that hypothesized for myasthenia gravis could be involved in Graves' disease. This disease is caused by the presence of thyroid-stimulating antibodies mimicking the effect of thyrotropin [77]. These antibodies could possibly arise as a consequence of immunization to bacteria, since it was shown that a substance present in *Yersinia enterocolitica* behaves like the thyrotropin receptor in binding thryrotropin [78]. This bacterial antigen could directly stimulate the formation of antireceptor antibodies. Furthermore, serologic evidence for infection with *Yersinia* has been obtained in a large proportion of Graves disease patients [78].

Is there any evidence that antigenic mimicry between mycobacteria and proteoglycans, as defined in the model of AA, could play a role in human pathology? As mentioned before, arthritis is seen sometimes in association with tuberculosis [28] and individuals repeatedly immunized with BCG in the course of cancer immunotherapy have been seen to develop arthritis in a significant number of cases [30]. Furthermore, in proliferation assays lymphocytes specifically obtained from patients with RA have been found to be sensitized to a fraction of MT rich in antigen cross-reactive with cartilage [56]. This sensitivity was noted in synovial fluid lymphocytes early in disease and later in the peripheral blood lymphocytes. The responses of the RA patients to streptococcal antigens and to mitogens were as in the controls.

Thus, not only in AA but also in RA, sensitization to determinants present in mycobacteria might indeed play a role. Moreover, some groups of arthritis patients also show cell-mediated immunity to cartilage proteoglycans [79]. These observations are compatible with the possibility that the same antigenic mimicry that seems crucial in the origin of AA may be etiologically connected to RA.

The presence in microbes of epitopes mimicking normal tissue epitopes is certainly not limited, as suggested by table 5, to bacteria. Viruses, associated with diseases such as diabetes mellitus and multiple sclerosis, have been found to carry such cross-reactive epitopes [80, 81]. With the advent of new techniques such as monoclonal antibodies and monoclonal populations of antigen reactive T cells, structural mimicry may well turn out to be a very common and general phenomenon.

Irrespective of its possible consequences, one might wonder what would be the origin of such an abundance of antigenic mimicries. It has been made clear that some parasites, and especially the more complex ones, do in fact use their mimicking epitopes as a protective disguise to their own benefit in order to evade the host immune defence [82].

However, since antibodies do see antigenic determinants composed of 4–6 amino acids or monosaccarides [83] and T cells see in some cases determinants as small as 7 amino acids [84], it is clear that any macromolecule with hundreds or thousands of aminoacids or sugars could have myriads of antigenic determinants. Consequently, the number of such determinants in a whole microorganism must be so large that some of them by chance might resemble host macromolecules. Therefore, one should keep in mind that the bulk of the mimicry is probably incidental and unavoidable.

Regulatory T Cells Restore Self Tolerance

In view of the wide prevalence of antigenic mimicry, one may ask why autoimmune disease is not a more common phenomenon. The answer may be that autoimmunity is common, but that its expression is actively down regulated. The immune system has its own built-in control mechanisms capable of turning off responses directed to dangerously self- cross-reactive epitopes and focussing its activity on the safely non-cross-reactive epitopes [85]. How this is achieved is subject to debate. The fact that selfrecognizing lymphocytes do exist in healthy individuals and that autoreactive lymphocytes can be aroused experimentally to produce autoimmune diseases of choice [57] seems to refute Burnet's hypothesis of the so-called 'forbidden' clones which were supposed to be eliminated during early ontogeny [86].

Alternatively, one might think of negative feedback signals, probably exerted by T suppressor cells, actively preventing self recognizing clones from responding to self antigens [87]. The fact that we have succeeded in vaccinating rats and mice against experimental autoimmune diseases [88, 89) indicates that the built-in control mechanisms can be activated specifically to desired ends. In the model of AA we recently obtained results that hint at the nature of the control mechanisms involved. As already mentioned, the A2 cell line could induce arthritis in irradiated rats. In nonirradiated recipients inoculation of A2 induced resistance to subsequent induction of AA by active immunization to MT [42]. Depending on the condition of the recipient, the A2 cell line could either induce disease or protection. To investigate the possibility that distinct subclones within A2 could be responsible for this bifunctional phenotype, A2 was cloned further in the search for specifically protective clones. And indeed a clone was isolated which was fully protective and not arthritogenic. This clone, called A2c, was protective in the sense that not only could we vaccinate with it, but also accellerate remission of disease in rats with existing active AA [43, 90]. We were apparently dealing with a T cell clone with the potential of preventing or therapeutically aborting the auto-immune process. Hence, we investigated in vitro the influence of the A2c protective clone on the proliferative responses of the arthritogenic A2b clone. When cultured together, the two clones did not appear to interact. When, however, draining lymph node cells obtained from rats primed with A2c were added to A2b, the A2b response to MT, was found to be completely abrogated. This phenomenon was not observed after priming with irrelevant control clones and was specific for the A2b responses. Abrogation of the response of an unrelated BP-specific cell line (Z1a) was seen in the comparable situation only when simultaneously the A2b clone and its antigen MT were present in the culture. These findings seem to indicate that the A2c clone was capable of recruiting in vivo one or more populations of cells that could suppress lymphocyte proliferation, depending on the specific presence of both the A2b clone and MT. Since the A2c has, like A2 and A2b, the helper/DTH phenotype [90], A2c could well be a suppressor inducer T cell. This then, would imply that a single suppressor inducer T cell clone might initiate a course of events leading to the specific control of an autoimmune disease and thus to restoration of self tolerance.

The clone capable of initiating all this, A2c, was isolated from the A2 cell line. This means that the A2c, and probably additional clones with similar properties, are activated during immunization with MT, together with the perniciously autoimmune population of cells. So, by immunizing with a complex antigen, like MT, cells of opposing functional characteristics can be activated. Screening of both the A2b and A2c for reactivity to a panel of different atypical mycobacteria indicated that the fine specificities of A2b and A2c were different [90]. It is likely that both clones recognized a different molecule or different epitopes on the same molecule present in MT. Reactivity for proteoglycans has not consistently been observed with A2c. The picture that arises from this is that immunization with a complex antigen not only leads to activation of clones with specificity for a range of different epitopes present on the immunogen, but also that at the same time clones are activated which initiate events devised to suppress the expansion of clones specific for certain, possibly dangerously cross-reactive, epitopes. It is attractive to assume that this way of restricting the responding repertoire is a general phenomenon in the immune response evoked by complex immunogens [89]. It could serve the desired purpose of helping the immune system to focus down on a few of the many potential epitopes available. Teleologically, this would also help avoid responding to the large number of self mimicking epitopes.

Also in the course of active AA restoration of self tolerance seems to occur naturally. As already mentioned, following a period of acute inflammation of the joints, rats recover spontaneously, at least macroscopically. After recovery, rats become refractory to potentially arthritogenic challenges with MT and no reactivation of the arthritic process is seen. Thus, not only self tolerance is restored following active AA, but also the protective regulatory mechanisms seem to be more alert. So, while in a naive susceptible recipient the balance of functionally competing clones seems to be easily tipped towards the temporary advantage of perniciously auto-immune clones, in an immune recipient, such is not the case.

Genetic Control of the Immune Response to Mycobacteria

Not all inbred strains of rats are equally susceptible to arthritis upon immunization with MT. Lewis rats are susceptible, but many other strains are not. The differential susceptibility for the disease in the rat was found to be influenced by MHC-linked Ir genes [91]. This is not surprizing since MHC-linked Ir genes are assumed to play a central role in the selection of epitopes for immune recognition [85, 92] and, furthermore, they are known to control regulatory cell interactions [93]. At this stage it is impossible to conclude whether in AA the MHC-linked control is operative at the level of epitope selection or regulation, or possibly both. The fact that in the EAE model, T cells recognizing BP could be isolated not only from susceptible but also both from protected and from genetically resistant animals [3, 4], argues for genetic control exerted at the level of regulation. However, to extrapolate from findings made in different models might be hazardous.

In humans also susceptibility to autoimmune diseases, both organ specific and non-organ specific, seems to a remarkable extent to be controlled by the MHC [94]. For no other group of diseases, HLA associations have been detected with more consistency than for the group of autoimmune disorders. This is likely to result from the key role played by the MHC in epitope selection and/or immune regulation. The polymorphism of the MHC is likely to be a consequence of evolutionary selection at the population level by infectious diseases [95, 96]. This would imply that the majority of MHC alleles have been selected for their usefulness in facilitating recognition of or regulating responses to epitopes critical in defences against microbial invaders. In some instances this might have happened at the expense of subtle immune regulation needed to avoid autoimmune reactivity. Taking this further, the potential for autoimmune reactivity can be seen to result from genes selected for their usefulness in antimicrobial immunity in general. The hypothesis that the physiological trigger of autoimmunity should be of microbial origin would fit this reasoning.

Leprosy is illustrative. Leprosy is a chronic infectious disease caused by *Mycobacterium leprae*. This bacterium itself is virtually nontoxic to its host. Most of the pathology seen in leprosy depends on the host immune response, which is highly variable. As a result, the clinical spectrum of the disease ranges from lepromatous leprosy, with multiple lesions, exuberant bacterial growth and a specific cellular anergy for *M. leprae* to tuberculoid leprosy, with few lesions containing few bacteria due to active cell-mediated immunity [97]. The cellular anergy characteristic of lepromatous leprosy is probably due to active suppression of specific responses caused by the presence of specific suppressor T lymphocytes [98]. More recently a phenolic glycolipid specifically present in *M. leprae* was shown to induce suppression in vitro [99]. In tuberculoid leprosy, despite the fact that some have reported the presence of suppressor T cells [100], cell-mediated immunity seems to be intact. Although peripheral nerves are involved in all forms of leprosy, especially in tuberculoid leprosy an inflammatory response in the nerves occurs in the virtual absence of bacteria, possibly representing autoimmune reactivity [101]. The characteristic variation in the clinical expression of leprosy has been found to be controlled, at least in part, by MHC-linked genes. In families with multiple cases of the same clinical type of leprosy, HLA haplotype segregation has been found to occur non-randomly [102–106]. Furthermore, at the population level, HLA class II alleles have been found to be associated with the distinct clinical forms of the disease [106, 107]. From those observations it may be concluded that the antimycobacterial immune response in leprosy is controlled, at least partly, by MHC-linked genes. Depending on the genes present, the immune response seems directed preferentially to either suppression-inducing epitopes, possibly located on the phenolic glycolipid, or to epitopes which evoke a response leading to destruction of nerves, possibly due to structural mimicry between these epitopes and self epitopes present in peripheral nerve tissue. Although this scheme of events is certainly simplified, it serves to illustrate the role of genetic polymorphism in the host immune response to mycobacteria. In some individuals the genes dictate non-responsiveness, leaving the microbe uninhibited in the host tissues, while in other individuals the genes give way to an effective immunological inhibition of bacterial growth with deleterious nerve damage for the host.

That the HLA system may influence the recognition of mycobacterial antigens has been shown also by more direct means. When healthy volunteers were skin tested with a battery of ultrasonicates of different species of mycobacteria [108], it turned out that HLA-DR3-positive individuals were absent from the population that did not respond to any of the mycobacteria tested, whereas DR3-positive individuals were frequently found among the individuals that responded to all mycobacteria [109]. Individuals reacting to all mycobacteria, including mycobacteria to which they had not been known to be immunized probably did so because they became sensitized to so-called mycobacterial common antigens. Thus, individuals carrying the DR3 allele seem to react preferentially to mycobacterial common antigens. This is especially of interest, because in some populations DR3 was shown to predispose to tuberculoid leprosy and to confer resistance to lepromatous leprosy [107]. From this one might hypothesize that reactivity to these common antigens ensures a preference for the responder type of leprosy, i.e. tuberculoid leprosy or, alternatively, that recognition of common antigens blocks the generation of effective suppression, characteristic of lepromatous leprosy.

An indication that patients with RA exhibit an unusual reactivity to certain mycobacterial antigens has been obtained, as discussed before [56]. Furthermore, RA is definitely associated with HLA-DR4 in European populations [94]. It is therefore remarkable, that by skin testing a group of Spanish leprosy patients, HLA-DR4-positive patients were seen to react strongly to tuberculin of MT [110]. Although this observation has not yet been made in healthy individuals, it might be a first indication that in the pathogenesis of RA the MHC plays a role in directing the immune system to respond to certain critical, and possibly self cross-reactive, epitopes.

Conclusion

Investigation of the model of AA has shown that structural mimicry between microbial antigens in the environment and self antigens in the individual may trigger autoimmune disease. It may do so by activating effector T cells with specificity for the self antigen. The generation of such effector T cells may be part of a legitimate defensive immune response targeted at microbial invaders. The avoidance of self reactivity seems regulated functionally and not sustained by elimination of 'forbidden clones'. This regulation seems to be controlled genetically, and at least in part by MHC-linked genes. Our findings, added to preexisting evidence for a role of microbes in arthritis and for the existence of structural mimicries between various microbes and self tissue elements, suggest that the information gathered from the model of AA may well be extrapolated to human autoimmune disease.

The model has also shown that the capacity of the immune system to regulate and to control destructive autoimmunity can be influenced positively. The clinical potential of these findings might well become apparent in the not too distant future.

References

1 Rosenberg, Y.J.: Autoimmune and polyclonal B cell responses during murine malaria. Nature, Lond. *274:* 170–174 (1978).

2 Gleichmann, E.; Pals, S.T.; Rolink, A.G.; Radaszkiewics, T.; Gleichmann, H.: Graft-versus – host reactions: clues to the etiopathology of a spectrum of immunological diseases. Immunol. Today *5:* 324–332 (1984).

3 Ben-Nun, A.; Cohen, I.R.: Spontaneous remission and acquired resistance to autoimmune encephalomyelitis (EAE) are associated with suppression of T cell reactivity. Suppressed EAE effector T cells recovered as T cell lines. J. Immun. *128:* 1450 (1982).

4 Ben-Nun, A.; Eisenstein, S.; Cohen, I.R.: Experimental autoimmune encephalomyelitis (EAE) in genetically resistant rats: PVG rats resist active induction of EAE but are susceptible to and can generate EAE effector T cell lines. J. Immun. *129:* 918 (1982).

5 Bodmer, W.F.: Evolutionary significance of the HLA-system. Nature, Lond. *237:* 139–145 (1972).
6 Dumonde, D.C.; Steward, M.W.: The role of microbial infection in rheumatic disease; in Copeman's, Textbook for rheumatic diseases, pp. 222–258, Churchill Livingstone, Edinburgh (1978).
7 Stollerman, G.H.: Streptococcal immunology: Protection versus injury, editorial. Ann. intern. Med. *88:* 422 (1978).
8 Taranta, A.; Kleinberg, E.; Feinstein, A.R.; Wood, H.F.; Tursky, E.; Simpson, R.: Relation of rheumatic fever recurrence rate per streptococcal infection to pre-existing clinical features of patients. Ann. intern. Med. *60:* suppl. 5, pp. 58–68 (1964).
9 Fox, A.; Brown, R.R.; Anderle, S.K; Chetty, G.; Cromartie, W.J.; Gooder, H.; Schwab, J.H.: Arthropatic properties related to the molecular weight of peptidoglycan–polysaccharide polymers of streptococcal cell walls. Infect Immun. *35:* 1003–1010 (1982).
10 Braun, D.G.; Holm, S.E.: Streptococcal anti-group A precipitins in sera from patients with rheumatoid arthritis and acute glomerulonephritis. Int. Archs Allergy appl. Immun. *37:* 216–222 (1970).
11 Toivanen, A.; Granfors, K.; Lahesmaa-Rnatala, R.; Leino, R.; Stahlberg, T.; Vuento, R.: Pathogenesis of Yersinia-triggered reactive arthritis: immunological, microbiological and clinical aspects. Immunol. Rev. *86:* 47–70 (1985).
12 Ebringer, R.W.; Cawdell, D.R.; Cowling, P.; Ebringer, A.: Sequential studies in ankylosing spondylitis: Association of *Klebsiella pneumoniae* with active disease. Ann. rheum. Dis. *37:* 146–1152 (1978).
13 Geczy A.F.; Alexander, K.; Bashir, H.V.; Edmonds, J.P.; Upfold, L.; Sullivan, J.: HLA-B27, Klebsiella and ankylosing spondylitis: biological and chemical studies. Immunol. Rev. *70:* 23–50 (1983).
14 Upfold, L.I.; Sullivan, J.S.; Prendergast, J.K.; Geczy, A.F.: HLA-B27: speculation on the nature of its involvement in ankylosing spondylitis. Prog. Allergy, vol. *36:* 177–190 (Karger, Basel 1985).
15 Prendergast, J.K.; Sullivan, J.S.; Geczy, A.; Upfold, L.I.; Edmonds, J.P.; Bashir, H.V.; Reiss-Levy, E.: Possible role of enteric organisms in the pathogenesis of ankylosing spondylitis and other seronegative arthropathies. Infect. Immunity *41:* 935–941 (1983).
16 Van Bohemen, C.G.; Grumet, F.C.; Zanen, H.C.: Identification of HLA-B27 M1 and -M2 cross-reactive antigens in Klebsiella, Shigella and Yersinia. Immunology *52:* 607–614 (1984).
17 Schachter, J.: Can chlamidial infections cause rheumatic disease? in Dumonde, Infection and immunology in the rheumatic diseases, pp. 151–158 (Blackwell, London 1975).
18 Delbarre, F.; Amor, B.: Ankylosing spondylitis and Reiter's syndrome: genetic and microbiological studies; in Dumonde, Infection and immunology in the rheumatic diseases, pp. 159–168 (Blackwell, London 1975).
19 Onion, D.K.; Crumpacker, C.S.; Gilliland, B.C.: Arthritis of hepatitis associated with Australia antigen. Ann. intern. Med. *75:* 29–33 (1971).
20 Kantor, T.G.; Tanner, M.: Rubella arthritis and rheumatoid arthritis. Arthritis Rheum. *5:* 378–383 (1962).

21 Ogra, P.L.; Herd, J.K.: Arthritis associated with induced rubella infection. J. Immun. *107:* 810–813 (1971).
22 Chantler, J.K.; Ford, D.K.; Tingle, A.J.: Persistent rubella infection and rubella associated arthritis. Lancet *i:* 1323–1325 (1982).
23 Chantler, J.L.; Tingle, A.J.; Petty, R.E.: Persistent rubella virus infection associated with chronic arthritis in children. New Engl. J. Med. *313:* 1117–1123 (1985).
24 Keat, A.: Reiter's syndrome and reactive arthritis in perspective. New Engl. J. Med. *309:* 1606–1615 (1983).
25 Friis, J.; Svejgaard, A.: Salmonella arthritis and HLA-27. Lancet *i:* 1350 (1974).
26 Steere, A.C.; Malawista, S.E.; Hardin, J.A.; Ruddy, S.; Askenase, P.W.; Andiman, W.A.: Erythema chronicum migrans and Lyme arthritis. The enlarging clinical spectrum. Ann. intern. Med. *86:* 685–698 (1977).
27 Greenwood, B.M.: Whitte, H.L.: The pathogenesis of meningococcal arthritis; in Dumonde, Infection and immunology in the rheumatic diseases, pp. 118–130 (Blackwell, London 1976).
28 Brav, E.A.; Hench, P.S.: Tuberculous rheumatism. J. Bone Jt Surg. *16:* 839–866 (1934).
29 Turk, J.L.; Belehu, A.: Immunological spectra in infectious diseases. Parasites in the immunized host. Ciba Found. Symp. *25:* 101–110 (1974).
30 Torisu, M.; Miyahara, T.; Shinohara, N.; Ohsato, K.; Sonozaki, H.: A new side effect of BCG immunotherapy – BCG-induced arthritis in man. Cancer Immunol. Immunother. *5:* 77–83 (1978).
31 Kalliomaki, J.L.; Halonen, P.: The role of viruses in the aetiology of connective tissue diseases. Ann. clin. Res. *7:* 129–135 (1975).
32 Steere, A.C.; Green, J.; Schoen, R.T.; Taylor, E.; Hutchinson, G.J.; Rhan, D.W.; Malawista, S.E.: Successful parenteral penicillin therapy of established Lyme arthritis. New Engl. J. Med. *312:* 869–874 (1985).
33 Johnston, Y.E.; Duray, P.H.; Steere, A.C.: Lyme arthritis: spirochetes found in synovial microangiopathic lesions. Am. J. path. *118:* 26–34 (1985).
34 Paterson, P.Y.; Drobish, D.G.; Hanson, M.A.; Jacobs, A.F.: Induction of experimental allergic encephalomyelitis in Lewis rats. Int. Archs Allergy appl. Immun. *37:* 26–36 (1970).
35 Vladutiu, A.O.; Rose, N.R.: Autoimmune murine thyroiditis: Relation to histocompatibility (H-2) type. Science *174:* 11137–1139 (1971).
36 Brown, C.A.; Carey, K.; Colvin, R.B.: Inhibition of autoimmune tubulointerstitial nephritis in guinea pigs by heterologous antisera containing anti-idiotype antibodies. J. Immun. *123:* 2101–2108 (1979).
37 Trentham, D.E.; Townes, A.S.; Kang, A.H.: Autoimmunity to type II collagen. An experimental model of arthritis. J. exp. Med. *146:* 857–868 (1977).
38 Pearson, C.M.: Development of arthritis, periarthritis and periostitis in rats given adjuvant. Proc. Soc. exp. Biol. Med. *91:* 95–101 (1956).
39 Pearson, C.M.; Wood, F.D.: Studies of polyarthritis and other lesions induced in rats by injection of mycobacterial adjuvant: 1 General clinical and pathologic characteristics and some modifying factors. Arthritis Rheum. *2:* 440–459 (1959).
40 Pearson, C.M.: Experimental models in rheumatoid disease. Arthritis Rheum. *7:* 80–86 (1964).

41 Whitehouse, D.J.; Whitehouse, M.W.; Pearson, C.M.: Passive transfer of adjuvant-induced arthritis and allergic encephalomyelitis in rats using thoracic duct lymphocytes. Nature, Lond. *224:* 1322 (1969).
42 Holoshitz, J.; Naparstek, Y.; Ben-Nun, A.; Cohen, I.R.: Lines of T lymphocytes induce or vaccinate against autoimmune arthritis. Science *219:* 56–58 (1983).
43 Cohen, I.R.; Holoshitz, J.; Eden, W. van; Frenkel, A.: T lymphocyte clones illuminate pathogenesis and affect therapy of experimental arthritis. Arthritis Rheum. *28:* 841–845 (1985).
44 Holoshitz, J.; Matitiau, A.; Cohen, I.R.: Arthritis induced in rats by clones of T lymphocytes responsive to mycobacteria but not to Collagen type II. J. clin. Invest. *73:* 211–215 (1984).
45 Ben-Nun, A.; Cohen, I.R.: Experimental autoimmune encephalomyelitis (EAE) mediated by T cell lines. Process of selection of lines and characterization of the cells. J. Immun. *129:* 303–308 (1982).
46 Naparstek, Y.; Ben-Nun, A.; Holoshitz, J.; Reshef, T.; Frenkel, A.; Rosenberg, M.; Cohen, I.R.: T lymphocyte lines producing or vaccinating against autoimmune encephalomyelitis (EAE). Functional activation induces PNA receptors and accumulation in the brain and thymus of line cells. Eur. J. Immunol. *13:* 418–423 (1983).
47 Holoshitz, J.; Naparstek, Y.; Ben-Nun, A.; Marquardt, P.; Cohen, I. R.: T-lymphocyte lines induce autoimmune encephalomyelitis, delayed hypersensitivity and bystander encephalitis or arthritis. Eur. J. Immunol. *14:* 729–734 (1984).
48 Trentham, D.E.; McCune, W.J.; Susman, P.; David, J.R.: Autoimmunity to collagen in adjuvant arthritis of rats. J. clin. Invest. *66:* 1109–1117 (1980).
49 Iizuka, Y.; Chang, Y.H.: Adjuvant polyarthritis. VII. The role of type II collagen in pathogenesis. Arthritis Rheum. *25:* 1325–1332 (1982).
50 Kaibara, N.; Hotokebuchi, T.; Takagishi, K.; Katsuki, I.; Morinaga, M.; Arita, C.; Yingushi, S.: Pathogenetic difference between collagen arthritis and adjuvant arthritis. J. exp. Med. *159:* 1388–1396 (1984).
51 Taurog, J.D.; Kerwar, S.S.; McReynolds, R.A.; Sandberg, G.P.; Leang, S.L.; Mahowald, M.L.: Synergy between adjuvant arthritis and collagen-induced arthritis in rats. J. exp. Med. *162:* 962–678 (1985).
52 Caplan, A.I.: Cartilage. Scient. Am. *251:* 82–90 (1984).
53 Van Eden, W.; Holoshitz, J.; Nevo, Z.; Frenkel, A.; Klajman, A.; Cohen, I.R.: Arthritis induced by a T lymphocyte clone that responds to Mycobacterium tuberculosis and to cartilage proteoglycans. Proc. natn. Acad. Sci. USA *82:* 5064–5067 (1985).
54 Maron, R.; Zerubavel, R.; Friedman, A.; Cohen, I.R.: T lymphocyte line specific for thyroglobulin produces or vaccinates against autoimmune thyroiditis in mice. J. Immun. *131:* 2316–2322 (1983).
55 Kolk, A.H.J.; Ho, M.L.; Klatser, P.R.; Eggelte, T.A.; Kuyper, S.; De Jonge, S.; Van Leeuwen, N.: Production and characterization of monoclonal antibodies to *Mycobacterium tuberculosis, M.bovis* (BCG) and *M.leprae.* Clin. exp. Immunol. *58:* 511–521 (1984).
56 Holoshitz, J.; Klajman, A.; Drucker, I.; Lapidot, Z.; Yaretzky, A.; Frenkel, A.; Van Eden, W.; Cohen, I.R.: T-lymphocytes of rheumatoid arthritis patients show

augmented reactivity to a fraction of mycobacteria cross-reactive with cartilage Lancet *ii:* 305–309 (1986).

57 Cohen, I. R.: Autoimmunity: physiologic and pernicious. Adv. intern. Med. *29:* 147–165 (1984).

58 Hushby, G.; Van de Rijn, I.; Zabriskie, J. B.; Abdin, Z. H.; Williams, R. C.: Antibodies reacting with cytoplasm of subthalamic and caudate nuclei neurons in chorea and acute rheumatic fever. J. exp. Med. *144:* 1094–1110 (1976).

59 Wood, J. N.; Hudson, L.; Jessel, T. M.; Yamamoto, M.: A monoclonal antibody defining antigenic determinants on subpopulations of mammalian neurones and *Trypanosoma cruzi* parasites. Nature, Lond. *296:* 34–38 (1982).

60 Van Eden, W.; Holoshitz, J.; Cohen, I. R.: Autoimmunity and the host-parasite relationship. Clin. Immunol. Allergy *6:* 113–126 (1986).

61 Kaplan, M. H.; Meyeserian, M.: An immunologic cross-reaction between group A streptococcal cells and human heart tissue. Lancet *i:* 706–707 (1962).

62 Dale, J. B.; Beachey, E. H.: Multiple, heart-cross-reactive epitopes of streptococcal M proteins. J. exp. Med. *161:* 113–122 (1985).

63 Fillet, H.; Damle, S. P.; Gregory, J. D.; Violin, C.; Poon-King, T.; Zabriskie, J.: Sera from patients with post-streptococcal glomerulonephritis contain antibodies to glomerular heparan sulfate proteoglycan. J. exp. Med. *161:* 277–289 (1985).

64 Bokisch, V. A.; Chiao, J. W.; Bernstein, D.; Krause, R. M.: Homogeneous rabbit 7S anti-IgG with antibody specificity for peptidoglycan. J. exp. Med. *138:* 1184–1193 (1973).

65 Lafer, E. M.; Rauch, J,; Andrezejewski, C. Jr.; Mudd, D.; Furie, B.; Furie, B.; Schwartz, R. S.; Stollar, B. D.: Polyspecific monoclonal lupus autoantibodies reactive with both polynucleotides and phospholipids. J. exp. Med. *153:* 897–909 (1981).

66 Shoenfeld, Y.; Rauch, J.; Massicotte, H.; Datta, S. K.; Schwartz, J. A.; Stollar, B. D.; Schwartz, R. S.: Polyspecificity of monoclonal lupus autoantibodies produced by human-human hybridomas. New Engl. J. Med. *308:* 414–420 (1983).

67 Koike, T.; Tomioka, H.; Kumagai, A.: Antibodies cross-reactive with DNA and cardioliplin in patients with systemic lupus erythematosus. Clin. exp. Immunol. *50:* 298–302 (1982).

68 Schleider, M. A.; Nachman, R. L.; Jaffe, E. A.; Coleman, M.: A clinical study of the lupus anticoagulant. Blood *48:* 499 (1976).

69 Rauch, J.; Tannenbaum, H.; Stollar, B. D.; Schwartz, R. S.: Monoclonal anticardiolipin antibodies bind to DNA. Eur. J. Immunol. *14:* 529–534 (1984).

70 Faaber, P.; Capel, P. J. A.; Rijke, G. P. M.; Vierwinden, G.; Van de Putte, L. B. A.; Koene, R. A. P.: Cross-reactivity of anti-DNA antibodies with proteoglycans. Clin. exp. Immunol. *55:* 502–508 (1984).

71 Fuchs, S.; Feingold, C.; Bardfield, E.: Molecular approaches to myasthenia gravis; in Schotland, Diseases of the motor unit, pp. 245–256 (Wiley, New York 1982).

72 Stefansson, K.; Dieperink, M. E.; Richman, D. P.; Gomez, C. M.; Marton, L. S.: Sharing of antigenic determinants between the nicotinic acetylcholine receptor and proteins in *Escherichia coli, Proteus vulgaris,* and *Klebsiella pneumoniae.* New Engl. J. Med. *312:* 221–225 (1985).

73 Edmonds, J.; Macanly, D,; Tyndall, A.; Liew, M.; Alexander, K.; Geczy, A.;

Bashir, H.: Lymphocytotoxicity of anti-Klebsiella antisera in ankylosing spondylitis and related arthropathies. Arthritis Rheum. *24:* 1–7 (1981).

74 Brewerton, D.A.; Caffrey, M.; Hart, F.D.; James, D.C.Q.; Nicholls, A.; Sturrock, R.D.: Ankylosing spondylitis and HLA-W27. Lancet *i:* 904–906 (1973).

75 Van Rood, J.J.; Van Leeuwen, A.; Ivany, P.; Cats, A.; Breur-Vriesendorp, B.S.; Dekkers-Saeijs, A.J.; Kijlstra, A.; Van Kregten, E.: Blind confirmation of Geczy factor in ankylosing spondylitis. Lancet *ii:* 943–944 (1985).

76 Geczy, A.F.; Alexander, K.; Bashir, H.V.; Edmonds, J.P.: Characterization of a factor(s) present in Klebsiella culture filtrates that specifically modifies an HLA-B27-associated cell-surface component. J. exp. Med. *152:* 331S–340S (1980).

77 Adams, D.D.: Thyroid-stimulating autoantibodies. Vitam. Horm. *38:* 159–203 (1980).

78 Weiss, M.; Ingbar, S.H.; Winblad, S.; Kasper, D.L.: Demonstration of a saturable binding site for thyrotropin in Yersinia enterocolitica. Science *219:* 1331–1334 (1983).

79 Glant, T.; Csongor, J.; Scucz, T.: Immunopathologic role of proteoglycan antigens in rheumatoid joint disease. Scand. J. Immunol. *11:* 247–252 (1980).

80 Fujinami, R.S.; Oldstone, M.B.A.; Wroblewska, Z.; Frankel, M.E.; Koprowski, H.: Molecular mimicry in virus infection: Cross-reaction of measles virus phosphoprotein or of herpes simplex protein with human intermediate filaments. Proc. natn. Acad. Sci. USA *80:* 2346–2350 (1983).

81 Tardieu, M.; Powers, M.L.; Hafler, D.A.; Hauser, S.L.; Weiner, H.L.: Autoimmunity following viral infection: demonstration of monoclonal antibodies against normal tissue following infection of mice with reovirus and demonstration of shared antigenicity between virus and lymphocytes. Eur. J. Immunol. *14:* 561–565 (1984).

82 Bloom B.R.: Games parasites play: how parasites evade immune surveillance. Nature, Lond. *279:* 21–26 (1979).

83 Talmon, J.; Ranghino, G.; Yonath, A.; Cohen, I.R.: Structural analysis of insulin determinants seen by T cells directed by H-2 genes. Immunogenetics *18:* 79–89 (1983).

84 Watts, T.H.; Gariepy, J.; Schoolnik, G.K.; McConnell, H.M.: T-cell activation by peptide antigen: effect of peptide sequence and method of antigen presentation. Proc. natn. Acad. Sci. USA *82:* 5480–5484 (1985).

85 Cohen, I.R.; Altmann, D.M., Friedman, A.: The advantage of being a low responder. Immunol. Today *6:* 147–148 (1985).

86 Burnet, F.M.: The clonal selection theory of acquired immunity (Vanderbilt University Press, Nashville 1959).

87 Nossal, G.J.V.: Cellular mechanisms of immunologic tolerance. A. Rev. Immunol. *1:* 33–62 (1983).

88 Cohen, I.R.; Holoshitz, J.; Maron, R.; Zerubavel, R.: Vaccination against autoimmune disease using lines of autoimmune T lymphocytes. Immunol. Today *4:* 227–230 (1983).

89 Cohen, I.R.: Prospects for the treatment of immunological diseases. Clins Immunol. Allergy *4:* 585–597 (1984).

90 Holoshitz, J.; Van Eden, W.; Reshef, T.; Cohen I.R.: Prevention and treatment of autoimmune arthritis by a T-lymphocyte clone (submitted).

91 Batisto, J.R.; Smith, R.N.; Bechman, K.; Sternlight, M.; Welles, W.L.: Susceptibility to adjuvant arthritis in DA and F344 rats. A dominant trait controlled by an autosomal gene locus linked to the major histocompatibility complex. Arthritis Rheum. *25:* 1194–1200 (1982).

92 Shevach, E.M.; Rosenthal, A.S.: The function of macrophages in antigen recognition by guinea pig T lymphocytes. II. Role of the macrophage in regulation of the genetic control of the immune response. J. exp. Med. *138:* 1213–1229 (1973).

93 Svejgaard, A.; Morling, N.; Platz, P.; Rijder, L.P.; Thomsen, M.: HLA and disease; in Fougereau, Dausset, Immunology 80, pp. 530–540 (Academic Press, London 1980).

95 De Vries, R.R.P.; Meera Khan, P.; Bernini, L.F.; Van Loghem, E.; Van Rood, J.J.: Genetic control of survival in epidemics. J. Immunogenet. *6:* 271–287 (1979).

96 Van Eden, W.; De Vries, R.R.P.; Van Rood, J.J.: The genetic approach to infectious disease with special emphasis on the MHC. Dis. Markers *1:* 221–242 (1983).

97 Godal, T.: Immunological aspects of leprosy–present status. Prog. Allergy, vol. 25, pp. 211–242 (Karger, Basel 1980).

98 Mehra, V.; Convit, J.; Rubinstein, A.; Bloom, B.R.: Activated suppressor T cells in leprosy. J. Immun. *129:* 1946–1951 (1982).

99 Mehra, V.; Brennan, P.J.; Rada, E.; Convit, J.; Bloom, B.: Lymphocyte suppression in leprosy induced by unique *M. leprae* glycolipid. Nature, Lond. *308:* 194–196 (1984).

100 Nath, I.; Von Rood, J.J.; Mehra, N.K.; Vaidya, M.C.: Natural suppressor cells in human leprosy. The role of HLA-D identical peripheral blood lymphocytes and macrophages in the in vitro modulation of lymphoproliferative responses. Clin. exp. Immunol. *42:* 203–210 (1980).

101 Crawford, C.L.; Evans, D.M.L., Evans, E.M.: Experimental allergic neuritis induced by sensory nerve myelin may provide a model for nonlepromatous leprosy. Nature, Lond. *251:* 223–225 (1974).

102 De Vries, R.R.P.; Lai-A-Fat, R.F.M.; Nyenhuis, L.E.; Van Rood, J.J.: HLA-linked genetic control of host response to Mycobacterium leprae. Lancet *ii:* 1328–1339 (1976).

103 Van Eden, W.; De Vries, R.R.P.; Mehra, N.K.; Vaidya, M.C.; D'Amaro, J.; Van Rood, J.J.: HLA segregation of tuberculoid leprosy: Confirmation of the DR2 marker. J. infect. Dis. *141:* 693–701 (1980).

104 Fine, P.E.M.; Wolf, E.; Pritchard, J.; Watson, B.; Bradley, D.J.; Festenstein, M.; Chacko, G.J.G.: HLA-linked genes and leprosy. A family study in Karigiri, South India. J. infect. Dis. *140:* 152–161 (1979).

105 Van Eden, W.; Gonzalez, N.M.; De Vries, R.R.P.; Convit, J.; Van Rood, J.J.: HLA-linked control of predisposition to lepromatous leprosy. J. infect. Dis. *151:* 9–14 (1985).

106 Van Eden, W.; De Vries, R.R.P.: HLA and leprosy: A reevaluation. Lepr. Rev. *55:* 89–104 (1984).

107 Van Eden, W.; De Vries, R.R.P.; D'Amaro, J.; Schreuder, G.M.Th.; Leiker, D.L.; Van Rood, J.J.: HLA-DR associated genetic control of the type of leprosy in a population from Surinam. Human Immunol. *4:* 343–350 (1982).

108 Paul, R.C.; Stanford, J.L.; Carswell, J.W.: Multiple skin testing in leprosy. J. Hyg. *75:* 57–68 (1975).

109 Van Eden, W.; De Vries, R. R. P.; Stanford, G. L.; Rook, G. A. W.: HLA-DR3 associated genetic control of response to multiple skin tests with new tuberculins. Clin. exp. Immunol. *51:* 207–292 (1983).
110 Ottenhoff, T. H. M.; Torres, P.; Terencio de las Aguas, J.; Fernandez, R.; Eden, W., Van; Vries, R. R. P., De; Stanford, J. L.: Evidence for an HLA-DR4 associated immune response (Ir) gene for Mycobacterium tuberculosis: a due to the pathogenesis of rheumatoid arthritis? Lancet *ii:* 310–313 (1986).

Dr. W. van Eden, MD, PhD, Department of Immunology, Veterinary Faculty, University of Utrecht, Yalelaan 1, NL-3584 CL Utrecht (The Netherlands)

Concepts Immunopathol., vol. 4, pp. 171–199 (Karger, Basel 1987)

Role of Cytokines in Rheumatological Inflammation

Paul Emery, D. James Williamson, Ian R. Mackay

Reid Memorial Laboratory, The Clinical Research Unit of The Walter and Eliza Hall Institute of Medical Research and The Royal Melbourne Hospital, Victoria, Australia

Introduction

Rheumatoid arthritis (RA) is one of mankinds most intensively investigated diseases. In regard to cause and pathogenesis, the pessimists would say that there is scarcely a glimmer of an understanding, with research activities orbiting around what is essentially a 'black hole' (fig. 1). The optimists on the other hand would say that the pathogenesis of RA is, in principle, solved by claiming that the disease is *initiated* by a transiently present infectious agent(s), *perpetuated* in genetically predisposed subjects by an uncontrolled immunological response in which the reactivity of anti-immunoglobulin and perhaps anti-collagen antibodies play an essential role, and with *effector* mechanisms depending on the activities of cytokines of various types, as will be described in this review.

The progression of disease in the rheumatoid synovium has been divided into several stages, but this is artificial since the rheumatoid process is a continuum dominated histologically by the accumulation in the joint of lymphocytes which generate cytokines capable of activating various cell types within the joint. Here we hope to capture part of the great upsurge in interest in effects of cytokines, concentrating particularly on their role in synovial inflammation. We define cytokines very simply as cellular products which act as chemical mediators of cell-cell interactions within a local microenvironment.

We propose to examine in detail the role of cytokines in rheumatoid inflammation and to specify how they may be implicated in marshalling the intrasynovial immune response and in activating effector cells, macrophages and granulocytes, to promote articular destruction. The cyto-

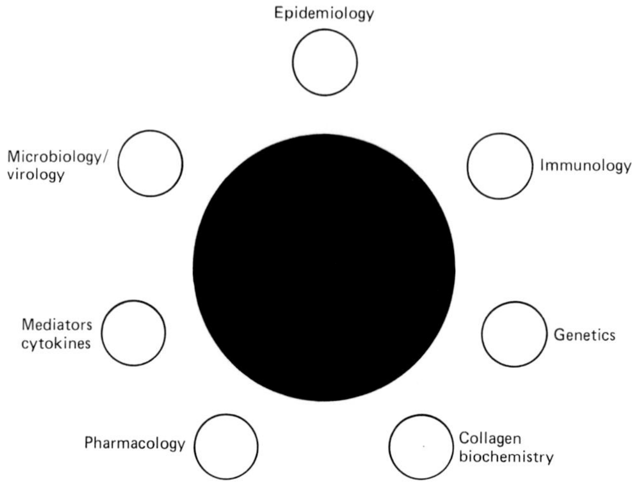

Fig. 1. There is no universally accepted explanation for rheumatoid arthritis, the pathogenesis of which remains a 'black hole', around which are orbiting the various disciplines which impinge on this enigmatic disease.

kines considered to be of particular relevance to RA are interleukin-1 (IL-1), interleukin-2 (IL-2), interferon-γ (IFN-γ), colony-stimulating factor (CSF), osteoclast-activating factor (OAF), and fibrogenic and vascularization factors.

Interleukin-1

Background

The term interleukin-1 was proposed in 1979 for a product of macrophages that activated T (and B) lymphocytes [Aarden et al., 1979]. Macrophage products with properties of IL-1 had been known under different names for many years and further macrophage-derived factors have since been isolated with structures similar to that of IL-1 but with different properties. It is now recognised that IL-1 comprises a family of molecules many of which had been given functional or descriptive labels such as lymphocyte-activating factor, mononuclear cell factor, leucocyte endogenous mediator, catabolin, proteolysis-inducing factor, endogenous pyrogen and epidermal cell activating factor [Duff, 1985].

Biochemistry

IL-1 was shown by several investigators to exist as two molecular species of molecular weights 15 and 35 kDa, both with two isoelectric points. Partial clarification ensued when two distantly related forms of human IL-1, IL-1-α of 271 amino acids and IL-1-β of 269 amino acids, were cloned and expressed [March et al., 1985], and the same workers provided evidence that the biological activity of IL-1 resided in the C-terminal region of about 150 amino acids. This supported the concept that human IL-1 molecules are synthesized as high molecular weight precursors that become cleaved to yield biologically active lower molecular weight forms. Murine IL-1 has been cloned and shows 62% amino acid sequence homology with human IL-1-α but only 26% with IL-1-β [Lomedico et al., 1984].

Sources and Actions of IL-1

Macrophages and monocytes synthesize and release IL-1 in response to infections, immunological stimuli including immune complexes, and other inflammatory stimuli [Dinarello, 1984; Arend et al., 1985]. The most important stimulators in an immunological context are T lymphocytes activated by interaction with specific antigen and Ia molecules on antigen-presenting cells [Durum et al., 1984]. Although macrophages are the major cellular source of IL-1, other cells such as synovial dendritic cells, keratinocytes and Langerhans cells [Durum et al., 1984] also have been shown, at least in vitro, to be IL-1 producers. The interpretation of work in vitro has been complicated by the fact that IL-1-producing cells can be activated during their preparation, particularly by minute quantities of lipopolysaccharide present in the culture medium [Duff and Atkins, 1982]. Although the receptor for IL-1 has not been identified, competition for binding of labelled molecules suggests that IL-1α and IL-1-β have, at least on the T lymphocytes, a shared receptor [Allison, 1985].

The actions of IL-1 are diverse but can be broadly grouped into local effects occurring at the site of production, and systemic effects. Local effects include activation of various types of cells, particularly T lymphocytes, and induction of mediators of cartilage, bone and connective tissue degradation. Systemic effects include fever, stimulation of acute phase reactants, alteration in serum cations and release of neutrophils from bone marrow (fig. 2). Recent observations indicate that certain actions of IL-1 are confined to one or other type of IL-1. Thus while the actions of

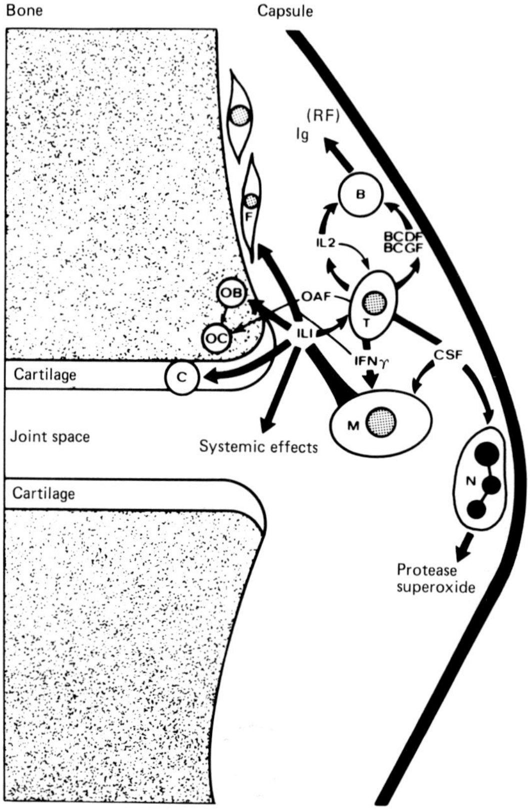

Fig. 2. Proposed immunopathology of the rheumatoid synovium. A key event is the interaction between the T lymphocyte (T) and the macrophage (M), each of which releases lymphokines, including from M, interleukin-1 (IL-1) which activates T cells to liberate various cytokines. Whether the various lymphokine-producing T cells belong to the same or different lineages is not addressed. The cytokines of T cell origin include IL-2, IFN-γ, CSF, OAF, and B cell growth/differentiation factors (BCGF/BCDF), the last-named driving B cells towards plasma cells which synthesize immunoglobulin (Ig), including rheumatoid factor (RF). The targets of cytokines are shown as neutrophils (N), fibroblasts (F), chondrocytes (C) and osteoblasts/osteoclasts (OB/OC).

IL-1α and IL-1-β on lymphocytes and cartilage degradation are similar, the effects on bone are predominately due to IL-1-β [Allison, 1985].

The mechanisms which regulate the actions and the production of IL-1 are not yet fully understood. Inhibitors of IL-1 activity were initially identified in the urine of febrile patients [Liao et al., 1984], and have also been found in serum and synovial fluid without being fully characterized

[Aelion et al., 1985; Maeda et al., 1985]. Interestingly, inhibition appears to affect the actions of IL-1 selectively with the activation of fibroblasts by IL-1 unaffected [Maeda et al., 1985], suggesting the selective inhibition of one of the IL-1 subtypes.

Assay

The activity of IL-1 is conventionally measured by augmentation of lectin-induced mouse thymocyte proliferation [Gery et al., 1972]. Subsequently, assays were developed using cultured cell lines [Gillis and Mizel, 1981] and have since been improved upon [Conlon, 1983; Simon et al., 1985]. Problems however remain with a lack of specificity of these assays, and the obscuring effects of inhibitors. An alternative assay exists, the leucocyte pyrogen test, that utilises the rise in temperature after IL-1 injection into rabbits or mice, but this is insensitive and rarely used [Dinarello, 1984].

IL-1 in Rheumatological Diseases

Synovial effusions from patients affected by RA [Fontana et al., 1982] and other diseases [Wood et al., 1983] have IL-1 activity in bioassays. Further, synovial cells [Wood et al., 1985] and rheumatoid synovial dendritic cells [Duff et al., 1985] extracted from the synovial membrane of patients with RA produce IL-1 in vitro. Peripheral blood mononuclear (PBM) cells from patients with RA when tested in vitro display an increased production of IL-1 compared to controls, but reduced production compared with that of paired samples of mononuclear cells from synovial fluid [Nouri et al., 1985a]. In contrast, PBM cells from patients with systemic lupus erythematosus (SLE) have a reduced production of IL-1 compared with that of cells from control groups [Linker-Israeli et al., 1983]. To annotate the fibrogenesis-inducing activity of IL-1, PBM cells from patients with scleroderma release IL-1 spontaneously in vitro [Alcocer-Varela et al., 1984], perhaps explaining the fibroblast proliferation in this disease, and also the diminished response of dermal fibroblasts to monocyte supernatants in vitro [Whiteside et al., 1985].

Local Effects. The potential importance of IL-1 in rheumatic diseases should be evident from its range of actions. Thus the stimulatory effects on T lymphocytes may be a major determinant of the intrasynovial proliferation of these cells which is characteristic of active synovitis. IL-1 also has a role in the interactions between cells of the immune system and effector processes within joints. IL-1 is a potent bone resorbing factor [Gowen et al., 1983] but, although capable of stimulating prostaglandin E_2 production, this is not the major pathway whereby IL-1 induces bone resorption [Gowan et al., 1985a], as described in the section on osteoclast-activating factor. Thus, IL-1 appears to act on osteoclasts indirectly via 'short-range' signals from osteoblasts [Thompson et al., 1985] and, in addition, IL-1 induces production of collagenase by the latter cells [Gowen et al., 1985b]. Likewise, chondrocytes [Saklatvala et al., 1983] together with fibroblasts and synovial cells [Mizel et al., 1981; Postlethwaite et al., 1983] are stimulated by IL-1 to produce collagenase and prostaglandins. As there is evidence that IL-1 can influence connective tissue matrix production [Schmidt et al., 1982], IL-1 can be viewed as a mediator of both destruction and repair of this tissue [Krane et al., 1982; Dingle et al., 1984].

There are known inhibitors of these local effects of IL-1. Thus, bone absorption induced by IL-1 is completely blocked by interferon-γ [Bertolini et al., 1985], and is apparently antagonised by cyclosporin A [Skjodt et al., 1985]. Retinoic acid and 1,25-hydroxy vitamin D_3 are inducers of bone resorption factors and both of these substances are claimed to enhance release of IL-1 and also to regulate release of IL-2 and IL-3 [Treschsel, 1985].

Systemic Effects. The systemic actions of IL-1 of relevance to rheumatological diseases are the reduction of serum cations especially iron [Kampschmidt, 1981], mediation of muscle proteolysis [Clowes et al., 1983] and stimulation of the production of acute phase proteins from the liver [Sipe et al., 1982]. Perhaps the variations in the acute phase response observed in different autoimmune diseases, exemplified by the normal levels of C-reactive protein in active SLE versus the abnormal levels in RA, reflect differing levels of IL-1 production: an explanation for such differences in these diseases would improve understanding of their pathogenesis. The failure to find a close correlation between acute phase responses and fever, given that IL-1 acts as an endogenous pyrogen, may relate to the existence of other pyrogens such as interferon-α [Dinarello et al., 1984] or to IL-1 molecular species without endogenous pyrogen activity [Allison, 1985].

In summary, the various actions of IL-1 explain several important clinical features of RA: moreover IL-1 is produced by cells isolated from the synovium and is detectable in synovial fluid. The activity of IL-1 could explain the persisting inflammation in a rheumatoid joint by a positive feedback mechanism as follows. The production of IL-1 from macrophages can be stimulated by IgG rheumatoid factor and immune complexes present in a rheumatoid joint, and it is postulated that production of these immunoglobulins in turn is increased as a result of IL-1 acting on B cells, probably mainly via T cells. A more primary role for IL-1, predicated on the high synovial levels of this cytokine, would involve the breaking of tolerance as recently described [Feldman et al., 1985; Green et al., 1985], so permitting responses to weakly immunogenic antigens such as collagen, and in turn promoting persistence of the immune response within the joint.

Even if IL-1 were to fall short of providing a full explanation for the initiation of the chain of pathogenic events, a high degree of relevance to the clinical manifestations of RA would remain. Turning again to SLE, and noting in this disease the infrequency of both joint effusions and long-term joint damage, we can annotate the low level of IL-1 production contrasting strikingly with that of diseases associated with active synovitis and joint destruction such as RA and gout [Woolf et al., 1985]. Finally, it has been convincingly demonstrated that progression of bone damage in RA continues in those patients with a persistent acute phase response, but halts in those patients in whom it can be controlled [Dawes et al., 1986; Pullar and Capell, 1986]. This work can be interpreted as suggesting that IL-1 levels in the serum correlate with those in the joint and that the latter determine joint disruption. If this proves to be correct then logically the suppression of IL-1 levels should become the 'gold standard' in the measurement of therapeutic success.

Interleukin-2

Background

About 10 years ago the maintenance and growth of T cells in vitro was shown to require the presence of spleen-derived conditioned medium. Purification allowed the isolation of a newly recognised factor termed T cell growth factor (TCGF) [Morgan et al., 1976] [reviewed in Gillis, 1983; Robb, 1984]. This lymphocyte product which stimulates T cell proliferation was named interleukin-2 at the same time as lymphocyte-activating factor was named interleukin-1 [Aarden et al., 1979].

Biochemistry

Human IL-2 is a 133 amino acid polypeptide containing a single intramolecular disulphide bridge. The amino acid sequence has been derived from an examination of cDNA from transformed and non-transformed cells [Taniguchi et al., 1983; Devos et al., 1983]. The approximate molecular weight of IL-2 is 15–16 kDa and there is heterogeneity in isoelectric points and degree of migration on SDS-PAGE. There is only a single copy of the human IL-2 gene [Seigel et al., 1984], so that the heterogeneity of IL-2 arises essentially from post-translational modification of the parent molecule. Recombinant IL-2 and the variably glycosylated natural forms have all been shown to have the same activity in vitro [Roifman et al., 1985].

Sources and Actions of IL-2

IL-2 is released by lymphocytes, the main source being cells of the CD4 'helper' subset [Pfizenmaier et al., 1984; Meuer et al., 1982] in response to antigen-presenting accessory cells which provide the requisite signals of antigen in association with class II MHC products and IL-1 [Smith, 1980]. Once released, IL-2 acts independently of antigen to stimulate any IL-2 receptor-bearing cells. The specificity of the immune response is maintained at the level of IL-2 receptor expression, this again requiring both antigen presentation by accessory cells and an IL-1 lymphokine signal. IL-2 binds to a specific high affinity cell surface receptor absent from resting cells; the IL-2 receptor is expressed after antigen or mitogen stimulation as these cells become responsive to IL-2. An antibody (anti-TAC) has been developed [Morgan et al., 1976; Uchiyama et al., 1981] which blocks IL-2 binding in a specific way [Leonard et al., 1982] and has been used to characterise the IL-2 receptor at various stages of differentiation. In mice several factors have been identified in serum which antagonise IL-2 or inhibit its actions [Hardt et al., 1981; Male et al., 1985; Hooton et al., 1985]. It is probable that similar factors exist in humans and may explain the absence of any identifiable IL-2 in blood.

IL-2 stimulates activated T cells possessing IL-2 receptors to progress from the late G1 phase of the cell cycle into the S phase [Klaus et al., 1984]. IL-2 induces such cells to produce both interferon-γ [Farrar et al., 1982] which can influence various non-T cells, and B cell growth and differentiation factors [Howard et al., 1983; Inaba et al., 1983]. IL-2 also causes an increase in NK activity above that attributable to interferon-γ [Henney et al., 1981]. IL-2 receptors have been identified on murine B cells in numbers equivalent to those on T cells [Lowenthal et al., 1985] and there is evidence that IL-2 has a direct stimulating effect on these cells [Miedema et al., 1985].

Assay

IL-2 is conventionally measured in a microassay by assessing the replication of responsive cells by tritiated thymidine incorporation. To minimize problems with variability and specificity, continuous IL-2-dependent murine or rodent tumor-specific cell lines are used. Alternative assays include the use of the IL-2-dependent cells induced after lectin stimulation of thymocytes or splenocytes, or of the short-term IL-2-responsive cells produced by IL-2 feeding of the lectin-stimulated cells. The latter does allow the use of human cells if desired, but both assays have problems with variability. A solid-phase radioimmunometric assay using a combination of a polyclonal serum and a monoclonal antibody has been described, but while overcoming problems of reliability, it is quite insensitive [Gehman and Robb, 1984].

IL-2 in Rheumatological Diseases

A characteristic feature of RA is the depressed cellular immune responses seen on skin testing [Waxman et al., 1973; Emery et al., 1984b] and a parallel reduction in blood lymphocyte transformation in vitro to antigens or mitogens [Silverman et al., 1976]. The addition to lymphocytes of exogenous IL-2 but not IL-1 or inhibitors of prostaglandin synthesis returns depressed lymphocyte transformation in RA to normal levels [Emery et al., 1984a; Alcocer-Varela et al., 1984] although another group found a less than complete response to IL-2 [Miyasaka et al., 1984]. Direct measurement of IL-2 produced by stimulated lymphocytes from patients with RA confirmed a reduced ability to produce IL-2 [Nouri et al., 1985b], and this reduction was greater for lymphocytes from the synovial membrane than for blood lymphocytes [Combe et al., 1985; Silver et al., 1983]. As for blood lymphocytes, the decreased production of IL-2 by synovial lymphocytes was improved by exposure of cells to exogenous IL-2 [Silver et al., 1983]. The decreased production by lymphocytes of IL-2 in RA appears to correlate with disease activity [Cathely et al., 1985].

Attempts to measure IL-2 in synovial fluid have been hampered by technical difficulties with the bioassy. IL-2 activity was found in synovial fluids from a significant proportion of RA patients in one study [Wilkins et al., 1983], and in all joint fluids examined including those from osteoarthritis patients in another, using a blast cell assay [Nouri et al., 1984). However, both ourselves [unpubl. observations] and others [Lund and Egeland, 1985] have been unable to detect IL-2 activity in synovial fluid using the conventional murine CTLL assay.

In SLE, stimulated blood lymphocytes produce less IL-2 in vitro than controls but, unlike RA, there is also a failure of cells to respond to exogenous IL-2 [Alcocer-Varela and Alarcon-Segovia, 1982; Linker-Israeli et al., 1983]. In Sjögren's syndrome there is a similar but less-marked defect than in SLE [Alcocer-Varela and Alarcon-Segovia, 1982] but, interestingly and in contrast to the behaviour of synovial lymphocytes of RA patients, lymphocytes from the salivary glands of patients with Sjögren's syndrome produced high levels of IL-2 and had increased staining of IL-2-like material detected by antibodies against synthesised peptides of IL-2 [Fox et al., 1985]. In systemic sclerosis alone among the rheumatological disorders, patients have blood lymphocytes which show an augmented release of IL-2 and this appears to correlate with the extent of skin involvement [Keystone et al., 1985].

In the mouse inhibitors of IL-2 are present in the blood during infection and this is associated with a generalized depression of cellular immune responses [Lelchuk et al., 1985]. Accordingly, when leukopheresis is used in RA, the simultaneous improvement in indices of disease activity and lymphocyte proliferative responses to antigens [Wahl et al., 1983] may be due to removal of inhibitors of IL-2. In studies from this Unit on cases of RA, we have found a marked inhibitory effect of synovial fluid on the conventional mouse CTLL IL-2 assay and this effect was abrogated by heating at 56 °C. Absorption of pre-formed IL-2 by RA blood lymphocytes has been demonstrated and this effect was more marked for lymphocytes from synovial fluid [Knobloch et al., 1985]. On the other hand, there have been identified suppressor factor(s) from allo-antigen stimulated murine spleen cells which appear to act on T lymphocytes by suppressing IL-2 release and preventing acquisition of IL-2 responsiveness [Kramer and Koszinowski, 1983]; since this factor is also thermolabile, it may be relevant to the IL-2 inhibitors identified in humans.

The explanation of the demonstrable abnormalities in RA of IL-2 production, and response to IL-2, is not clear. The defective production in RA of IL-2 in vitro by T lymphocytes may be explained by these cells being pre-activated in vivo so rendering them resistant to further activation. In support of this is the high proportion of T lymphocytes which are activated, as judged by Ia/DR positivity within the synovial membrane and fluid [Burmester et al., 1981]. But, paradoxically, when synovial fluid and synovial membrane are examined for the presence of IL-2 using monoclonal antibodies, staining is relatively scanty [Husby and Williams, 1985]. The histological appearance of the synovial membrane, in which activated helper T cells and antigen presenting cells exist in close association [Janossy et al., 1981], should be associated with abundant IL-2 production; hence the scanty staining, given that it may not reflect actual turnover of IL-2, is a surprise. In another study on synovial cells, the finding was of T lymphocytes with marked Ia expression but reduced expression of receptors for IL-2 and transferrin, indicative of an absence of terminal effector cells which could result in a failure of 'down-regulation' of the immune system, and so act as a perpetuating influence on the disease [Konttinin et al., 1985]. There is evidence that the level of IL-2 at the time of antigen presentation is critical in determining the option of tolerance or immunological response [Malkovsky and Medawar, 1984], which may be another means by which IL-2 could influence the outcome of an immunopathic disease.

Despite the clear indications in RA of abnormalities of the IL-2 system, it is still not apparent whether there is a deficiency or excess of IL-2 within the rheumatoid joint, but a deficiency seems likely. Perhaps the relative amounts of IL-2 and its regulators, at the time of initial antigen presentation, play a critical role in determining the magnitude of the immune response and hence disease outcome. This effect may be separable from the reduced production of IL-2 by lymphocytes which, in RA at least, seems to correspond to disease activity [Cathely et al., 1985].

Interferon-γ

Background

IFN was discovered in 1957 as a substance produced by virally infected cells which could protect other cells from viral infection. Interferon was subsequently subclassified as interferon-α if produced by leucocytes and interferon-β if produced by fibroblasts. A closely related interferon species, interferon-γ [Wheelock, 1966], was later shown to be released from lymphocytes in vitro by stimuli which included specific antigens and mitogens [Gresser, 1977].

Biochemistry

There is a single IFN-γ gene situated on the long arm of chromosome 12 coding for a 144 amino acid protein [Gray et al., 1982] which is quite unrelated to the sequence of either IFN-α or IFN-β. The molecular weight of IFN-γ is 17 kDa, and post-translational glycosylation results in products of molecular weights of 20 or 25 kDa which may aggregate to form random dimers.

Sources and Actions of IFN-γ

The main source of IFN-γ is T cells stimulated by antigen or mitogen. The 'helper' subset of T lymphocytes is the major source after stimulation by antigens [Biondi et al., 1984]. Such cells also release IFN-α in response to viral infection [Pasternack et al., 1984]. Both IL-1 and IL-2 increase IFN-γ production by T lymphocytes [Farrar et al., 1982]. Another producer of IFN-γ is the NK cell, and this is the major source when IL-2 is added in vitro to non-activated lymphoid cells which lack high affinity IL-2 receptors [Trinchieri et al., 1984]. Separate receptors exist for the β and γ species of IFN, although the presence of IFN-γ causes down-regulation of the other receptors. Subsequent to occupation of the receptor there is synthesis of RNA and various polypeptides, some common to all IFNs but several unique to IFN-γ. The receptor for IFN-γ has been characterised [Celada and Schreiber, 1985; Finbloom et al., 1985].

Of rheumatological interest, IFN-γ increases proliferation of synovial fibroblasts [Brinckerhoff and Guyre, 1985], and appears to effect suppression of hemopoiesis [Linch, 1985]. Other actions of IFN-γ are essentially stimulatory [Trichieri and Perussia, 1985] except for a debated role in growth inhibition of cells and blockade of the IL-1 effect on bone. IFN-γ induces the appearance of new surface markers associated with differentiation and, in the case of T and possibly NK cells, proliferation also. Expression of class I MHC antigens is enhanced, and IFN-γ induces or enhances expression of class II MHC antigen expression in a wide variety of cells, this occurring after the rapid induction of mRNA [Collins et al., 1984]. IFN-γ also induces myelomonocytic cells to become activated and differentiated, and induces cells of the monocyte-macrophages lineage to become efficient mediators of antibody-dependent cytotoxicity. IFN-γ has macrophage activating factor (MAF) activity, and induces macrophages to release IL-1 [Arenzana-Seisdos et al., 1985] and become capable of antigen presentation. Also, IFN-γ induces high affinity Fc receptors for monomeric Ig on myelomonocytic cells [Perussia et al., 1983]. IFN-γ may be responsible for the fusion of osteoclast precursor cells [Weinberg et al., 1984]. There is evidence that IFN-γ has a role in B cell activation synergistically with that of other B cell-activating factors [Leibson et al., 1984].

Assay

Measurement of IFN-γ depends upon its ability to inhibit viral damage to human cell lines, either in a plaque inhibition assay or in other assays which measure the inhibition of viral cytopathic effect [Finter, 1981]. The units of activity of IFN are expressed in relation to the activity of a reference preparation of IFN-γ. Determination of the IFN type being measured requires the use of either neutralizing antibodies, or utilisation of physical properties since IFN-γ specifically is both acid-labile and heat-labile. Recently radioimmunoassays (RIA) have been developed.

Studies of IFN in Rheumatological Diseases

Studies on levels of IFN-γ in RA and other rheumatological diseases, using paired samples of synovial fluid and serum, showed the highest incidence of detectable IFN-γ in RA [Cesario et al., 1983; Degre et al., 1983], but there was little correlation between synovial and serum levels. When a RIA rather than a biological assay was used, no IFN-γ was detected in either serum or synovial fluid from a variety of rheumatological conditions including RA [Ridley et al., 1986]. Production of IFN-γ by PBM cells from patients with RA has been shown to be defective when measured by bioassay [Hasler et al., 1986; Combe et al., 1985] but normal when assayed by RIA [Ridley et al., 1986]. On the other hand, measurement by RIA of IFN-α revealed both raised levels and an apparent insensitivity of peripheral blood mononuclear cells to IFN-α (as judged by an inhibitory effect on EBV-induced DNA synthesis) [Hasler et al., 1986]. The known actions of IFN-γ are compatible with this cytokine playing a significant role in synovial inflammation. One striking feature of the synovial membrane in RA is the increased expression of HLA-DR, especially on dendritic cells [Janossy et al., 1981] but also on synovial cells, fibroblasts and activated T and B cells. In vitro experiments have confirmed the effectiveness, in RA, of IFN-γ as an inducer of MHC expression; HLA DR+ synovial cells cultured without IFN-γ ceased transcription of mRNA for MHC class II gene products, and Ia expression became weak. Addition of IFN-γ to the culture system induced re-expression of MHC class II antigens [Pujol et al., 1985]. Therefore, IFN-γ could contribute to the perpetuation of the synovial immune response by inducing expression of HLA-DR which in turn would facilitate antigen presentation to helper T lymphocytes, so augmenting the stimulation of such cells and further production of IFN and other cytokines. The presumed homeostatic controls over this mechanism have not been elucidated. It is relevant that IFN-γ has been implicated in the initiation of other autoimmune diseases, especially those involving the thyroid gland [Bottazzo et al., 1983], by inducing HLA-DR expression on target cells – thyrocytes in the case of thyroiditis – so facilitating autoantigen presentation by these cells. The same model of induction by IFN-γ of aberrant expression of HLA-DR could pertain in RA. The above theories obviously depend on the presence of IFN-γ in affected joints; but as yet this has not been clearly established. It may be that new cytokines, with activities currently attributed to IFN-γ, such as the macrophage activating factor activity described by Andrew et al. [1984] may prove to be relevant to RA.

The sera of 50% of patients with SLE was shown to contain acid-labile IFN but the type was not defined [Prebble et al., 1982]. Others report difficulties in defining the IFN type present in serum of patients with SLE [Hooks et al., 1982], and in a further study a correlation existed between disease activity and IFN levels, but the characteristics of the IFN suggested it was IFN-α [Ytterberg and Schitzner, 1983]. Production in vitro of IFN-γ by stimulated PBM cells from most patients with SLE is normal [Sibbet et al., 1984] although a subgroup with deficient PHA-induced production of IFN-γ was observed by another group [Tsokas et al., 1982].

Colony-Stimulating Factors (CSFs)

Background

The colony-stimulating factors [Metcalf, 1984] comprise a group of glycoproteins that control the proliferation and differentiation of hemopoietic progenitor cells and which may be classified according to the specific lineages on which they exhibit their most obvious effects. Their characterization stemmed from the initial observation [Bradley and Metcalf, 1966; Ichikawa et al., 1966] that the growth of hemopoietic progenitor cells to form colonies in vitro depended on the presence of exogenous factors. The intervening 20 years have seen considerable progress in this field. Human granulocyte-macrophage CSF (GM-CSF), granulocyte CSF (G-CSF) and macrophage CSF (CSF-1, human urinary CSF) have been purified and their genes have been cloned and expressed [Nicola et al., 1979; Wong et al., 1985; Nicola et al., 1985; Nomura et al., 1986; Nagata et al., 1986; Kawasaki et al., 1985]. Unlike the murine counterpart (M-CSF), this last molecule has no direct proliferative effect on human macrophage progenitors but can stimulate the release of other CSFs from mature monocytes [Ishizaka et al., 1986]. At present human analogues of murine multi-lineage CSF (multi-CSF, interleukin-3) [Ihle et al., 1982; Cutler et al., 1985]; and eosinophil CSF (eosinophil differentiation factor) [Lopez et al., 1986a; Sanderson et al., 1986] have not been unequivocally identified but their existence is strongly suspected.

Biochemistry

The polypeptide backbone of GM-CSF contains 127 amino acids and has a molecular weight of 14 kDa (Wong et al., 1985]. Differences in glycosylation would account for the variable molecular weights of purified GM-CSF which have been reported. Purified recombinant GM-CSF produced from COS cells is glycosylated, has a molecular weight of 19 kDa and a specific activity of 4–16 × 10^7 U/mg protein [Metcalf et al., 1986a]. G-CSF is a relatively hydrophobic glycoprotein comprising 177 amino acids with a molecular weight of 19 kDa [Nagata et al., 1986]. From a comparison of known sequence data, it is probably closely-related to pluripoietin, which was initially thought to be the human analogue of murine multi-CSF [Welte et al., 1985]. Human urinary CSF, unlike the other known CSFs except for the homologous murine M-CSF, is a dimer and has a molecular weight of 45 kDa [Das and Stanley, 1982]. There is no significant homology between the protein-coding regions of different CSFs from the same species.

Sources and Actions

Known cellular sources of CSFs include activated T cells, macrophages, fibroblasts and endothelial cells which are all well-represented in the rheumatoid synovium. The potential importance of CSFs to the understanding of inflammatory joint diseases lies not in their ability to stimulate the proliferation of hemopoietic progenitor cells but in their ability to stimulate the functional activity of mature cells of the appropriate lineage [Vadas and Lopez, 1984]. The effects of GM-CSF on human peripheral blood neutrophils include enhancement of degranulation and superoxide production in response to chemotactic stimuli, increased antibody-dependent cytotoxicity and inhibition of migration [Gasson et al., 1984; Weisbart et al., 1985; Metcalf et al., 1986a; Lopez et al., 1986] which together would serve to trap and activate these cells at sites of inflammation. Similar examples of functional activation of murine macrophages by M-CSF [Hamilton et al., 1980] and GM-CSF [Handman and Burgess, 1979] have been described but human GM-CSF, in contrast to IFN-γ, failed to stimulate human macrophages to secrete H_2O_2 or kill toxoplasma [Nathan et al., 1984].

Assays

The standard assays for CSF depend on their characteristic property of inducing the clonal growth of colonies from single hemopoietic precursor cells in semi-solid agar or methylcellulose cultures. Usually, the concentration of stimulus which results in the growth of 50% of the maximum colonies is ascribed an activity of 50 U/ml, although other definitions have been used. Developments of the original assays include some which depend on the proliferation of factor-dependent cell lines, and the induction of differentiation in responsive cell lines, e.g. murine and human G-CSF acting on the myelomonocytic leukaemia cell line WEHI-3B D^+. For futher information about these assays, see Metcalf [1984].

CSFs Rheumatological Diseases

Colony-stimulating activity has recently been detected in synovial fluid and was shown to be CSF by demonstration of its direct proliferative action on hemopoietic progenitor cells. However, a range of assays indicated that it could not be attributed to any one of the known CSFs acting in isolation [Williamson et al., in preparation]. The presence of celluar sources and targets of CSF in relation to the inflammed joint and the detection of CSF in the synovial fluid, lend support to this putative pathogenic mechanism and it may be that CSFs have as important a role to play in activating effector cells at sites of inflammation as they do in controlling hemopoiesis in the bone marrow. Certainly one of the most striking consequences of injecting recombinant murine CSFs into the peritoneal cavity of mice was a marked increase in both the number of peritoneal monocytes/macrophages and their phagocytic capacity [Metcalf et al., 1986b].

Non-Immunological Effects of Cytokines

Fibrosis

The factors influencing fibroblast activity and which thereby determine fibrosis are complex. Fibroblasts are stimulated by products from T cells (including interferon-γ) and macrophages (IL-1), with ensuing collagen production. Recently, attention has been focussed on the interaction of mast cells and fibrosis [Claman, 1985]. Mast cells have been circumstantially closely associated with chronic fibrotic conditions [Fernex, 1986], and histamine present in mast cell granules has been shown to stimulate fibroblast growth [Russell et al., 1977]. There are increased numbers of mast cells in the synovium of patients with RA, and there is an association between the numbers of these cells and the level of inflammation [Crisp et al., 1984; Godfrey et al., 1984]. The role of the mast cell as a mediator of inflammation in the rheumatoid synovium has been recently reviewed [Wasserman, 1984].

In early scleroderma there has been shown to be an increased number of mast cells in involved skin compared to that of non-involved skin [Hawkins et al., 1985]. In vitro work has shown that supernatants from peripheral blood lymphocytes of patients with scleroderma selectively induce collagen stimulation [Cathcart and Krakauer, 1981]. A primary vascular hypothesis for the cause of scleroderma has been proposed [Campbell and Leroy, 1975] which sees the initial abnormality as excessive intimal fibroblast activity (see also section on IL-1). It is of interest therefore that lymphocyte supernatants from certain patients with scleroderma induce angiogenesis [Majewski et al., 1985] and that tumor angiogenesis factor produces a strong mast cell reaction. This may therefore provide an explanation for the inter-relationship of mast cells, angiogenesis and fibrosis in this disease.

Angiogenesis

The existence of tumor angiogenesis factor was postulated by Folkman who later isolated it and demonstrated its action in inducing new blood vessels in the chorioallantoic membrane assay [Folkman et al., 1983]. Angiogenesis factors have been found also in synovial fluid [Kumar et al., 1985]. Recently, a tumor angiogenesis factor has been purified and cloned [Fett et al., 1985]; it is a single chain basic protein with a molecular weight of 14.4 kDa. Studies using transmission electron microscopy of the synovium of rheumatoid arthritis joints have shown that there were similarities between the new vessels seen in tumors and those from synovium [Kumar et al., 1985]. An angiogenesis factor was isolated from the synovial fluids and was immunologically identical to tumor-angiogenesis factor but different from a macrophage angiogenesis factor. Hyaluronic acid was also found to be a powerful stimulator of neovascularization [West et al., 1985]. As abundant blood vessel formation is found in both rheumatoid arthritis and osteoarthritis, the clarification of the role of angiogenesis factor, which should occur with the use of recombinant angiogenin, will be of interest for rheumatology.

Osteoclast-Activating Factor

The biological activity of osteoclast activation is the final pathway by which bone destruction occurs and probably represents the net effect of a number of immune cell products. Recombinant preparations of lymphotoxin and tumor necrosis factor, which share 64% DNA homology [Pennica et al., 1984], and IL-1 all stimulate bone resorption in organ culture [Gowen et al., 1985]. However, work on disaggregated osteoclasts suggests that, in the case of IL-1 at least, this effect is indirect; IL-1-stimulating osteoclasts via 'short-range' signals released from osteoblasts [Thompson et al., 1985]. The nature of this signal is not resolved, although it is known that bone absorption induced by IL-1 is not significantly inhibited by blockade of arachidonic acid metabolism [Gowen et al., 1985a], and that IL-1 has both prostaglandin dependent and independent effects on bone formation [Canalis, 1985]. It has been suggested that colony-stimulating factors including GM-CSF may cause bone resorption as they increase differentiation of osteoclast precursor cells [MacDonald et al., 1985]. Finally, OAF activity induced by lymphokines can be inhibited by IFN-γ, whereas bone resorption mediated by parathormone and 1,25-hydroxy vitamin D_3 appears to be unaffected [Gowen et al., 1985b]. This indicates that there are two pathways mediating bone resorption. This could be particularly important clinically as inhibition of bone resorption is a major therapeutic aim in rheumatology.

Conclusion

The above review gives a selective and somewhat speculative interpretation of the role of what are judged to be the most important cytokines in rheumatological inflammation. Most published work has had to rely on less than ideal methodologies, predominantly bioassays. The advent of recombinant DNA technology, the cloning of the genes of these cytokines, and subsequent development of genetic probes will enable more precise information to be acquired. Consequently in this transitory period provisional data which may soon be superceded has not been dwelt upon at length; rather, new and in some cases unsubstantiated data has been reviewed to give signposts to the paths of future research.

There are several messages that are worthy of emphasis. First, and obviously, there are fundamental disturbances in the regulation of cytokines in the rheumatological disorders. Second, because of their actions, these cytokines must have a profound effect on the inflammatory processes in these diseases. Third, the characteristic cytokine profile of a disease will probably correspond to its clinical expressions – for example, the IL-1-induced muscle wasting, osteoporosis and acute phase response of RA in contrast to the absence of these features in SLE. Fourth, the identification of cytokine abnormalities provides the possibility of therapeutic intervention at a more fundamental level than has previously been possible.

References

Aarden, L. A.; Burner, T. K.; Cerrotini, J. C.; et al.; Revised nomenclature for antigen non-specific T cell proliferation and helper factors. J. Immun. *123:* 2928 (1979).

Aelion, J. A.; Endres, R. O.; Postlethwaite, A. E.: Characterisartion of an interleukin 1 inhibitor derived from human synovial fluid (Abstract). Arthritis Rheum. *28:* suppl. 79, D21 S79 (1985).

Alcocer-Varela, J.; Alarcon-Segovia, D.: Decreased production of and response to interleukin 2 by cultured lymphocytes from patients with systemic lupus erythematosus. J. clin. Invest. *69:* 1388–1392 (1982).

Alcocer-Varela, J.; Laffón, A.; Alarcón-Segovia, D.: Differences in the production of and/or the response to interleukin 2 by T lymphocytes from patients with the various connective tissue diseases. Rheumatol. Int. *4:* 39–44 (1984).

Alcocer-Varela, J.; Martinez-Codero, E.; Alarcon-Segovia, D.: Spontaneous production of and defective response to IL-1 by peripheral blood mononuclear cells from patients with scleroderma. Clin. exp. Immunol. *59:* 666–672 (1985).

Allison, A. C.; The interleukin-1 family of molecules. Bioessays *3:* 260–263 (1985).

Andrew, P. W.; Rees, A. D. M.; Scoging, A.; Dobson, N.: Secretion of a macrophage activating factor distinct from IFN-γ by human T cell clones. Eur. J. Immunol. *14:* 962–964 (1984).

Arend, W. P.; Joslin, F. G.; Massoni, R. J.: Effects of immune complexes on production by human monocytes of interleukin 1 or an interleukin 1 inhibitor. J. Immun. *134:* 3868–3875 (1985).

Arenzana-Seisdos, F.; Virchzier, J.L.; Fiers, W.: Interferons as macrophage activating factors. III. Preferential effects of interferon γ on the interleukin 1 secretory potential of fresh or aged human monocytes. J. immun. *134:* 2444–2449 (1985).

Bertolini, D.R.; Nedwin, G.; Bringman, T.: Evidence that recombinant human lymphotoxin possesses OAF activity (Abstract). Am. Soc. Bone Min. Res. *69* (1985).

Biondi, A.; Roach, J.A.; Schlossman, S.F.; Todd, R.F., III: Phenotypic characterisation of human T lymphocyte population producing macrophage activating factor (MAF) lymphokines. J. Immun. *133:* 281–285 (1984).

Bottazzo, G.F.; Pujol-Borrell, R.; Hanafusa, T.; Feldman, M.: Hypothesis: role of aberrant HLA-DR expression and antigen presentation the induction of endocrine autoimmunity. Lancet *ii:* 1115–1119 (1983).

Bradley, T.R.; Metcalf, D.: The growth of mouse bone marrow cells in vitro. Aust. J. exp. Biol. med. Sci. *44:* 287–300 (1966).

Brinckerhoff, C.E.; Guyre, P.M.: Increased proliferation of human synovial fibroblasts treated with recombinant immune interferon. J. Immun. *134:* 3142–3146 (1985).

Burmester, G.; Yu, D.T.Y.; Irani, A.M.; Kunkel, H.G.; Winchester, R.J.: Ia^+ T cells in synovial fluid and tissues of patients with rheumatoid arthritis. Arthritis Rheum. *24:* 1370–1376 (1981).

Campbell, P.M.; Leroy, E.C.: Pathogenesis of systemic sclerosis a vascular hypothesis. Semin. Arthritis Rheum. *4:* 351–368 (1975).

Canalis, E.: Interleukin-1 has prostaglandin dependent and independent effects on bone formation in vitro. Calcif. Tissue int. *84:* suppl. (1985).

Cathcart, M.K.: Krakauer, R.S.: Immunologic enhancement of collagen accumulation in progressive systemic sclerosis (PSS). Clin. Immunol. Immunopathol. *21:* 128–133 (1981).

Cathely, G.; Amor, B.; Kahan, A.; Fournier, C.: Abnormalities of IL-2 production and regulation in rheumatoid arthritis: relationship with disease activity (Abstract). Proc. Eur. Soc. Immunol. *26:* (1985).

Celada, A.; Schreiber, R.D.: Demonstration of a specific interferon-gamma (IFN-γ) receptor on human monocytes (mo), U937 and HL60 (Abstract). Fed. Proc. *44:* 1698 (1985).

Cesario, T.C.; Andrews, B.S.; Martin, D.A.; Jason, M.; Treadwell, T.; Friou, G.; Tilles, J.G.: Interferon in synovial fluid and serum of patients with rheumatic diseases. J. Rheumatol. *10:* 647–650 (1983).

Claman, H.N.: Mast cells, T cells and abnormal fibrosis. Immunol. Today *6:* 192–195 (1985).

Clowes, G.H.A., Jr.; George , B.C.; Villee, C.A., Jr.; Saravis, C.A.: Muscle proteolysis induced by a circulating peptide in patients with sepsis or trauma. New Engl. J. Med. *308:* 545–552 (1983).

Collins, T.; Korman, A.J.; Wake, C.T.; Boss, J.M.; Kappes, D.J.; Fiers, W.; Ault, K.A.; Gimbrone, M.A.; Strominger, J.L.; Prober, J.S.: Immune interferon activates multiple class II major histocompatibility complex genes and the associated invariant chain gene in human endothelial cells and dermal fibroblasts. Proc. natn. Acad. Sci. USA *81:* 4917–4921 (1984).

Combe, B.; Pope, R.M.; Fishbach, M.; Darnell, B.; Baron, S.; Talal, N.: Interleukin 2 in rheumatoid arthritis: production of and response to interleukin 2 in rheumatoid synovial fluid, synovial tissue and peripheral blood. Clin. exp. Immunol. *59:* 520–528 (1985).

Conlon, P.J.: A rapid biologic assay for the detection of interleukin 1. J. Immun. *131:* 1280–1282 (1983).

Crisp, A.J.; Chapman, C.M.; Kirkham, S.E.; Schiller, A.L.; Krane, S.M.: Articular mastocytosis in rheumatoid arthritis. Arthritis Rheum. *27:* 845–851 (1984).

Cutler, R.L.; Metcalf, D.; Nicola, N.A.; Johnson, G.R.: Purification of a multipotential colony stimulating factor from pokeweed mitogen-stimulated mouse spleen cell conditioned medium. J. biol. Chem. *260:* 6579–6587 (1985).

Das, S.K.; Stanley, E.R. Structure-function studies of a colony stimulating factor (CSF-1). J. biol. Chem. *257:* 13679–13684 (1982),

Dawes, P.T.; Fowler, P.D.; Clarke, S.; Fisher, J.; Lawton, A.; Shadforth, M.F.: Rheumatoid activities: treatment which controls the reactive protein and ESR reduces radiological progression. Br. J. Rheumatol. *25:* 44–49 (1986).

Degre, M.; Mellbye, O.J.; Clarke-Jenssen, O.: Immune interferon in serum and synovial fluid in rheumatoid arthritis and related disorders. Ann. rheum. Dis. *42:* 672–676 (1983).

Devos, R.; Plaetinck, G.; Cheroute, H.; Simons, G.; Degrave, W.; Tavernier, J.; Remout, E.; Fiers, W.: Molecular cloning of human interleukin 2 cDNA and its expression in *E. coli.* Nucl. Acid Res. *11:* 4307–4323 (1983).

Dinarello, C.A.: Interleukin-1 and the pathogenesis of the acute-phase response. New Engl. J. Med. *311:* 1413–1418 (1984).

Dinarello, C.A.; Bernheim, H.A.; Duff, G.W.; Le, H.V.; Nagabhushan, T.L.; Hamilton, N.C.; Coceani, F.: Mechanisms of fever induced by recombinant interferon. J. clin. Invest. *74:* 906–913 (1984).

Dingle, J.T.: The role of cellular interactions in joint erosions. Clin. Orthop. rel. Res. *182:* 24–30 (1984).

Duff, W.G.: Many roles for interleukin 1. Nature, Lond. *313:* 352–353 (1985).

Duff, W.G.; Atkins, E.: The detection of endotoxin by in vitro production of endogeneous pyrogen. Comparison with limulus amebocyte lysate gelation. J. Immunol. Methods *13:* 323–331 (1982).

Duff, G.W.; Forre, O.; Waalen, K.; Dickens, E.; Nuki, G.: Rheumatoid arthritis synovial dendritic cells produce interleukin 1. Br. J. Rheumatol. *24:* suppl. 1, pp. 94–97 (1985).

Durum, S.K.; Higuchi, C.; Ron, Y.: Accessory cells and T cell activation. The relationship between two components of macrophage accessory cell function Ia and IL-1. Immunobiology *168:* 213–231 (1984).

Duram, S.K.; Schmidt, J.A.; Oppenheim, J.J.: Interleukin 1. An immunological perspective. A. Rev. Immunol. *3:* 263–287 (1985).

Emery, P.; Panayi, G.S.; Nouri, A.M.E.: Interleukin 2 reverses deficient cell mediated immune responses in rheumatoid arthritis. Clin. exp. Immunol. *57:* 123–129 (1984a).

Emery, P.; Panayi, G.S.; Symmons, D.; Brown, G.: Mechanisms of depressed delayed type hypersensitivity in rheumatoid arthritis. The role of protein energy malnutrition. Ann. rheum. Dis. *43:* 430–434 (1984b).

Farrar, J.J.; Benjamin, W.R.; Hilfiker, M.L.; Farrar, W.L.; Fuller-Farrar, J.: The biochemistry, biology, and role of interleukin-2 in the induction of cytotoxic

T cell and antibody-forming B cell responses. Immunol. Rev. *63:* 129–166 (1982).

Feldman, M.; Essery, G.; Londei, M.; Austin, P.; Trowsdale, J.; Bodmer, W.; Lamb, J.R.: Role of IL-1 in the activation and inactivation of human T cell clones. Relevance to rheumatological disease. Br. J. Rheumatol. *24:* suppl. 1, pp. 102–104 (1985).

Fernex, M.: The mast cell system: its relationship to atherosclerosis fibrosis and eosinophils (Williams & Wilkins, Baltimore 1986).

Fett, J.W.; Strydom, D.J.; Lobb, R.R.; Alderman, E.M.; Bethune, J.L.; Riordan, J.R.; Vallez, B.L.: Isolation and characterisation of angiogenesis and angiogenic protein from human carcinoma cells. Biochemistry *24:* 5480–5486 (1985).

Finbloom, D.S.; Hoover, D.; Wahl, L.: Binding of human recombinant interferon gamma to its receptor on human monocytes and U937 and HL60 cell lines (Abstract). Clin. Res. *33:* 375A (1985).

Finter, N.B.: Interferon assays and standards, interferons, pp. 87–103 (North Holland, Amsterdam 1981).

Folkman, J.; Langer, R.; Linhardt, R.J.; Handenschild, C.; Taylor, S.: Angiogenesis inhibition and tumor regression caused by heparin or a heparin fragment in the presence of cortisone. Science *221:* 719–725 (1983).

Fontana, A.; Hengartner, H.; Weber, E.; Fehr, K.; Grob, P.J.; Cohen, G.: Interleukin 1 activity in the synovial fluid of patients with rheumatoid arthritis. Arthritis Rheum. *2:* 49–53 (1982).

Fox. I.R.; Theofilopoulos, A.N.; Altman, A.: Production of interleukin 2 (IL-2) by salivary gland lymphocytes in Sjogren's syndrome. Detection of reactive cells by using antibody directed to synthetic peptides of IL-2. J. Immun. *135:* 3109–3115 (1985).

Gasson, J.C.; Weisbart, R.H.; Kaufman, S.E.; Clark, S.C.; Hewick, R.M.; Wong, G.G.: Purified human granulocyte-macrophage colony-stimulating factor: direct action on neutrophils. Science *226:* 1339–1342 (1984).

Gehman, L.O.; Robb, R.J.: An ELISA-based assay for quantitation of human interleukin-2. J. immunol. Methods *16:* 39–47 (1984).

Gery, I.; Gershon, R.K.; Waksman, B.H.: Potentiating of the T lymphocyte response to mitogens. I. The responding cell. J. exp. Med. *136:* 128–142 (1972).

Gillis, S.: Interleukin-2. Biology and biochemistry. J. clin. Immunol. *3:* 1–13 (1983).

Gillis, S.; Mizel, S.B.: T-cell lymphoma model for the analysis of interleukin-1 mediated T-cell activation. Proc. natn. Acad. Sci. USA *78:* 1133–1137 (1981).

Godfrey, H.P.; Icardi, C.; Engber, W.; Graziano, F.M.: Quantitation of human synovial mast cells in rheumatoid arthritis and other rheumatic diseases. Arthritis Rheum. *27:* 852–885 (1984).

Gowen, M.; Nedwin, G.; Mundy, G.R.: Preferential inhibition of cytokine-stimulated bone resorption by recombinant interferon gamma (Abstract). Am. Soc. Bone Min. Res. *69:* (1985).

Gowen, M.; Russell, R.G.G.; Mundy, G.R.: Studies on the control of IL-1 stimulated bone resorption. J. Leucocyte Biol. *37:* 708 (1985a).

Gowen, M.; Wood, D.D.; Ihrie, E.J.; McGuire, M.K.B.; Russell, R.G.G.: An interleukin 1 like factor stimulates bone resorption in vitro. Nature, Lond. *306:* 378–380 (1983).

Gowen, M.; Wood, D. D.; Russell, R. G. G.: Stimulation of the proliferation of human bone cells in vitro by human monocyte products with interleukin-1 activity. J. clin. Invest. *75:* 1223–1229 (1985b).

Gray, P. W.; Leung, D. W.; Pennica, D.; Yelverton, E.; Najarian, R.; Simonsen, C. C.; Derynck, R.; Sherwood, P. J.; Wallace, D. M.; Berger, S. C.; Levinson, A. D.; Goeddel, D. V.: Expression of human immune interferon cDNA in E. coli and monkey cells. Nature, Lond. *295:* 503–508 (1982).

Green, D. R.; Chue, B.; Ferguson, T. A.; Beaman, K. D.; Flood, P. M.: Production of an antigen-specific component of suppressor inducer factor by a helper T-cell line. Possible role for IL-1 at the interface of immunity and tolerance. Br. J. Rheumatol. *24:* suppl. 1, pp. 105–111 (1985).

Gresser, I.: On the varied biologic effects of interferon. Cell. Immunol. *34:* 406–415 (1977).

Hamilton, J. A.; Stanley, E. R.; Brugess, A. W.; Shadduck, R. K.: Stimulation of macrophage plasminogen activator activity by colony-stimulating factors. J. Cell Physiol. *103:* 435–445 (1980).

Handman, E.; Burgess, A. W.: Stimulation by granulocyte-macrophage colony-stimulating factor of *Leishmania tropica* killing by macrophages. J. Immun. *122:* 1134–1137 (1979).

Hardt, C.; Rollinghoff, M.; Pfizenmeier, K.; Mosman, H.; Wagner, H.: Lyt $2\text{–}3^{+}$ cyclophosphamide-sensitive cells regulate the activity of an IL-2 inhibitor in vivo. J. exp. Med. *154:* 262–274 (1981).

Hawkins, R. A.; Claman, H. N.; Clark, R. A. F.; Steigerwald, J. C.: Increased dermal mast cell populations in progressive systemic sclerosis. A link in chronic fibrosis? Ann. intern. Med. *102:* 182–186 (1985).

Hasler, F.; Laubscher, A. H.; Rentsch, H. U.; Gerber, N. J.: Alpha interferon abnormalities in rheumatoid arthritis (Abstract). Br. J. Rheumatol. *25:* 118 (1986)

Henney, C. S.; Kuribayashi, K.; Kern, D. E.; Gillis, S.: Interleukin-2 augments natural killer cell activity. Nature, Lond. *291:* 335–338 (1981).

Hooks, J. J.; Moutsopoulos, H. M.; Geis, S. A.; Stahl, N. I.; Decker, J.; Notkins, A. L.: Immune interferon in the circulation of patients with autoimmune disease. New Engl. J. Med. *301:* 5–8 (1979).

Hooks, J. J.; Jordan, G. W.; Cupps, T.; Moutsopoulos, H.; Fauci, A. S.; Notkins, A. L.: Multiple interferons in the circulation of patients with systemic lupus erythematosus and vasculitis. Arthritis Rheum. *25:* 396–399 (1982).

Hooton, J. W. L.; Reindau, D.; Paetkau, V.: Is IL-2 regulated by a serum inhibitor. Cell. Immunol. *95:* 311–321 (1985).

Howard, M.; Matis, L.; Malek, T. R.; Shevach, E.; Kell, W.; Cohen, D.; Nakanishi, K.; Paul, W. E.: Interleukin-2 induces antigen-reactive T cell lines to secrete BCGF-1. J. exp. Med. *158:* 2024–2039 (1983).

Husby, G.; Williams, R. C., Jr.: Immunohistochemical studies of interleukin 2 and γ interferon in rheumatoid arthritis. Arthritis Rheum. *28:* 174–181 (1985).

Ichikawa, Y.; Pluznik, D. H.; Sachs, L.: In vitro control of the development of macrophage and granulocyte colonies. Proc. natn. Acad. Sci. USA *56:* 488–495 (1966).

Ihle, J. N.; Keller, J.; Henderson, L.; Klein, F.; Palaszynski, E.: Procedures for the purification of interleukin 3 to homogeneity. J. Immun. *129:* 2431–2436 (1982).

Inaba, K.; Ganelli-Piperno, A.; Steinman, R. M.: Dendritic cells induce T lymphocytes to release B cell-stimulating factors by an interleukin-2 dependent mechanism. J. exp. Med. *158:* 2040–2057 (1983).

Ishizaka, Y.; Motoyoshi, K.; Hatake, K.; Saito, M.; Takaku, F.; Miura, Y.: Mode of action of human urinary colony-stimulating factor. Exp. Hematol. *14:* 1–8 (1986).

Janossy, G.; Panayi, G.S.; Duke, O.; Bofill, M.; Poulter, L.; Goldstein, G.: Rheumatoid arthritis. A disease of T lymphocyte/macrophage immunoregulation. Lancet *ii:* 839–842 (1981).

Kampschmidt, R.F.: Leukocytic endogenous mediator/endogenous pyrogen; in Powanda, Canonico, The physiologic and metabolic responses of the host, pp. 55–75 (Elsevier/North Holland, Amsterdam 1981).

Kawasaki, E.S.; Ladner, M.B.; Wang, A.M.; Van Arsdell, J.; Warren, M.K.; Coyne, M.Y.; Schweickart, V.L.; Lee, M.-T.; Wilson, K.J.; Boosman, A.; Stanley, E.R.; Ralph, P.; Mark, D.F.: Molecular cloning of a complementary DNA encoding human macrophage-specific colony-stimulating factor (CSF-1). Science *230:* 291–296 (1985).

Kessler, D.A.; Langer, R.S.; Pless, N.A.; Folkman, J.: Mast cells and tumour angiogenesis. Int. J. Cancer *18:* 703–709 (1976).

Keystone, E.C.; Shore, A.; Jaglal, S.; Ramsden, M.; Lee, P.; Gladman, D.: IL-2 production by peripheral mononuclear cells from patients with diffuse scleroderma is enhanced and is highly correlated with extent of skin involvement (Abstract). Arthritis Rheum. *28:* suppl. D34 (1985).

Klaus, G.G.B.; Hawrylowicz, C.M.: Cell cycle control in lymphocyte stimulation. Immunol. Today *5:* 15–19 (1984).

Knobloch C.; Schlesier, M.; Drager, R.; Gartner, M.; Peter, H.H.: Quantitative absorption of interleukin 2 by peripheral blood and synovial fluid lymphocytes from patients with rheumatoid arthritis. Rheumatol. int. *5:* 133–139 (1985).

Konttinen, Y.; Bergroth, V.; Nykänen, P.: Lymphocyte activation in rheumatoid arthritis synovial fluid in vivo. Scand. J. Immunol. *22:* 503–507 (1985).

Kramer, M.D.; Koszinowski, U.H.: Regulatory counteraction to IL-2 activity. Lymphokine Res. *2:* 77–82 (1983).

Krane, S.M.; Goldring, S.R.; Dayer, J.M.: Interactions among lymphocytes, monocytes and synovial cells in the rheumatoid synovium. Lymphokines *9:* 75–136 (1982).

Kumar, P.; Erroi, A.; Sattar, A.; Kumar, S.: Weibel-Palade bodies as a marker for neovascularisation induced by tumor and rheumatoid angiogenesis factors. Cancer Res. *45:* 4339–4348 (1985).

Leibson, H.J.; Gefter, M.; Zlontnick, A.; Marrack, P.; Kappler, J.W.: Role of γ interferon in antibody producing responses. Nature, Lond. *309:* 799–801 (1984).

Lelchuk, R.; Playfair, J.H.L.: Serum IL-2 inhibitor in mice. I. Increase during infection. Immunology *56:* 113–118 (1985).

Leonard, W.J.; Depper, J.M.; Uchimaya, T.; Smith, K.A.; Waldmann, T.A.; Green, W.L.: A monoclonal antibody that appears to recognize the receptor for human T-cell growth factor; partial characterization of the receptor. Nature, Lond. *300:* 267–269 (1982).

Liao, Z.; Grimshaw, R.S.; Rosenstreich, D.C.: Identification of a specific interleukin 1 inhibitor in the urine of febrile patients. J. exp. Med. *159:* 126–136 (1984).

Linch, D.C.: Activated suppressor T cells and the role of interferon in aplastic anaemia. Immunol. Today *6:* 155–156 (1985).

Linker-Israeli, M.; Bakke, A.S.; Kitridou, R.C.; Gendler, S.; Gillis, S.; Horwitz, D.A.: Defective production of IL-1 and IL-2 in patients with SLE. J. Immun. *130:* 2651–2655 (1983).

Lomedico, P.T.; Gubler, U.; Hellmann, C.P.; Dukovich, M.; Giri, J.G.; Pan, Y.C.E.; Collier, K.; Semionow, R.; Chua, A.O.; Mizel, S.B.: Cloning and expression of murine interleukin-1 cDNA in E. coli. Nature, Lond. *312:* 458–462 (1984).

Lopez, A.F.; Begley, C.G.; Williamson, D.J.; Warren, D.J.; Vadas, M.A.; Sanderson, C.J.: Murine eosinophil differentiation factor. An eosinophil-specific colony stimulating factor with activity for human cells. J. exp. Med. *163:* 1085–1098 (1986).

Lopez, A.F.; Williamson, D.J.; Gamble, J.R.; Begley, C.C.; Harlan, J.M.; Klebanoff, S.J.; Waltersdorph, A.; Wong, G.; Clark, S.C.; Vadas, M.A.: A recombinant human granulocyte-macrophage colony-stimulating factor (rH GM-CSF) stimulates in vitro mature human neutrophil and eosinophil function, surface receptor expression and survival J. clin. Invest. (in press, 1986).

Lowenthal, J.W.; Zubler, R.H.; Nabholz, M.; MacDonald, H.R.: Similarities between IL-2 receptor number and affinity on activated B and T lymphocytes. Nature, Lond. *315:* 669–672 (1985).

Lund, H.; Egeland, R.: Immunoregulatory lymphokines in rheumatoid arthritis production of IL-2 in rheumatoid joints (Abstract). Scand. J. Immunol. *22:* 448 (1985).

MacDonald, B.R.; Mundy, G.R., Clark et al.: Recombinant human hemopoietic colony stimulating factor increases the number of osteoclast like cells in long-term marrow culture. Am. Soc. Bone Mineral Res. (abstract) *143* (1985).

Maeda, S.; Akahoshi, T.; Kashiwazaki, S.: Interleukin 1 and IL-1 inhibitor in the patients with rheumatoid arthritis. XVIth Int. Congr. Rheumatol., 1985, abstracts, P280, 258.

Majewski, S.; Scopinska-Rozewska, E.; Jablonska, S.; Polakowski, I.; Pawinska, M.; Marczak, M.; Szmurlo, A.; Modulatory effect of sera from scleroderma patients on lymphocyte-induced angiogenesis. Arthritis Rheum. *28:* 1133–1139 (1985).

Male, D.; Lelchuk, R.; Curry, S.; Pryce, G.; Playfair, J.H.L.: Serum IL inhibitor in mice. II. Molecular characteristics. Immunology *56:* 119–125 (1985).

Malkovsky, M.; Medawar, P.B.: Is immunological tolerance (non-responsiveness) a consequence of interleukin-2 deficit during the recognition of antigen. Immunol. Today *5:* 340–343 (1984).

March, C.J.; Mosley, B.; Larsena-Cerretti, D.P.; Braedt, G.; Price, V.; Gillis, S.; Henney, C.S.; Kronheim, S.R.; Grabstein, K.; Conlon, P.J.; Hopp, J.P.; Cosman, D.: Cloning sequence and expression of two distinct human interleukin-1 complementary DNAs. Nature, Lond. *315:* 641–647 (1985).

Metcalf, D.: The hemopoietic colony stimulating factors (Elsevier, Amsterdam 1984).

Metcalf, D.; Begley, C.G.; Johnson, G.R.; Nicola, N.A.; Vadas, M.A.; Lopez, A.F.; Williamson, D.J.; Wong, G.G.; Clark, S.C.; Wang, E.A.: Biologic properties in vitro of a recombinant human granulocyte-macrophage colony-stimulating factor. Blood *67:* 37–45 (1986a).

Metcalf, D.; Begley, C.G.; Johnson, G.R.; Nicola, N.A.; Lopez, A.F.; Williamson, D.J.: Effects of purified bacterially-synthesized murine multi-CSF (IL-3) on hemopoiesis in normal adult mice. Blood *68:* 46–57 (1986b).

Meuer, S.C.; Hussey, R.E.; Penta, A.C.; Fitzgerald, K.A.; Stadler, B.M.; Schlossmann, S.F.; Reinherz, E.L.: Cellular origin of interleukin-2 (IL-2) in man: evidence for stimulus restricted IL-2 production by$T4^+$ and $T8^+$ T lymphocytes. J. Immun. *129:* 1076–1079 (1982).

Miedema, F.; Melief, C.J.M.: T cell regulation of B cell activation: a re-appraisal of the role of IL-2. Immunol. Today *6:* 258–259 (1985).

Miyasaka, N.; Nakamura, T.; Russell, I.J.; Talal, N.: Interleukin-2 deficiencies in rheumatoid arthritis and systemic lupus erythematosus. Clin. Immunol. Immunopathol. *31:* 109–117 (1984).

Mizel, S.B.; Dayer, J.M.; Krane, S.M.; Mergenhagen. S.E.: Stimulation of rheumatoid synovial cell collagenase and prostaglandin production by partially purified lymphocyte activating factor (interleukin 1). Proc. natn. Acad. Sci. USA *78:* 2474–2477 (1981).

Morgan, D.A.; Ruscetti, F.W.; Gallo, R.: Selective in vitro growth of T lymphocytes from normal human bone marrows. Science *193:* 1007–1008 (1976).

Nagata, S.; Tsuchiya, M.; Asano, S.; Kaziro, Y.; Yamazaki, T.; Yamamoto, O.; Hirata, Y.; Kubota, N.; Oheda, M.; Nomura, H.; Ono, M.: Molecular cloning and expression of cDNA for human granulocyte colony-stimulating factor. Nature, Lond. *319:* 415–418 (1986).

Nathan, C.F.; Prendergast, T.J.; Wiebe, M.E.; Stanley, E.R.; Platzer, E.; Remold, H.G.; Welte, K.; Rubin, B.Y.; Murray, H.W.: Activation of human macrophages. Comparison of other cytokines with interferon-γ. J. exp. Med. *160:* 600–605 (1984).

Nicola, N.A.; Begley, C.G.; Metcalf, D.: Identification of the human analogue of a regulator that induces differentiation in murine leukaemic cells. Nature, Lond. *314:* 625–628 (1985).

Nicola, N.A.; Metcalf, D.; Johnson, G.R.; Burgess, A.W.: Separation of functionally distinct human granulocyte-macrophage colony-stimulating factor. Blood *54:* 614–626 (1979).

Nomura, H.; et al.: Eur. molec. Biol. Org. J. (Submitted).

Nouri, A.M.E.; Panayi, G.S.; Goodman, S.M.: Cytokines and the chronic inflammation of rheumatic disease. II. The presence of interleukin-2 in synovial fluid. Clin. exp. Immunol. *58:* 402–409 (1984).

Nouri, A.M.E.; Panayi, G.S.; Goodman, S.M.; Waugh, A.P.W.: Cytokines in Rheumatoid Arthritis: Production of IL-1. Br. J. Rheumatol. *24:* suppl. 1, pp. 191–196 (1985a).

Nouri, A.M.E.; Panayi, G.S.; Waugh, A.P.W.: Deficient IL-2 production by rheumatoid arthritis lymphocytes. XVIth Int. Congr. Rheumatology, 1985b, abstracts, F181, p. 140.

Pasternack, M.S.; Bevan, M.J.; Klein, J.R.: Release of discrete interferons by cytotoxic T lymphocytes in response to immune and non-immune stimuli. J. Immun. *133:* 277–280 (1984).

Pennica, D.; Nedwin, G.E.; Hayflick, J.S.; Seeburg, H.; Dcrynck, R.; Palladino, M.A.; Kohr, W.J.; Aggarwal, B.B.; Goeddel, D.V.: Human tumour necrosis factor. Precursor structure expression and homology to lymphotoxin. Nature, Lond. *312:* 724–729 (1984).

Perussia, B.; Dayton, E.T.; Lazarus, R.; Fanning, V.; Trinchieri, G.: Immune interferon induces the receptor for monomeric IgG1 on human monocytic and myeloid cells. J. exp. Med. *158:* 1092–1113 (1983).

Pfizenmaier, K.; Scheurich, P.; Daubener, W.; Kronke, M.; Rollinghoff, M.; Wagner, H.: Quantitative representation of all T cells committed to develop into cytoic effector cells and/or interleukin 2 activity-producing helper cells within murine T lymphocyte subsets. Eur. J. Immunol. *14:* 33–39 (1984).

Postlethwaite, A.E..; Lachman, L.B.; Mainardi, C.L.; Kang, A.H.: Interleukin-1 stimulation of collagenase production by cultured fibroblasts. J. exp. Med. *157:* 801-806 (1983).

Prebble, O.T.; Black, R.J.; Friedman, R.M.; Klippel, J.; Vilcek, J.: Systemic lupus erythematosus: presense in human serum of the unusual acid labile leukocytes interferon. Science *216:* 429–431 (1982).

Pujol, J.P.; Loyan, G.; Charron, D.J.: HLA-DR DQ and DP expression on synovial living cells from rheumatoid arthritis: A molecular and quantitative study (Abstract), Immunogenetics *22:* 135–136 (1985).

Pullar, T.; Capell, H.A.: Can treatment really influence the radiological progression of rheumatoid arthritis. Br. J. Rheumatol. *25:* 2–6 (1986).

Ridley, M.G.: Panayi, G.S.; Nicholas, N.S.; Murphy, J.: Mechanisms of macrophage activation in rheumatoid arthritis (RA) the role of interferon gamma. Clin. exp. Immunol. (in press, 1986).

Robb, R.J.: Interleukin-2. The molecule and its function. Immunol. Today *5:* 203–209 (1984).

Roifman, C. M.; Mills, G.B.; Chu, M.; Gelfand, E.N.: Functional comparison of recombinant interleukin-2 with IL-2 preparations derived from cultured cells. Cell. Immunol. *95:* 146–156 (1985).

Russell, J.D.; Russell, S.B.; Trupin, K,M.: The effect of histamine on the growth of cultured fibroblasts isolated from naval and keloid tissue. J. Cell Physiol. *93:* 389–393 (1977).

Saklatvala, J.; Curry, V.A.; Sarsfield, S.J.: Purification to homogeneity of pig leucocyte catabolin, a protein that causes cartilage resorption in vitro. Biochem. J. *215:* 385–392 (1983).

Sanderson, C.J.; O'Garra, A.; Warren, D.J.; Klaus, G.G. B.: Eosinophil differentiation factor also has B-cell growth factor activity. Proposed name interleukin-4. Proc. natn. Acad. Sci. USA *83;* 437–440 (1986).

Schmidt, J.A.; Mizel, S.B.; Cohen, D.; Green, I.: Interleukin-1, a potential regulator of fibroblast proliferation. J. Immun. *128:* 2177–2182 (1982).

Seigal, L.J.; Harper. M.E.; Wong-Staal, F.; Gallo, R.C.; Nash, W.G.; O'Brien, S.J.: Gene for T-cell growth factor. Location on human chromosome 4q and feline chromosome B1. Science *223:* 175–178 (1984).

Sibbitt, W.L.; Gibbs, D.L.; Kenny, C.; Bankhurst, A.D.; Searles, R.P.; Ley, K.D.: Relationship between circulating interferon and anti-interferon antibodies and impaired natural killer cell activity in systemic lupus erythematosus. Arthritis Rheum. *28:* 624–629 (1985).

Silver, R.M.; Redelman, D.; Zvaifler, N.J.: Studies of rheumatoid synovial fluid lymphocytes. II. A comparison of their behaviour with blood mononuclear cells in the autologous mixed lymphocyte reaction and response to TCGF. Clin. Immunol. Immunopathol. *27:* 15–27 (1983).

Silverman, H. A.; Johnson, J. S.; Vaughan, J. H.; McGlamory, J. C.: Altered lymphocyte reactivity in rheumatoid arthritis. Arthritis Rheum. *19:* 509–515 (1976).

Simon, P. L.; Laydon, J. T.; Lee, J. C.: A modified assay for interleukin-1. J. immunol. Methods *84:* 85–94 (1985).

Sipe, J. D.; Vogel, S. N.; Sztein, M. B.; Skinner, M.; Cohen, A. S.: The role of interleukin-1 in acute phase serum amyloid A and serum amyloid P biosynthesis. Ann. N. Y. Acad. Sci. *389:* 137–150 (1982).

Skjødt, H.; Crawford, A.; Elford, P. R.: Cyclosporin A modulates interleukin 1 activity on bone in vitro. Br. J. Rheumatol. (in press, 1986).

Smith, K. A.: T cell growth factor. Immunol. Rev. *51:* 337–357 (1980).

Taniguchi, T.; Matsui, H.; Fujita, T.; Takaoka, C.; Kashima, N.; Yoshimoto, R.; Hamuro, J.: Structure and expression of a cloned cDNA for human interleukin-2. Nature, Lond. *302:* 305–310 (1983).

Thompson, B. M.; Saklatvala, J.; Chambers, T. J.: The effect of pig interleukin-1 (catabolin) on bone resorption by osteoclasts disaggregated from rat bone. Br. J. Rheumatol. *24:* suppl. 1, pp. 140–142 (1985).

Trechsel, U.; Evequoz, B.; Hodler, B.; et al.: Similarity of the effects of 1,25 $(OH)_2D_3$ and retinoic acid on interleukin 1, 2 and 3 production. (abstract) Am. Soc. Bone Mineral Res. *279* (1985).

Trinchieri, G.: Matsumoto-Kobayashi, M.; Clark, S. V.; Sheera, J.; London, L.; Perussia, B.: Response of resting human peripheral blood natural killer cells to interleukin-2. J. exp. Med. *160:* 1147–1169 (1984).

Tsokos, G. C.; Rook, A. H.; Djeu, J. V.; Balow, J. E.: Natural killer cells and interferon responses in patients with systemic lupus erythematosus. Clin. exp. Immunol. *50;* 239–245 (1982).

Trinchieri, G.; Perussia, B.: Immune interferon. A pleiotropic lymphokine with multiple effects. Immunol. Today *6:* 131–136 (1985).

Uchiyama, T.; Nelson, D. L.; Fleisher, T. A.; Waldmann, T. A.: A monoclonal antibody (anti-Tac) reactive with activated and functionally mature human T cells. II. Expression of Tac antigen on activated cytotoxic killer T cells, suppressor cells, and on one of two types of helper T cells. J. Immun. *126:* 1398–1403 (1981).

Vadas, M. A.; Lopez, A. F.: Regulation of granulocyte function by colony-stimulating factors. Lymphokine Res. *3:* 45–50 (1984).

Wahl, S. M.; Gately, C. L.: Modulation of fibroblast growth by a lymphokine of human T cell and continuous T cell line origin. J. Immun. *130;* 1226–1230 (1983).

Wahl, S. M.; Wilder, R. L.; Katona, I. M.; Wahl, L. M.; Allen, J. B.; Scher, I.; Decker, J. L.: Leukopheresis in rheumatoid arthritis. Arthritis Rheum. *26:* 1076–1084 (1983).

Wasserman, S.: The mast cell and synovial inflammation. Arthritis Rheum. *27:* 841–844 (1984).

Waxman, J.; Lockshin, M. D.; Schnapp, J. J.; Doneson, I. N.: Cellular immunity in rheumatic diseases. I. Rheumatoid arthritis. Arthritis Rheum. *16:* 499–506 (1973).

Weinberg, J. B.; Hobbs, M. M.; Misukonis, M. M.: Recombinant human interferon induces human monocyte polykaryon formation. Proc. natn. Acad. Sci. USA *81:* 4554–4557 (1984).

Weisbart, R.H.; Golde, D.W.; Clark, S.C.; Wong, G.G.; Gasson, J.C.: Human granulocyte-macrophage colony-stimulating factor is a neutrophil activator. Nature, Lond. *314:* 361–363 (1985).

Welte, K.; Platzer, E.; Lu, L.; Garbilove, J. L.; Levi, E.; Mertelsman, R.; Moore, M.A.S.: Purification and biochemical characterization of human pluripotent hematopoietic colony-stimulating factor. Proc. natn. Acad. Sci. USA *82:* 1526–1530 (1985).

West, D.C.; Hampson, I.N.; Arnold, K.; Kumar, S.: Angiogenesis induced by degradation products of hyaluronic acid. Science *228:* 1324–1326 (1985).

Wheelock, E.F.: Interferon-like virus inhibitor induced in human leucocytes by phytohemagglutinin. Science *149:* 310–311 (1966).

Whiteside, T.L.; Worral, J.G.; Prince, R.K.; Buckingham. R.B.; Rodnan, G.P.: Soluble mediators from mononuclear cells increase the synthesis of glycosaminoglycan by dermal fibroblast cultures derived from normal subjects and progressive systemic sclerosis patients. Arthritis Rheum. *28:* 188–197 (1985).

Wilkins, J.A.; Warrington, R.J.; Sigurdson, S.L.; Rutherford, W.J.: The demonstration of an interleukin-2 like activity in the synovial fluid of rheumatoid arthritis patients. J. Rheumatol. *10:* 109–113 (1983).

Wong, G.G.; Witek, J.S.; Temple, P.A.; Wilkens, K.M.; Leary, A.C.; Luxenberg, D.P.; Jones, S.S.; Brown, E.L.; Kay, R.M.; Orr, E.C.; Shoemaker, C.; Golde, D.W.; Kaufman, R.J.; Hewick, R.M.; Wang, E.A.; Clark, S.C.: Human GM-CSF: molecular cloning of the cDNA and purification of the natural and recombinant proteins. Science *228:* 810–815 (1985).

Wood, D.D.; Ihrie, E.J.; Dinarello, C.A.; Cohen, P.L.: Isolation of an interleukin-1 like factor from human joint effusions. Arthritis Rheum. *26:* 975–983 (1983).

Wood, D.D.; Ihrie, E.J.; Hamerman, D.: Release of interleukin-1 from human synovial tissue in vitro. Arthritis Rheum. *28:* 853–862 (1985).

Woolf, A.D.; Nouri, A.M.E.; Woo, P.; Richter, M.B.; Panayi, G.S.; Gibson, T.: Interleukin-1 and the acute phase response in acute crystal synovitis. Br. J. Rheumatol. *24:* Suppl. 1, pp. 203–208 (1985).

Yoneda, T.; Mundy, G.R.: Prostaglandins are necessary for osteoclast activating factor production by activated peripheral blood leukocytes. J. exp. Med. *139:* 279–283 (1979).

Ytterberg, S.; Schnitzer, T.: Serum interferon levels in patients with systemic lupus erythematosus. Arthritis Rheum. *25:* 401–406 (1983).

Paul Emery, MD, Reid Memorial Laboratory, The Clinical Research Unit of The Walter and Eliza Hall Institute of Medical Research and The Royal Melbourne Hospital, Post Office, Royal Melbourne Hospital, Parkville,
Victoria 3050 (Australia)

Concepts Immunopathol. vol. 4, pp. 200–214 (Karger, Basel 1987)

Autoimmunity in Rheumatoid Arthritis

A Qualitative and Quantitative Approach to the Role of Ia Antigens[1]

Dominique Charron, Luc Teyton

Laboratoire d'Immunogénétique moléculaire, Département d'Hématologie du CHU Pitié Salpêtrière, Institut des Cordeliers, Paris, France

Introduction

Along with the immune disorders observed in the peripheral blood of patients with rheumatoid arthritis (RA) a variety of immune reactions take place within the synovial membrane and the synovial fluid which play a leading role in the destruction of the joints [1]. Hyperexpression of Ia antigens represents a feature common to both the adherent and nonadherent cell populations present in the synovium pannus of RA [2, 3]. In view of the central role of HLA molecules in inducing and regulating immune responses of all types [4], the study of HLA expression became pertinent to a better understanding of the mechanisms involved in the induction and perpetuation of the disease. Evidence has accumulated over the past 10 years to consider the HLA-D region in the human and its equivalent in the mouse, the I region, as controller of the immune response and the products of this region (the Ia antigens) as the effector molecules: such a pivotal role is further supported by the fact that Ia antigen expression is inducible and highly regulated in physiological as well as in pathological states [5, 6]. Aberrant and/or unexpected expression of Ia antigens on cells not normally expressing them has been documented in several autoimmune states in which it appears to be a driving force in the autoimmune process [7, 8].

[1] This work was supported by grants from Inserm, CNRS, LNCC, ARC. We thank S. Goyert, J. Silver, F. Bach for the gift of monoclonal antibodies and M. Brandel for expert secretarial assistance.

The HLA-D region is vastly more complex than originally thought. At least, three subregions are recognized, namely HLA-DR, DQ and DP each encoding one or several transmembrane MHC class II glycoproteins composed of a 34-Kdalton alpha-chain noncovalently associated with a 28-Kdalton beta-chain [9]. Moreover, the observed differential expression of DR, DQ, and DP molecules in different cell types and/or activation states may reflect subtle differences in their functions [10,11]. It is thus critical in evaluating the role of Ia antigens in pathological states to take fully into account both the qualitative and quantitative aspects of their molecular expression in the involved tissues.

The importance of HLA class II antigens in RA is further emphasized by the finding that particular haplotypes of the HLA-D region contain susceptibility genes which increase the relative risk for the disease [12]. One can therefore postulate the presence of unique response gene within the HLA-D region which is the basis for the disease susceptibility by allowing recognition of foreign or autoantigen. This in turn would produce a proliferation and/or cytotoxic state leading to the lesional attack of the tissues in which the process takes place. Indeed, class II antigens can be considered either as target antigen or restriction element for foreign (and auto) antigen (or both) and their expression may be essential in altering the immune responses toward autoimmunity. However, one should not only consider the causative effect of Ia expression since it could also represent a secondary effect beneficial in eliminating infected or autoreactive cells.

In this article we will provide an interpretative review of some of the data concerning the influence of the HLA-D region in disease susceptibility to RA and the expression of Ia antigens in RA and will present an in vitro model of cultured synovial lining cells which offers a new tool to investigate the rôle of HLA class II molecules in the physiopathology of RA and possibly in evaluating future therapeutic approaches.

HLA Class II Haplotypes and Susceptibility to RA

The genetic polymorphism of the HLA-D region has been extensively studied in recent years in normal and patient populations. Initially defined by a cellular technique, the mixed lymphocyte reaction [13], the HLA-D region antigens were subsequently recognized on B lymphocytes by selected alloantisera which allowed serological analysis to be performed on large groups of individuals [14]. Association of RA was initially shown in a Caucasian with DR4 [15] (serologically defined antigen) as well as with DW4 (the corresponding cellular specificity) [16]. DR4 was present in 75% of patients with RA for a normal frequency around 25% leading to a relative risk over 4. In addition to DR4, and particularly in non-Caucasians, DR1 was shown to be potentially important in marking susceptibility to RA [17]. In recent work, Duquesnoy et al. [18] have defined a new serological specificity named MC1 (a determinant in strong linkage desequilibrium with DR1 and DR4 in the normal population) which is significantly increased in RA in adults (93.5% vs. 47% in controls) leading to a relative risk of 16.1. The MC1 epitope represents thus far the strongest disease-associated determinant in RA and this is not only in Caucasians but also in Blacks. It would be of great interest to study other ethnic populations such as Ashkenazi Jewish patients (which display a significant increase of DR1 without an increase of DR4) to determine whether or not the high frequency of DR1 reflects an even higher frequency of MC1 (which is in strong linkage desequilibrium with DR1). In such cases the MC1 determinant should be considered as the closest to the true disease-susceptibility gene in RA. It remains to be determined which gene encodes and which class II molecule bears the MC1 epitope. The data on MC1 illustrate how a more precise definition of epitopes (here obtained by serological analysis) allows delineation of the RA-specific immune response gene.

Such a goal can also be approached by cellular and molecular methods. The HLA-DR haplotypes have been further subdivided by mixed lymphocyte reaction (MLR) typing in at least five cellular clusters namely DW4, DW10, DW13, DW14, DW15, and preferential association of RA was demonstrated to occur with one of these DW types: DW4 [19]. All together the serological and cellular data imply that the DR4 haplotypes are strongly implicated in the association. Since the genes and the products of the genes of these various DR4 haplotypes are not yet completely identified and because of a strong linkage desequilibrium between loci, it is still too early to identify with certainty the 'RA' specific determinant(s), its sequence and the class II product(s) on which it is expressed. However, biochemistry and molecular biology technics have provided, over the past years, some insights to these questions. Two-dimensional gel electrophoresis (2D PAGE) of MHC class II molecules is able to recognize distinct HLA D region products [20, 21] and detects molecular variants within complex haplotypes [22, 23]. Extensive studies by

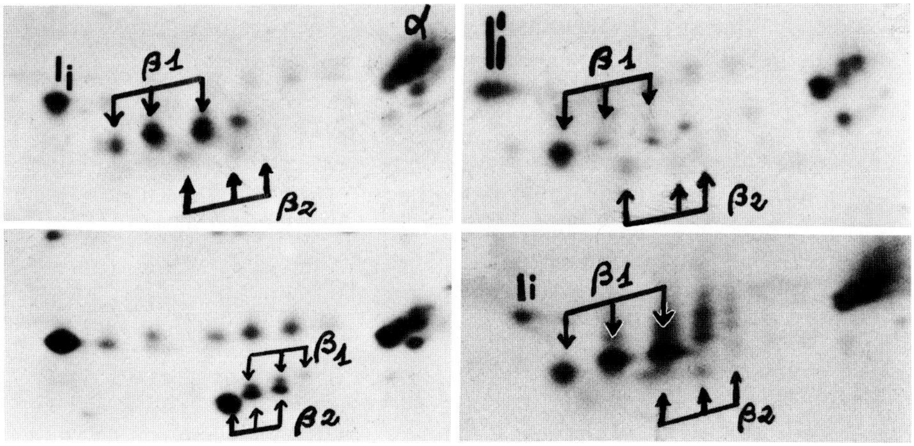

a b c d

Fig. 1. 2D PAGE of HLA DR molecules from a DR4/DW4 homozygous cell line from a patient with RA *(a)*. Two DR β-chains are observed (DRβ1 and DRβ2) associated with the α-chain. The DRβ2-chain is common to several other DR4 subtypes while the DRβ1-chain varies in these subtypes. As shown in panel *(b)* the DR4/DW10 β1-chain is more acidic while the DR4–DW15 β1-chain is slightly more basic *(c)*, the DRβ2-chain is also present in DR7/DW7 individuals as shown in *(d)*. The DRβ-chain commonly associated with RA is the DRβ1-chain shown in *(a)*.

Nepom et al. [24] using the resolving power of 2D PAGE have revealed the existence of five distinct DR β chains and three DQβ-chains among HLA-DR 4 haplotypes. The complexity and the diversity of the various HLA-DR haplotypes is increased at the product level by the number of expressed DRα-β-complexes. Some haplotypes may express only one DR molecule (DRαβ1) others two (DRαβ1 + DRαβ2) and even three (DRαβ1 + DRαβ2 + DRαβ3). As shown in figure 1, two DRβ-chains can be detected in the 2D gel patterns from two distinct DR4 homozygous cells belonging to two distinct DW subtypes (DW4 and DW15). The DRβ1-chain is electrophoretically different in the two cells while the DRβ2-chain which is more weakly expressed is common to the two cells. Additionally, this same DRβ2-chain can be detected in DR7 cells and thus is likely not to be relevant by itself for increased susceptibility to RA since no association has been documented with DR7 in this disease. Whether the DRβ1-chain is the critical element in the increased susceptibility to RA is debatable. In fact, the immune response gene effect may require the presence of one chain in association with another yet unknown element encoded within the same haplotype (CIS association) or in the other haplotype (TRANS complementation). Such a model may be proposed in the case of seropositive juvenile rheumatoid arthritis (JRA). Although clinically different from adult RA, seropositive JRA is strongly associated with DR4 with a relative risk over 7. This association has been recently investigated at the structural level. 2D PAGE analysis of seropositive JRA reveals a very restricted pattern for DRβ- and DQβ-chains which contrast with the heterogeneity found in the unselected normal population [25]. These data suggest that these molecular variants might play a role in disease susceptibility while the DR4 determinant (serologically defined) by itself is not an important marker for the disease. A more intriguing observation in this study comes from the analysis of HLA-DR homozygous individuals with JRA. While the patients are serologically homozygous (DR4/DR4), most of them are heterozygous by cellular (DW) typing and biochemical (2D PAGE) analysis [25]. The preponderance of DW4/DW10 patients results in an enormous heterozygous effect for disease susceptibility since DW4/DW10 individuals present a relative risk of 116 while it is much lower for DW4 or DW10 individuals. A similar situation is known for susceptibility to insulin dependent diabetes mellitus (IDDM) with early onset in which the relative risk for DR3/4 heterozygotes is vastly greater than for either DR3 or DR4 homozygous [26]. These results in the two diseases strongly suggest that combinatorial determinants contribute to the increased susceptibility. Indeed, hybrid class II molecules can be formed in heterozygous individuals by the associative combination of an α-chain from one haplotype and a β-chain from the other haplotype [27]. We have demonstrated this phenomenon to occur for DQ molecules in several haplotypic combinations [28, Teyton and Charron, unpubl.]. The number of such hybrid molecules, which may vary depending on both composing haplotypes, as well as the type of new determinants created de novo by this mechanism would explain the heterozygous effect observed. Moreover, hybrid determinants may be spatially mimicked by other hybrid determinants, a situation impossible to predict from serology data. This could account for the cases in which the DR4 haplotype is not present in the case of RA. It is not known whether some cells or tissues may allow more hybrid molecules to be formed and whether lymphokines which regulate class II expression affect the balance of hybrid vs orthodox class II molecules. These possibilities are presently studied using quantitative analysis of class II molecules in stimulated cell populations as well as in cells transfected with class II genes.

An additional tool was introduced a few years ago in the field of HLA and disease: genomic DNA digested with restriction enzymes generates restriction fragments which can be probed after electrophoresis with specific HLA class II probes. Polymorphism of these fragments (RFLP) are intensively studied for disease association purposes. At the present time no data is available in RA but it is predictable that one or several 'allogenotopes' [29] will be identified which will circumscribe the involved RA susceptibility genes. Whether these RA specific RFLP patterns will represent the coding sequence for RA specific epitopes or involve noncoding sequence (introns or pseudogenes) will be determinant in understanding their pathophysiological relevance. In any case it will remain of critical importance to evaluate the RA specific epitopes at the level where they operate by cellular and biochemical approaches.

HLA Class II Expression in RA

Since several aspects of HLA class II antigen expression appear to be disturbed in RA, it is likely that class II expression contributes by itself to the abnormal immune response in this disease.

Aberrant expression of Ia antigens on nonimmune cells not expressing Ia antigens normally, increased Ia expression on cells normally Ia-positive, and differential expression of the three distinct HLA class II subsets (DR, DQ and DP) have all been documented in RA using cell surface detection by monoclonal anti-HLA class II antibodies, either on isolated cells or tissues. Previous reports have shown that *firstly* the percentage of Ia-positive peripheral T cells is higher in RA than in normal individuals [30]. *Secondly,* hyperexpression of class II is detected locally in the synovial pannus by immunohistochemical methods [3]. These two features could be related to the ability of synovial tissue from RA to induce with high efficiency MLR and AMLR [31].

A better understanding of the involvement of class II antigens in RA requires more precise assessment of the quantitative and qualitative biochemical aspects of MHC class II expression in the involved tissues.

For this purpose we have developed an in vitro culture system for non-adherent synovial cells.

Synovial membranes are harvested during hip or knee joint arthroplasty replacement. The synovium is individualized by dissection with microsurgical tools, minced and dissociated by enzymatic treatment. Adherent and nonadherent synovial lining cells were separated at 24 h of culture. We used only primary cultures which yield limited size samples ($5-15 \times 10^5$ cells) and are heterogenous, containing three main populations of cells: fibroblast-like cells (40–60 %), dentritic-like cells (30–50 %) and macrophages (10–20 %). To study the quantitative aspect of Ia expression on such size-limited samples, particular techniques were needed.

We have developed Western-blot and dot immunobinding assays for proteins [32] and quick-blot for m-RNAs [33] using HLA class II specific monoclonal antibodies (Mab) able to discriminate DR, DQ and DP molecules, and a battery of cDNA probes specific for α- or β-chains of DR, DQ or DP gene, and for the invariant chain (Ii) [34].

As demonstrated by immunocytochemistry at 24 h of culture, all three HLA-D region products were expressed on ASLC from normal donors (20–40 % of positive cells) or from RA patients (40–65 % of positive cells). As shown in figure 2 by Western-Blot and by quick-blot both normal and RA ASLC expressed Ia antigens. Considering the level of Ia antigen expression, a clear-cut difference between normal and RA synovial cells is observed. Thus, a quantitative increase of class II antigens is one important feature of RA ASLC. No dissociation of DR, DQ, DP expression was observed either at the mRNA or at the protein levels in normal and RA ASLC and thus it is unlikely that DR, DQ and DP have distinct functions in ASLC.

Despite a quantitative difference, the kinetics of disappearance of Ia antigens were the same on normal or RA ASLC. Ia proteins and Ia-specific mRNAs became undetectable at day 4 by the methods we used. At the same time the level of expression of HLA class I antigens appreciated by the binding of the W6-32 MoAb (directed against monomorphic determinants of HLA A, B and C) on ASLC was dramatically decreased. This coordinated down-regulation of all the HLA products was also evidenced by radioactive synthetic labeling and immunoprecipitation.

Fig. 2. Kinetic of disparition of HLA class II expression on adherent synovial lining cells (ASLC).
a Western blot technique: Cell lysate from 5×10^5 was run in each track of a 10.5 % SDS-PAGE gel in denaturing conditions and transferred on a nitrocellulose sheet (12 V/h, 16h). After a saturation step (1 h, 3 % BSA-TBS) the incubation was done overnight with two anti class II monoclonal antibodies (Mab): SG-520 specific for β-chain and DA-6-147 specific for α-chains. The binding was revealed by a biotinylated antimouse antibody and a peroxidase labeled streptavidine complex (Amersham).

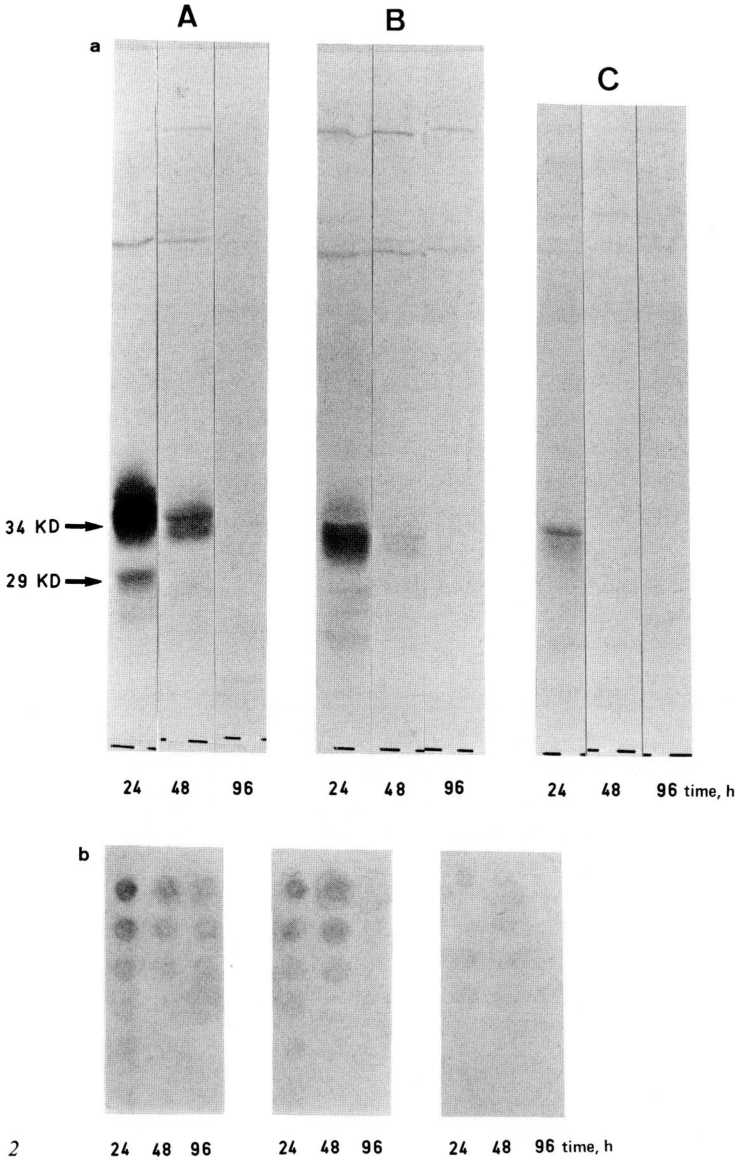

2

b Quick-blot mRNA technique: Serial dilutions of cell extract (starting from 2.5×10^5 cells by spot) were mixed with 12.2 *M* sodium iodide and spotted onto a nitrocellulose sheet. The specific hybridization was done (as in Northern-blot) with a DQ-alpha-chain-specific c-DNA probe (p DCH 1). A, B = Rheumatoïd arthritis; C = arthrotics patient.

Table I. IFN γ production by nonadherent synovial lining cells tested on Wish cells

Case No.	NS	PHA	PMA	PHA+PMA
RA				
1	< 3	96	<3	384
2	< 3	6	< 3	24
3	< 3	18	< 3	48
OA 4	< 3	48	< 3	144
5	< 3	4,5	< 3	36

NS = nonstimulated; RA = rheumatoid arthritis; OA = osteoarthritis.

From these first data we could conclude that in vivo HLA expression on ASLC is controlled by positive signals which disappear in in vitro culture. Although we are not yet able to identify the lymphokines which are active in vivo both in normal and in RA synovial membrane, interferon gamma (IFN γ) appears as a likely candidate. We therefore investigated IFN γ production by non-adherent synovial cells as shown in table I. While no IFN γ could be detected in the basal state IFN γ production was obtained after co-stimulation by PHA and PMA of the nonadherent cell population. Since IFN γ may be one of the in vivo acting lymphokines, we used it as an in vitro agent able of inducing Ia antigen in further studies. The IFN γ used was fully comparable with human IFN γ because its production was carried out in mammalian cells (chinese hamster ovary cells). Similar to that found in many systems, IFN γ at doses higher than 5 IU/ml was able to induce HLA class II mRNAs from Ia-negative ASLC (fig. 3) and to stimulate the transcription of HLA class I genes. Maximal effects were obtained for doses over 100 IU/ml.

Two features were important to notice:

firstly, all the three HLA-D products were induced by IFN γ and exhibited a similar sequence of appearance as well as Ii mRNA,

secondly, in the large number of cases we have tested, the maximum level of Ia expression reached, for a similar dose of IFNγ, was identical if the synovium came from normal individuals, arthritic patients or RA.

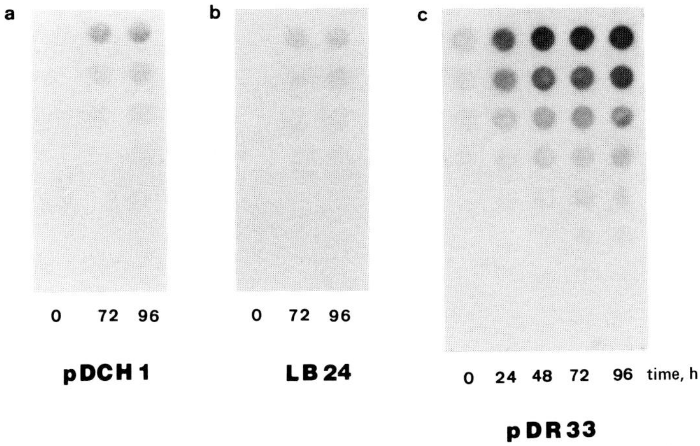

Fig. 3. Induction of specific HLA class II mRNA by IFN γ (50 UI/ml) on Ia-negative ASLC, tested by quick blot mRNA technique. *a* pDCH 1: Specific cDNA probe for DQ alpha-chain. *b* LB-24: Specific cDNA probe for DP alpha-chain. *c* p33DR: Specific cDNA probe for invariant chain. Serial dilutions (1:2) starting from 2.5×10^5 cells were spotted on nitrocellulose membrane (BA 85, Schleicher and Schuell).

Thus, the responsiveness to IFNγ is the same for all the ASLC and the ability to synthesize high levels of Ia antigens appears not to be a particular intrinsic property of ASLC from RA.

Qualitative appreciation of class II antigens was examined by 2D gel electrophoresis of immunoprecipitated radioactively labeled material. Using the opportunity of inducing Ia antigens, we were able to perform biochemical analysis of HLA class II molecules synthesized in ASLC. As control we used the PBL (Ficoll-Hypaque separated cells) from the same donor and processed in the same way.

ASLC and PBL were stimulated in culture by IFN γ at a dose of 50 IU/ml, for 4 days and labeled for 16 h by ^{35}S-methionine. Immunoprecipitation and 2D gels were carried out as previously reported [35]. The concluding remarks of this biochemical analysis are that α- and β-chains exhibit the same pattern on ASLC as on PBL, while the most basic spots of invariant chain are abnormally sialylated on ASLC compared with PBL (fig. 4).

As the invariant chain is clearly involved in transport to the membrane and in the glycosylation of α- and β-chains of Ia antigens, as re-

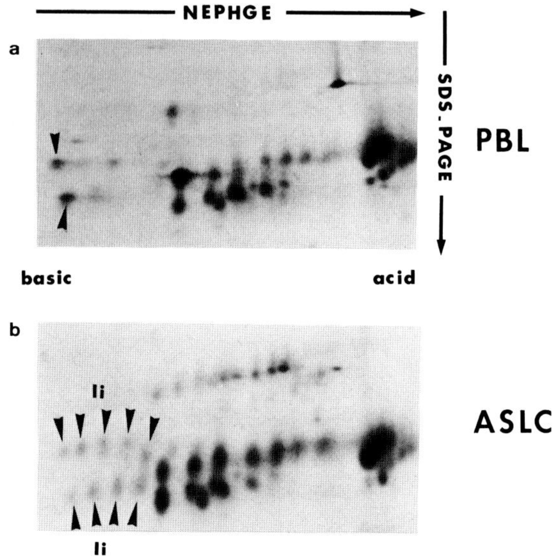

Fig. 4. 2D gel dectrophoresis analysis of HLA class II antigens expressed under IFN γ induction on PBL and ASLC from a rheumatoid arthritis patient. After 96 h of IFN γ stimulation (50 IU/ml) the cells were labeled with ^{35}S-methionine for 16 h and lysed in 0.5% NP 40. Immunoprecipitation was done by staphylococcus A after the binding of a specific anti-HLA class II Mabs *(a, b)* SG-520. The first dimension was a nonequilibrium pH gradient gel electrophoresis; the second dimension was a 10% polyacrylamide SDS-PAGE gel. Dried gels were exposed with X-Omat S film (Kodak) for 1 week. Class II molecules from PBL constituted the internal control. Arrows indicate the additional spots of invariant chain shown on ASLC.

cently demonstrated [36], such abnomalies of Ii chain on ASLC could lead to an impaired process of Ia antigens, particularly of their glycosylations. We are presently investigating this point especially in the view that glycosylations of Ia antigens could be discriminated by T cells [37] and that Ia glycosylation differences have been observed in different cell types [38].

A recently described feature of the biochemistry of HLA class II antigens is of great speculative interest in rheumatic diseases.

A proteoglycan of considerable size heterogeneity (MW = 40,000–70,000) was shown to be associated with Ia antigens [39]. This molecule belongs to the chondroitin-sulfate (CS) class of proteoglycans and its core protein is the invariant chain itself. The biological significance of this alternatively processed form of Ii is not known but it could be related to the secretion of CS proteoglycan of small size (CS = 70,000–170,000) by lymphocytes and monocytes [40]. Since the chondrocytes, which were shown to be Ia positive in certain diseases [41], particularly RA, specialize in cartilage chondroitin sulfate synthesis, this could interfere with Ii processing and function and possibly with Ia metabolism.

Concluding Remarks

The long-term postulated role of Ia antigens in immunopathology and autoimmunity begins to be progressively demonstrated in both in vivo and in vitro models. Genetic, cellular and molecular tools have been developed recently which allow more precise elucidation of the functions and molecular diversity of class II antigens. In this context it becomes increasingly important not only to detect class II expression at the cell surface but to quantitate expression and biosynthesis for the various molecular forms of class II molecules and analyze the post translational modifications (glycosylation, acylation, phosphorylation) and the various associated molecules (invariant chain, proteoglycan, membrane receptors) in the involved tissues. Each of these parameters may affect the impact of HLA class II molecules in induction and perpetuation of the disease. Moreover, such approaches are critical in evaluating in the future a possible beneficial effect of anti-Ia therapy as first proposed and demonstrated in murine models by H. O. McDevitt.

References

1 Janossy, G.; Duke, O.; Poulter, L.W.; Panayi, G.; Boffil, M.; Goldstein, G.: Rheumatoïd arthritis. A disease of T-lymphocyte/macrophage immunoregulation. Lancet *Oct. 17:* 839 (1981).

2 Burmester, G.R.; Yu, D.T.; Irami, A.M.; Kunkel, H.G.; Winchester, R.J.: Ia+ T cells in synovial fluid and tissues of patients with rheumatoïd arthritis. Arthritis Rheum. *24:* 1370 (1981).

3 Lindbla, D.S.; Klareskog, L.; Hedfors, E.; Forsum, U.; Sundstrom, C.: Phenotypic characterization of synovial tissue cells in situ in different types of synovitis. Arthritis Rheum. *26:* 1321 (1983).

4 Dausset, J.: The major histocompatibility complex in man. Science *213:* 1469 (1981).

5 King, D.; Jones, P.: Induction of Ia and H2 antigens on a macrophage cell line by immune interferon. J. Immun. *131:* 315 (1983).

6 Radka, S.; Charron, D.J.; Brodsky, F.: Class II molecules of the major histocompatibility complex considered as differentiation markers. Human Immunol. (in press, 1986).

7 Bottazzo, G.F.; Pujol-Borell, R.; Hanafusa, T.: Rôle of aberrant HLA DR expression and antigen presentation in induction of endocrine auto immunity. Lancet *Nov. 12:* 1115 (1983).

8 Londei, M.; Lamb, J.; Bottazzo, G.; Feldmann, M.: Epithelial cells expressing aberrant MHC class II determinants can present antigen to cloned human T cells. Natur, Lond. *312:* 639 (1984).

9 Kaufmann, J.F.; Auffray, C.; Korman, A.J.; Shackelford, D.A.; Strominger, J.: The class II molecules of the human and murine major histocompatibility complex. Cell *36:* 1 (1984).

10 Gonwa, T.A.; Picker, L.J.; Raff, H.V.; Goyert, S.M.; Silver, J.; Stobo, J.D.: Antigen presenting capabilities of human monocytes correlates with their expression of HLA-DS, an Ia determinant distinct from HLA-DR. J. Immun. *130:* 706 (1983).

11 Faille, A.; Turmel, P.; Charron, D.J.: Differential expression of HLA-DR and HLA-DC/DS molecules in a patient with hairy cell leukemia. Restoration of HLA-DC/DS expression by (12-0-tetradecanoyl phorbol-13-acetate), 5-acacytidine, and sodium butyrate. Blood *64:* 33 (1984).

12 Dausset, J.; Svejgaard, A.: HLA and disease (Munksgaard, Copenhagen 1976).

13 Bach, F.H.; Voynow, N.K.: One way stimulation in mixed leucocyte cultures. Science *153:* 545 (1966).

14 Winchester, R.J.; Fu, S.; Wernet, P.; Kunkel, H.G.; Dupont, B.; Jersild, C.: Recognition by pregnancy serums of non HLA-A allo antigens selectively expressed on B lymphocytes. J. exp. Med. *141:* 924 (1975).

15 Stasny, P.: Association of the B cell allo antigen DRW4 with rheumatoïd arthritis. New Engl. J. Med. *298:* 869 (1978).

16 McMichael, A.J.; Sasasuki, T.; McDevitt, H.O.: Increased frequency of HLA-CW3 and HLA DW4 in rheumatoïd arthritis. Arthitis Rheum. *20:* 1037 (1977).

17 Christiansen, F.T.; Kelly, H.; Dawkins, R.L.: Rheumatoïd arthritis; in Albert et al. Histocompatibility testing 1984, p. 378 (Springer, Berlin 1984).

18 Duquesnoy, R.J.; Marrari, M.; Hackbarth, S.; Zeevi, A.: Serological and cellular definition of a new HLA-DR associated determinant MC1, and its association with rheumatoïd arthritis. Human Immunol. *10:* 165 (1985).

19 Zoschke, D.; Segall, M.: DW subtypes of DR4 in rheumatoïd arthritis. Evidence for a preferential association with DW4. Human Immunol. *15:* 118 (1986).

20 Charron, D.J.; McDevitt, H.O.: Characterization of HLA DR region antigens by two dimensional gel electrophoresis: molecular genotyping. J. exp. Med. *152:* 18s (1980).

21 Goyert, S.; Shively, J.E.; Silver, J.: Biochemical characterization of a second family of human Ia molecules HLA-DS, equivalent to murine I-A sub-region molecules. J. exp. Med. *156:* 550 (1982).

22 Groner, J.; Watson, A.; Bach, F.H.: DW/LD related molecular polymorphism of DR4 β-chains. J. exp. Med. *157:* 1687 (1983).

23 Haziot, A.; Lepage, V.; Freidel, A.; Betuel, L.; Degos, L.; Charron, D.J.: Biochemistry of HLA-DRw6: Evidence for seven distinct haplotypes. J. Immun. (in press, 1986).
24 Nepom, G.T.; Nepom, B.S.; Antonelli, P.; Mickelson, E.; Silver, J.; Goyert, S.M.; Hansen, J.A.: The HLA-DR4 family of haplotypes consists of a series of distinct DR an DS molecules. J. exp. Med. *159:* 394 (1984).
25 Nepom, B.; Nepom, G.; Mickelson, E.; Schaller, J.; Antonelli, P.; Hansen, J.: Specific HLA-D-R4 associated histocompatibility molecules characterize patients with sero positive juvenile rheumatoïd arthritis. J. clin. Invest. *74:* 287 (1984).
26 Svejgaard, A.; Platz, P.; Ryder, L.P.: HLA and disease 1982. A survey. Immunol. Rev. *70:* 193 (1983).
27 Jones, P.P.; Murphy, D.B.; McDevitt, H.O.: Two gene control of the expression of a murine Ia antigen. J. exp. Med. *148:* 925 (1978).
28 Charron, D.J.; Lotteau, V.; Turmel, P.: Hybrid HLA-DC antigens provide molecular evidence for gene trans-complementation. Nature, Lond. *312:* 157 (1984).
29 Cohen, D.; Le Gall, I.; Marcadet, A.; Font, M.P.; Lalouel, J.M.; Dausset, J.: Clusters of HLA class II β-restriction fragments describe allelic series. Proc. natn. Acad. Sci. USA *81:* 7870 (1984).
30 Yu, D.T.Y.; Cune, J.M.; Fune, S.M.; Winchester, M.J.; Kunkel, H.G.: Two types of Ia positive T cells: synthesis and exchange of Ia antigens. J. exp. Med. *152:* 895 (1980).
31 Klareskog, L.; Forsum, U.; Kabelitz, D.; Ploen, L.; Sundstrom, C.; Nilsson, K.; Wigren, A.; Wigzell, H.: Immune functions of human synovial cells; phenotypic and T cell regulatory properties of macrophage-like cells that express HLA-DR. Arthitis Rheum. *25:* 488 (1982).
32 Teyton, L.; Lotteau, V.; Boyer, B.; Charron, D.J.: A quantitative dot immunobinding assay for human HLA class II antigens using nitrocellulose membrane filters. J. immunol. methods (in press, 1986).
33 Bresser, J.; Doering, J.; Gillepsie, D.: Quick-blot: selective mRNA or DNA immobilisation from whole cells. NA *2:* 243 (1983).
34 Piatier-Tonneau, D.; Turmel, P.; Auffray C.; Charron, D.J.: Construction of chain and locus specific HLA class II DNA probes. Study of HLA class II transcripts in leukemias. J. Immun. (in press, 1986).
35 Charron, D.J., McDevitt, H.O.: Analysis of HLA-D region associated molecules with monoclonal antibodies. Proc. natn. Acad. Sci. USA *76:* 6567 (1979).
36 Claesson-Welsh, L.; Peterson, L.: Implications of the invariant chain on the intracellular transport of HLA class II histocompatibility antigens. J. Immun. *135:* 355 (1985).
37 Cowing, C.; Chapdelaine, J.M.: T Cells disseminate between Ia antigens expressed on allogenic accessory cells and B cells. A Potential function for carbohydrate side chains on Ia molecules. Proc. natn. Acad. Sci. USA *80:* 6000 (1983).
38 Neel, D.; Giner, M.; Turmel, P.; Goussault, Y.; Charron, D.J.: Analysis of HLA-DR antigens glycosylation by serial lectin affinity chromatography. Molec. Immunol. *22:* 1053 (1985).
39 Sant, A.J.; Cullen, S.E.; Schwartz, B.D.: Identification of a sulfate bearing molecule associated with HLA class II antigens. Proc. natn. Acad. Sci. USA *81:* 1534 (1984).

40 Levitt, D.; Ho, P. L.: Induction of chondroitin sulfate proteoglycan synthesis and secretion in lymphocytes and monocytes. J. Cell. Biol. *97:* 351 (1983).

41 Burmester, G. R.; Menche, D.; Merryman, P.; Klein, M.; Winchester, R.: Application of monoclonal antibodies to the characterization of cells eluted from human articular cartilage. Arthritis Rheum. *26:* 1187 (1983).

Dominique Charron, MD, Laboratoire d'Immunogénétique moléculaire, Département d'Hématologie du CHU Pitié Salpêtrière, Institut des Cordeliers, 15, rue de l'Ecole de Médecine, F-75000 Paris (France)

Concepts Immunopathol., vol. 4, pp. 215–242 (Karger, Basel 1987)

Autoimmunity of the Ear[1]

T. J. Yoo, T. Ishibe

Departments of Medicine, Microbiology and Immunology, and Neurosciences Program, University of Tennessee, Memphis, Tenn., USA

Introduction

The pathogenesis of autoimmunity involves various genetic, immunologic and viral factors interacting through complicated mechanisms still poorly understood. Recent evidence suggests that at least immunological disturbances are associated with many causes of auditory dysfunction. There are several diseases associated with hearing loss that include Ménière's disease, otosclerosis, autoimmune sensory hearing loss and other forms of sudden hearing loss (table I).

Cogan's syndrome interstitial keratitis and vestibuloauditory disorder progressing to profound hearing loss, was well described in 1945 by Cogan [1]. In 1960, Cody and Williams implied this was a collagen disease. Their treatment included high doses of corticosteroid pointing out that the improvement of hearing produced by this drug was lost when the doses were reduced.

Lehnhardt [2] reported cases of bilateral sudden hearing loss and proposed an etiological hypothesis that the degenerated organ of Corti could induce anticochlear antibody which would react with another intact organ of Corti. Kikuchi [3] reported several cases of hearing loss as sympathetic otitis in which hearing in the opposite ear had been markedly influenced by the operation of the other ear. Beickert [4] was the first to publish the experimental data concerning autoimmune reaction in

[1] This research was supported by grants from the Deafness Research Foundation, American Otologic Society, National Hearing Association, and Medical Research Funds granted by the Veterans Administration.

Table I. Ear diseases with immunologic features

External ear	auricular chondritis relapsing polychondritis
Tympanic membrane	tympanosclerosis
Eustachian tube	autoimmune salpingitis
Middle ear	otosclerosis secretory otitis media necrotizing otitis media cholesteatoma
Inner ear	autoimmune sensorineural hearing loss Ménière's disease otosclerosis cochlear vasculitis sudden hearing loss
Retrocochlea	autoimmune CNS disease

Table II. Collagen-induced ear disease

Sensorineural hearing loss
Vestibular dysfunction
Spiral ganglion degeneration
Atrophy of organ of Corti
Cochlear vasculitis
Salpingitis and chondritis
Ostospongiosis-like lesion
Endolymphatic hydrops

the cochlea. He injected an anti-guinea pig cochlear antibody, produced in the duck, into a guinea pig. Sasaki and Terayama [5] produced experimental allergic labyrinthitis in guinea pigs by the immunization of guinea pig cochlea emulsified with Freund's adjuvant. They found degenerative changes in the spiral ganglia and stria vascularis, hemorrhages in the scala tympani and disintegration of the organ of Corti. They noted acoustic threshold shifts, although they could not demonstrate any anticochlear antibody.

In the past 5 years, a unique animal model of ear disease has been developed and partially characterized. Animals immunized with native type II collagen developed sensory hearing loss, vestibular dysfunction, degeneration in the spiral ganglion, crista ampullaris, vacuolar degeneration in the utricles, endolymphatic hydrops and otospongiosis-like lesions [6–13] (table II). Preliminary data suggest that this is associated with both cellular and humoral immune response to native type II collagen. In addition, the immunopathological changes in this model are parallel to human conditions. Furthermore, we are able to transfer this pathology by serum or lymphoid cells thus fulfilling the requirement of autoimmune phenomena.

Type II Collagen Autoimmune Response as a Basic Pathogenesis of Ear Lesions

Well-established criteria for immunologists who wish to determine the relationship of immunologic phenomena to disease etiology include the following: (1) the autoimmune response must be regularly associated with the disease; (2) a replica of the disease must be inducible in laboratory animals; (3) immunopathologic changes in the natural and experimental disease should parallel each other, and (4) transfer of the autoimmune illness should be possible by the transfer of serum or lymphoid cells from the diseased individual to a normal recipient. Though our studies are preliminary, we feel we have fulfilled these criteria for certain ear diseases as immunologic phenomena as seen in the following evidence.

Although there are several ear diseases in which an immunologic reaction might play a role, it is not clear at this time to what extent autoimmune responses are responsible for human ear lesions.

However, type II collagen autoimmunity was proven to exist in relapsing polychondritis in which auricular chondritis and cochlear and vestibular lesions also occur in approximately 50% of patients [14]. About 20% of patients with autoimmune sensorineural hearing loss (AISNHL) showed either type II ore type IV collagen immunitiy [15]; they also had positive responses in a migration inhibition assay when labyrinthine membranes were used as antigens [15, 16]. Though the exact biochemical properties of these labyrinthine antigens have not been characterized, preliminary studies show that they might contain type II collagens [16, 17]. This speculation is based on three studies performed in our laboratory: the presence of hydroxyproline and proline in amino acid analysis of this tissue (table III), and immunoperoxidase or immu-

Table III. Amino acid composition of human labyrinthine membrane (residues calculated/1,000)

	Parts per
Hydroxyproline	42.6
Asparagine	79.3
Threonine	28.4
Serine	39.6
Glutamine	95.8
Proline	95.1
Glycine	216.0
Alanine	102.9
Cysteine/2	6.2
Valine	45.9
Methionine	10.2
Isoleucine	25.6
Leucine	51.1
Tyrosine	12.9
Phenylalanine	31.4
Hydroxylysine	7.8
Lysine	43.4
Histidine	13.2
Arginine	47.9

These results indicate that 45% of the proteins are collagen in nature because of the presence of hydroxyproline residues. If they were all collagens, then we would have about 20 residues of hydroxylysine.
Therefore, these data are not incompatible with the presence of type II collagen (which contains enough hydroxylysine) in the samples. Immunofluorescence or immunoperoxidase data show the presence of type II collagen using monoclonal antibody against type II collagen.

nofluorescent staining using monoclonal antibodies against type II collagens [18, 19] and transblot technique [19].

The underlying causes for AISNHL must be multiple because at least some of these patients have type II collagen autoimmunity. We now have preliminary evidence that some experimental animals developed AISNHL without type II collagen autoimmunity and showed autoantibodies to other tissue components.

Some otosclerosis patients were shown to have type II collagen autoimmunity [8] and the presence of immune complexes in their lesions [20] which are also found in some patients with an idiopathic form of

Ménière's disease [21]. We found that the levels of antibodies to type II collagen were markedly higher in Ménière's disease, suggesting a possible role for type II collagen autoimmunity in the etiology of Ménière's disease [8]. Histopathologic study of the membranous labyrinth of the guinea pig hydrops model showed fluorescent deposits on the epithelium lining, indicating the presence of immune complexes in this area [11, 21].

This simultaneous occurrence of Ménière's disease and otosclerosis seems to support type II collagen autoimmunity [22]. Autoimmune responses to type II collagen in inner ear tissue could result in the deposition of immunoglobulin, complement, and other immune injuries in the endolymphatic duct which could impair the resorption mechanism of the endolymph, resulting in endolymphatic hydrops.

While the importance of the antibodies to type II collagen in Ménière's disease patients is not known, it appears that antibodies to type II collagen can cause hearing loss and endolymphatic hydrops in guinea pigs. The stimulus for the natural development of autoimmunity in this type of pathology remains unknown.

Animal Models

Collagen-Induced Ear Disease Model for the AISNHL, Spiral Ganglion Degeneration and Cochlear Vasculitis

Autoimmune sensorineural hearing loss was induced in rats by immunizing them with native bovine type II collagen. Type I, III and denatured type II collagen, administered by an identical immunization procedure, did not induce disease. Evidence of SNHL was obtained by measuring the brainstem evoked potential and observing the histopathological changes consisting of cochlear nerve degeneration and perineural vasculitis in affected animals. Immunized animals had high levels of antibodies to native type II collagen. Some had mild atrophy of the organ of Corti [10]. This also occurred in chinchillas [23], guinea pigs [11], and monkeys [24]. Female inbred Lewis and outbred Wistar rats, Hartley and Strain 13 guinea pigs and DBA-1 mice were also used [13].

After measuring the ABR and obtaining sera for antibody determinations, the temporal bones were examined.

Perivascular abnormalities were observed in the cochlear arteries. A large number of mononuclear cells had infiltrated around the artery; the

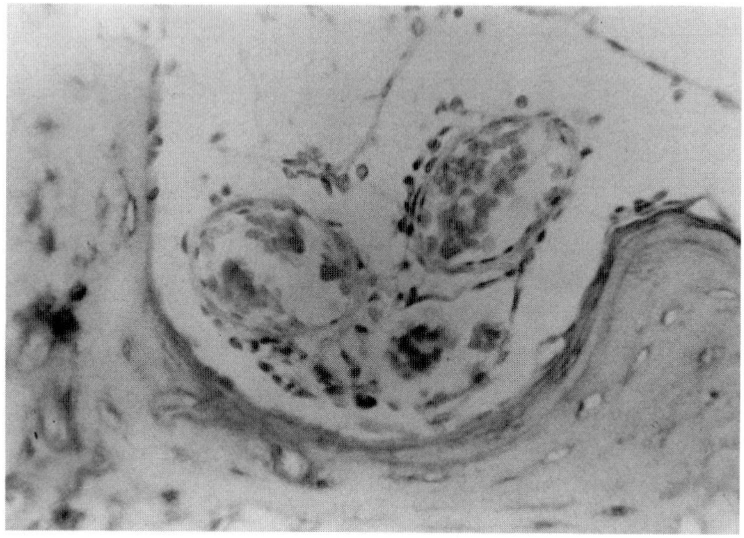

1a

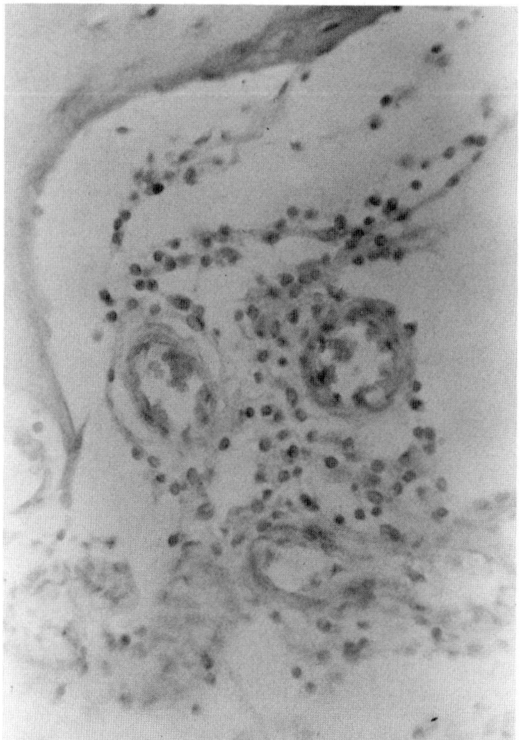

1b

vessel was thickened and the endothelial cells were increased. Mild fibrosis was found in the perivascular area (fig. 1a, b).

Immunofluorescence revealed the deposition of green fluorescent substances in the vessel wall, perivascular fibrous tissue, and surrounding bone tissue of the cochlear artery in all rats. Spiral ganglion cell degeneration was also observed. There was vacuolar degeneration of the cochlear neurons throughout most of the cochlea of the type II collagen-immunized rats. The ganglion cell bodies were swollen, the cytoplasm was clear, and the nuclei were pyknotic and displaced toward the axonal poles of the cells (fig. 2a, b) Nerve fibers showed slight atrophic changes.

Pathological changes were relatively conspicuous in the apical turn relative to the basal turn. Immunofluorescence studies did not show pathology in the area of the spiral ganglion. The organ of Corti, stria vascularis, and the cochlear nerve also had normal histologies revealed on both regular HE-stained and immunofluorescence sections.

These results are from the animals immunized for less than 1 month's duration. However, when these animals were examined two or three months after the initial immunization, mild atrophic changes were observed in the cochlear nerve, organ of Corti, and stria vascularis. Hair cells were still present but slightly atrophied. No apparent pathological changes were observed in the vestibular sensory organ and nerve other than those previously mentioned.

The ABR of the control rats and immunized rats showed that the amplitude and latency differed significantly. This also occurred in chinchillas, guinea pigs, and monkeys.

Guinea Pig Model of Autoimmune Hydrops and Saccular Degeneration

Endolymphatic hydrops were induced in guinea pigs by immunizing them with native bovine type II collagen. Histopathologic changes consisted of a moderate distension of Reissner's membrane, spiral ganglion degeneration, atrophied organ of Corti, and a mild atrophy of the surface epithelium in the endolymphatic duct [25]. These findings suggest that an immune response directed against type II collagen – a type of collagen found in the membranous labyrinth, subepithelial layer of the endolym-

---

Fig. 1 a Cochlear arteries and veins from normal rat. *b* Inflamed cochlear artery in autoimmune sensorineural hearing loss in rat. HE. × 144. Micrograph × 2,300.

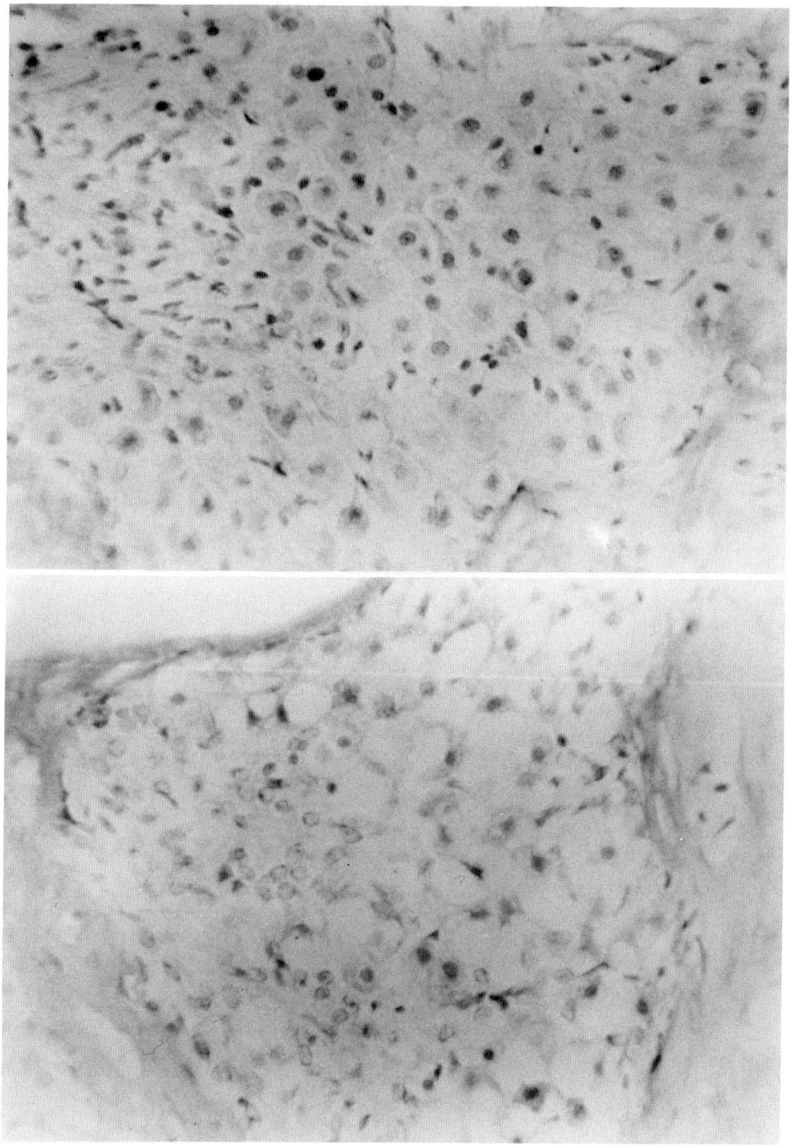

a

b

Fig. 2a Spiral ganglion from normal ear. *b* Degenerated spiral ganglion in ear with autoimmune sensorineural hearing loss. Neurons show vacuolate degeneration in which cell bodies are swollen, cytoplasm is clear, and nuclei are pyknotic and displaced toward two axonal poles of cells. Nerve fiber shows slight decrease in number × 1,500.

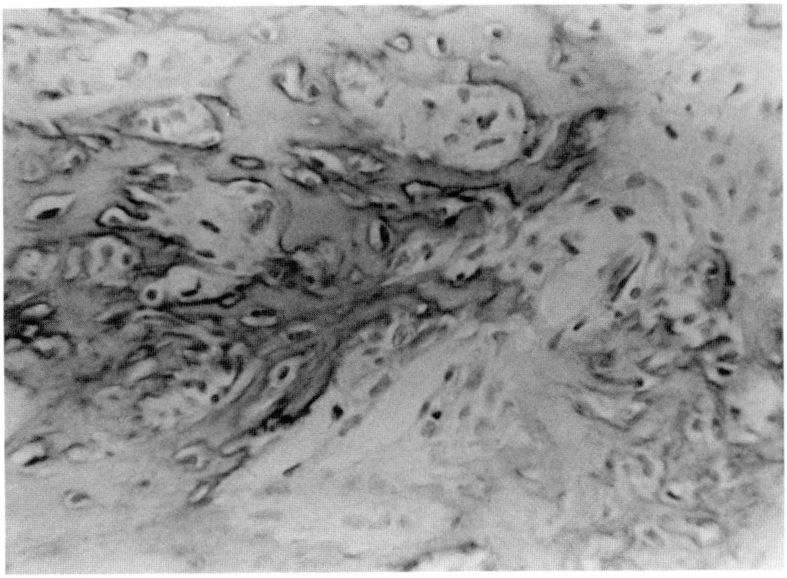

Fig. 3 External meatus bone from type II collagen immunized rat. Otospongiotic bone is characterized by dark staining due to alteration of chemical ground substance. Vascular spaces are wide and contain fibrous tissues. Large number of fibroblasts and osteoblasts are seen. Bone absorption and new bone formation are visible × 431.

phatic duct, spiral ligament, and enchondral layer of the capsule – may induce endolymphatic hydrops [25] (fig. 3).

Our animal model for hydrops has some limitations. The histology of the saccule and utricle is normal, except for some vacuolar degeneration in a few of the animals which could represent an early lesion. Most animals showed atrophy of the neurosensory elements of the inner ear which might not exist in patients with Ménière's disease.

The guinea pig is the only species which shows endolymphatic hydrops. We have tested a limited number of the following animal species without finding hydrops: mice, rats, chinchillas, rabbits, monkeys, gerbils, and cats.

Though our model has the intrinsic limitations, it still might be useful in defining the pathogenesis of human Ménière's disease. This model provides a new theory for the mechanism of the Ménière's attack [7].

Our experimental results, using animal models, indicate that the inner ear fluid from immunized animals has antibody activity against collagen type II antigen [12]. Type II collagen might be responsible for some

Table IV. Correlation of antibody levels and pathologic changes in the inner ear of guinea pigs immunized with type II collagen

Guinea pig strain	Number of animals	Weeks after Immunization with type II collagen	ELISA (absorbance) (mean = SD)	Endolymphatic hydrops	Degeneration of spiral Ganglion cells		Atrophy of organ of Corti	Atrophy of stria vascularis
					apical turn	nasal turn		
Hartley	7	2	0.324±0.078	–	–	–	–	–
	8	4	0.829±0.087	+	++	+	++	+
Strain 13	9	2	0.676±0.192	–	+	+	+	+
	9	4	1.037±0.170	+	++	++	+	+

No lesion indicated by '–'; mild lesion '+'; severe lesion '++'.
[1] ELISA background less than 0.009.

Table V. Guinea pig skin test reaction

Type	Immunizing antigen	Skin testing antigen	Size of skin reaction mm
Strain 13			
1	nCII	nCII	15×17
2	nCII	nCII	12×14
3	nCII	nCII	17×25
4	nBII	nBII	6× 9
5	nBII	nBII	6× 6
6	nBII	nBII	10×10
Hartley			
7	nCII	nCII	16×20
8	nCII	nCII	16×16
9	nCII	nCII	17×18
10	nBII	nBII	12×12
11	nBII	nBII	9× 8

nCII = Native chick type II collagen; nBII = Native bovine type II collagen.

of the immune injuries associated with inner ear disease. Immunologic findings observed in this model include elevated antibodies against type II collagen. The correlation of antibody levels and pathologic changes in the inner ear are seen in table IV. Results of the skin test for the measurement of cell-mediated immunity correlated well with the pathologic changes [11] (table V).

Animal Model for Degeneration of the Crista Ampullaris and Vestibular Dysfunction

In this model, the animal developed vacuolar degeneration of the crista ampullaris with vestibular dysfunction. Type II collagen exists in the crista ampullaris [9, 11].

Otospongiosis-like Lesions. Otosclerosis is a poorly understood pathological condition which causes hearing loss by affecting the otic capsules of the labyrinth and the stapes. Characteristic histopathologic changes of otosclerosis have been described in fetuses and in very young children as well as in adults of all ages. Although genetic and basic histologic patterns have been identified in otosclerosis, there is no agreement as to its etiology or precise pathogenesis [26].

We described an experimental model of otospongiosis-like lesion in rats caused by immunization with native type II collagen. Immunized rats developed spongiotic changes in the external meatal bone near the tympanic annulus and in the middle layer of the cochlear capsule. It was proposed that these changes are the result of collagen autoimmunity in this animal model and may shed some new light on the possible pathogenesis of human otosclerosis.

Spongiotic changes were observed in the anterior border of the external meatus bone near the tympanic annulus of the type II collagen-immunized rat. No lesions were found in the rats immunized with type I collagen. In normal rats this area consists of woven and lamellar bone. In type II collagen-immunized rats there were spongiotic vascular lesions characterized by numerous osteocytes and osteoblasts (dark staining was probably due to chemical alteration of ground substance) and wider vascular spaces with fibrosis (fig. 3). These distinctive pathological features resembled the spongification of bone which is seen in human otosclerosis.

The early lesion of spongiotic change was observed in the middle layer of the cochlear capsule. It shows the higher magnification of the blood vessel in the cochlear capsule. Macrophages and osteoclastic cells invaded the widely vascular space and eroded perivascular bone. Surrounding interstitial bone was acellular, nonviable, and contained degenerated lacunae. However, spongiotic changes were not clearly recognized in the oval window and other areas.

Immunofluorescence studies demonstrated that the fluorescent substances were deposited on the bone matrix and vessel wall within the area of spongiosis, which was separated with a defined boundary from other normal bone. There were no fluorescent substances in the adjacent bone or in the temporal bone of control animals. The temporal bones of rats with collagen-immunized spongiosis were further characterized by a strong deposition of green fluorescent substances on the enchondral layer of the otic capsule. In normal rats, there were no fluorescent substances on the same area. In the sections stained with H and E, there were no differences between the control and collagen-immunized rats except the thin blue staining on the surface of the lacunae and canaliculae. In addition, the walls of the vascular channels were slightly more prominent in immunized as compared to normal rats. These results were confirmed by other investigators [27].

Ossicular maxillary joints of immunized and control rats had normal histology in both H and E and immunofluorescence sections, whereas in the immunofluorescence sections, the bone tissue of ossicles from the type II collagen-immunized rats had a deposition of green fluorescent substances around lacunae, canaliculae, and vascular channels.

Human Ear Disease and Immunopathology in the CIAED (Collagen-Induced Autoimmune Ear Disease) Model

Though the animal models we presented in the previous section are somewhat artificial in that they were immunized with type II collagen, there is a certain similarity between the clinicopathologic picture of human ear disease and our animal models [3–5, 28–31]. In certain aspects, immunopathologic changes in humans paralleled experimental animal findings very closely. Experimental findings could also represent several different human ear diseases occurring at the same time in one animal model. However, a better understanding of the immunologic mechanisms seen in the rat, guinea pig, and monkey models (e.g. the presence/absence of joint lesions, presence/absence of endolymphatic hydrops) might be of great value to explain the role of immune responses in human autoimmune ear diseases.

Transfer of Disease

Cell Transfer of CIAED

We attempted to transfer these ear diseases by a passive transfer of immunocytes from the donor animals which were sensitized by type II collagen. Guinea pigs were used in our studies, and 1×10^8 spleen cells from sensitized strain 2 or sensitized strain 13 guinea pigs were given to the corresponding strain of guinea pigs. From sensitized Hartley guinea pigs, 4×10^7 cells were given to healthy Hartley guinea pigs. These animals were killed between 30 and 50 days after cell transfer. The temporal bone pathology was examined, and antibody activity against type II collagen was also measured. The most prominent finding from the guinea pig experiment was the degeneration of spiral ganglion cells. One animal developed mild to moderate endolymphatic hydrops in all turns. The saccule and crista ampullaris showed degeneration of sensory hair cells with vacuolization. The vessel walls of the modiolus seemed to be thicker than those of the controls. The lesions were more prominent in the guinea pigs that received cells from donors with high antibody titers against native bovine type II collagen. Immunofluorescence studies of the guinea pig showed anti-Ig or anti-C3 fluorescent deposits on the otic capsule, footplate of stapes (1 animal), perivascular area, and the subepithelial area of the endolymphatic duct. One animal had endolymphatic hydrops. The antibody level in the recipient guinea pigs showed a mild elevation [32]. Control animals that received normal lymphocytes did not have these lesions.

Thus, these studies showed that ear lesions can be transferred by sensitized cells and that lesions are due to injury mediated by immunologic mechanisms. Further studies are necessary to define the precise role of the components of the immune system (cellular versus humoral) in the production of ear immune injury. The following are the pathologic lesions observed in the recipient guinea pigs.

Cochlea. The organ of Corti showed degeneration in the upper turns of the cochlea where the outer hair cells were missing. In the lower turns, although the supporting cells sometimes showed a vacuolated degeneration, the hair cells were relatively well preserved.

Spiral Ganglion. Spiral ganglion cells showed severe vacuolated degeneration in which the cell bodies were swollen. The cytoplasm was clear, and the nuclei were pyknotic and displaced toward two axonal poles of cells. Nerve fibers showed atrophic changes. The degeneration of spiral ganglion was more extensive in the upper turns than in the lower turns. In the upper turns, more than 50% of the ganglion cells were degenerated. These ganglion cells were surrounded by ear structures which contained type II collagen.

Cochlear Vessels. Cochlear vessels showed a thickening of their walls in which endothelial cells seemed to increase. Moderate fibrosis was found in the perivascular area.

Saccule. The saccular macula showed a slight vacuolated degeneration in which the cell bodies were swollen and the cytoplasm was clear.

Serum Transfer of CIAED in Rats

To fulfill the immunologic criteria of autoimmune disease, we performed a transfer of CIAED in animals using serum. Wistar rats were immunized with native bovine type II collagen. Antisera were fractionated with ammonium sulfate, dialyzed, lyophilized, and reconstituted into a quarter of the volume of the original antisera. About 2.5–3 ml of this gamma-globulin fraction were given intravenously.

Fifty days later, the recipient animals were killed for histologic examination. The recipients had a mildly elevated antibody titer (0.125 + 0.095 by the ELISA assay). Some spiral ganglion cells showed a mild vacuolated degeneration in which the cytoplasm was clear, and the nuclei were pyknotic and necrotic. The cochlear vessels showed a thickening of their walls. Several mononuclear cells were observed around the vessels, and a mild fibrosis was found in the perivascular area. The organ of Corti had mild changes in which some supporting cells seemed to be swollen, but the hair cells were preserved. In the saccule, there was a loss of approximately half of the hair cells and supporting cells. The crista ampullaris seemed almost normal. Thus, CIAED which was transferable by immune sera fulfilled one of the immunologic criteria of ear disease. We have not done this experiment in guinea pigs.

Induction of Tolerance

We were able to induce tolerance by pretreating rats with type II collagen in varying doses prior to immunization with the antigen in an attempt to induce lesions. Four months after type II collagen immunization, these rats had not developed ear disease. These phenomena, so far, are antigen-specific, thus indicating another support of an immunologic mechanism for the induction of inner ear disease in these animal models [33].

Anatomic Basis of Type II Collagen Autoimmune Injury in the Ear

The occurrence of diverse ear lesions in the animal models can be understood if we assume that the immunization produced sensitized lymphocytes and antibodies capable of attacking the region where type II collagen is an important structural component. With this in mind, we studied extensively the distribution of type II collagen in the ears of humans, monkeys, cats, rats, chinchillas, mice, gerbils, guinea pigs, frogs, and guinea pig fetuses. The following are the results of these studies.

Collagen Distribution in the Middle and Inner Ear

Type II collagen-specific hybridoma monoclonal antibody was applied to localize type II collagen in the inner and middle ear. In the cochlea, positive staining to type II collagen was observed in the enchondral layer, globuli interossei in the cochlear capsule, cribriform base and Rosenthal canal in the modiolus, spiral ligament, and limbus. In the vestibule, staining occurred in the enchondral layer and globuli interossei in osseous labyrinth, macula utriculi and sacculi, semicircular canal membrane, the crista ampullaris, and the subepithelials connective tissues in the endolymphatic duct. In the external and middle ear, positive staining to type II collagen was observed in the meatus and tympanic annulus and in the interossicular joints, stapes footplate, enchondral layer and globuli interossei in the otic capsules, and the eustachian tube cartilage. The facial nerve, outer layers of tympanic membare, middle ear muscles, mucose and glands did not stain. None of the control sections showed specific staining in this study. These findings, as seen in the rats, were similar to findings observed in the guinea pig. Human stapes bones also showed similar results. However, so far, only the human temporal bone shows the presence of the fissure antefenestrum as a type II collagen structure. It was never found in the other animals tested.

Collagen Distribution in the Guinea Pig Fetus

The guinea pig fetus was stained with a monoclonal antibody against type II collagen. In the 20-day fetus, positive staining to type II collagen was observed in the primitive temporal bone, primitive ossicles, primitive otic capsule, primitive cochlear duct, primitive spiral ganglion area, semicircular canal membrane, crista ampullaris, utricle, and saccular macula. In the 30-day fetus, in addition to the findings in the 20-day fetus, staining occurred in the cartilage plate in the auricle and external ear meatus, tympanic membrane, endolymphatic duct, limbus, spiral ligament and the basilar membrane. In addition to the findings in the 30-day fetus, the 50-day fetus showed staining of the tympanic annulus, eustachian tube cartilage, Rosenthal canal, cribriform base, interossicular joint, the endochondral layer, and the globuli interossei in the otic capsule. Because cartilage develops into bone in the otic capsule, the ossicles, and the primitive temporal bone, the positive and negative staining are mixed in these areas. Thus, these studies indicate the presence of type II collagens in various locations of ear tissue [19].

Monoclonal antibody against streptococcal M protein was used as a negative serum.

Antigenic Structural Basis of the Induction of CIAED

Epitope of Type II Collagen

The preliminary finding of cyanogen bromide-cleaved peptide (CB-11) from type II collagen produced by cyanogen bromide cleavages seems to play an important role in the collagen-induced arthritis in mice [34]. The role of the peptide CB-11 or other peptides (CB-6, 7, 8, 9, 10, and 13) in the production of CIAED is being investigated. These studies might shed some light on the epitope-related phenomena in the production of CIAED. If, indeed, one or several different epitopes are responsible for the production of arthritis and CIAED, CIAED alone, or arthritis alone, it would add a great deal of understanding to these immunologic phenomena.

Cyanogen bromide peptides were made according to the method of Miller [35]. Cyanogen bromide was added to type II collagen and isolated by column chromatography. This denatured protein was renatured by stepwise cooling according to the methods of Igarashi et al [36].

These peptides were used for ELISA assays. The CB-11 peptides correlated with the production of arthritis in mice [34]. Preliminary studies with mice sera showed that, with CIAED, they indeed contained antibodies reacting against CB-11 peptides. The differential binding results with these peptides in various animals with different anatomic lesions (e.g. joint and ear diseases) could answer difficult questions about the relationship of concurrent disease.

In order to identify the epitope on the type II collagen molecule which induced autoimmune ear disease, electrophysiological and histological studies were carried out in DBA/IJ mice immunized with native chick type II collagen (CIIn) and cyanogen bromide (CNBr) peptide 11 (CB-11 peptide) which was cleaved from chicken type II collagen with CNBr digestion. Four months after immunization, 3 out of 6 CIIn-immunized mice and 5 out of 6 CB-11 peptide-immunized mice developed moderate hearing loss. No control animals showed hearing loss. The pattern of hearing loss was characteristic of progressive deafness. Further, the immunized mice showed temporal lesions involving atrophy of the Corti organ and degeneration of the spiral ganglion, in proportion to the

Table VI. Time-course of hearing level

Animal No.	Duration of follow-up, months 4 5 6
IFA treatment	
1	55-----50
2	50------------50------------50
3	50------------55------------60
4	55------------50------------50
5	55------------55------------55
CIIn+IFA treatment	
6	65------------85
7	65----------†
8	95----115
9	100-----------115------†
10	125-----------125†-------†
11	60---------†
CB11+IFA treatment	
12	75-----------115----------125†
13	80-----------115-----
14	95----110-----125-----
15	90-----------115------†
16	90-----------115---------†
17	60------------60

† Indicates spontaneous death.

level of the hearing loss. Since similar inner ear lesions were induced by immunization with CIIn and CB-11 peptide, CB-11 peptide was concluded to be one of the epitopes on the chick type II collagen molecule involved in pathogenesis of autoimmune ear disease.

The time sequence of thresholds in ABR is represented in table VI. Four months after the immunization, 5 out of 6 CB-11 peptide-immunized mice developed hearing loss over 65 dB pe SPL, while the threshold of controls were still within 60 dB pe SPL. Representative ABRs from

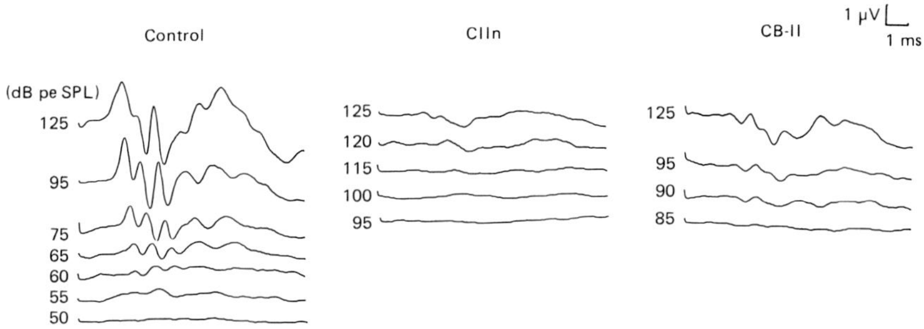

Fig. 4 Comparison of ABR records between control, CIIn-immunized and CB-11 peptide-immunized mice (4 months of follow-up). Control animals showed good response at the intensity of acoustic stimuli over 60 dB pe SPL. Note the elevation of threshold and the decrease of ABR responses in the immunized mice. The latencies of ABR of immunized mice were slightly delayed. × 79.

the three groups are presented in figure 4. The control animal (animal No. 5) showed good response in intensity over 65 dB pe SPL, and wave II was still identified in the low intensity of 55 dB pe SPL. On the other hand, a decrease of amplitude and an elevated threshold were noted in the mice immunized with either CB-11 peptide (animal No. 15) or CIIn (animal No. 9). Latencies of individual waves were slightly delayed in immunized mice with hearing loss. The auditory disorders became more marked with time. Six months after immunization, 4 out of 5 CB-11 peptide-immunized animals developed hearing loss over 115 dB pe SPL. In the CIIn-immunized group, 2 out of 3 mice developed the same level of hearing loss, however, these animals did not survive 10 months after the immunization. Control mice maintained good ABR responses 10 months after the immunization and the threshold remained within 60 dB pe SPL.

For the histological study, the remaining animals were sacrificed 10 months postimmunization. There was no sign of middle ear infection in any of the histological sections examined. Striking morphological changes were localized in the organ of Corti, stria vascularis and spiral ganglion cells including cochlear nerve of the temporal bones from the collagen immunized animals.

A comparison between histological changes and hearing levels at sacrifice are summarized in table VII. In controls, no changes were found in the inner ear tissues during this 10 month study period. A CIIn-immunized mouse (animal No. 8) sacrificed 5 months after immunization, showed mild atrophy in the organ of Corti, including missing outer hair

Table VII. Comparison between hearing level and histological change

Animal No.	Duration of follow-up months	Organ of Corti		Loss of hair cell	Decrease of cochlear nerve	Loss of spiral ganglia	Atrophy of stria vascularis
		hearing level when sacrificed dB pe SPL	precipitation of Corti organ				
IFA treatment							
1	5	50	–	–	–	–	–
2	10	50	–	–	–	–	–
3	10	60	–	–	–	–	–
4	10	50	–	–	–	–	–
5	10	55	–	–	–	–	–
CIIn+IFA treatment							
6	6	85	+	±	±	–	–
8	5	115	++	+	+	±	–
CB11-IFA treatment							
12	10	125	+	#	++	++	++
14	5	110	++	+	+	±	–
17	6	60	–	–	–	–	–

– = normal; ± = questionable; + = slight; ++ = moderate; # = severe.

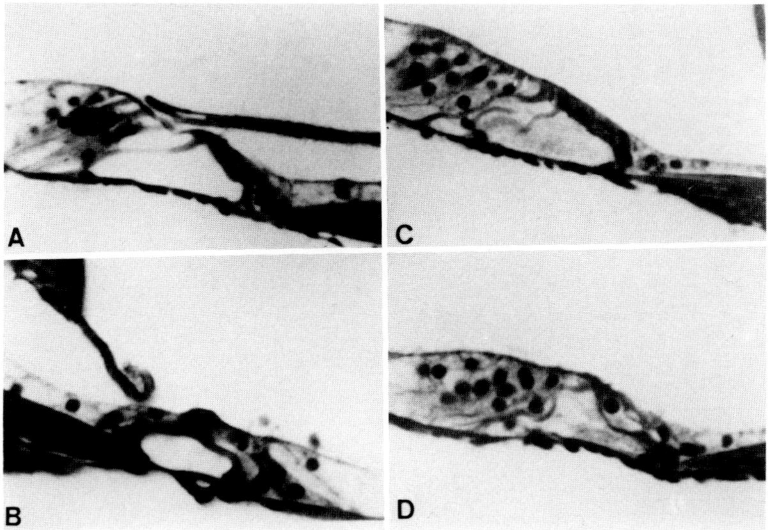

Fig. 5 Comparison of the Corti organ between control, CIIn-immunized and CB-11 peptide-immunized mice. *A* The organ of Corti in the control mouse (animal No. 5). × 256. *B* The organ of Corti in the basal turn of the CIIn-immunized mouse (animal No. 8). The organ of Corti is mildly atrophied and the outer hair cells of the second and third row were missing. × 256. *C* The organ of Corti in the upper turn of the CIIn-immunized mouse (animal No. 8). Note the precipitates in the tunnel of Corti. Both outer and inner hair cells were preserved in this turn. × 256. *D* The organ of Corti in the upper turn of CB-11 peptide-immunized mouse (animal No. 14). Similar precipitates were seen in the tunnel of Corti of this mouse.

cells of the second and third rows in the basal turn (fig. 5B). A slight decrease in the cochlear nerve fibers was observed in the basal turn of the CIIn-immunized mouse. In addition to these findings, eosinophilic precipitates were densely deposited in the tunnel of the Corti in the upper turn (fig. 5C). Such precipitates were never detected in the perilymphatic and the endolymphatic spaces. Similar changes were also seen in a CB-11 peptide-immunized mouse (animal No. 14) which was sacrificed at the same time (fig. 5D). Although both mice showed moderately elevated threshold at 110 dB pe SPL, no unusual changes were recognized in the spiral ganglion and stria vascularis.

Six months after immunization, a CIIn-immunized mouse (animal No. 6) with a slightly elevated threshold of 85 dB pe SPL, developed the same histological changes in the temporal bone, but the degree of the le-

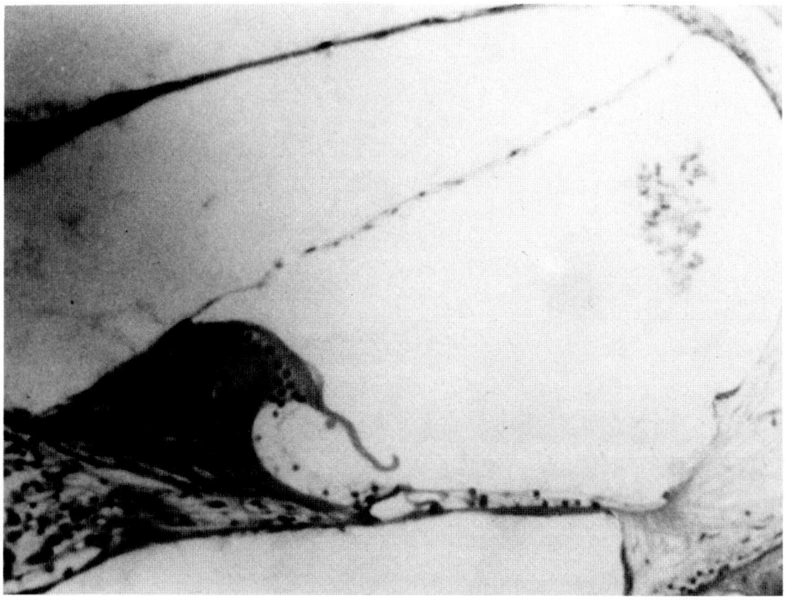

Fig. 6 Cochlear duct in the upper turn of the CB-11 peptide-immunized mouse (animal No. 12). Note the atrophic organ of Corti and total loss of the outer hair cells. The stria vascularis was also atrophied. × 64.

sions was parallel with the level of hearing loss. A CB-11 peptide-immunized mouse (animal No. 17) with normal hearing showed no morphological change in the inner ear in spite of long-term follow-up.

Ten months after immunization, a CB-11 peptide-immunized mouse (animal No. 12) with severe hearing loss over 125 dB pe SPL showed the most marked changes in the temporal bone, that is, severe atrophy of the organ of Corti and the stria vascularis (fig. 6). Further, all outer hair cells were missing in the upper turn. These changes were more severe in the basal turn. In the basal turn, the organ of Corti was completely atrophied and both inner and outer hair cells were totally missing (fig. 7A, B).

Precipitation was noted in both perilymph and endolymph, although not localized in the tunnel of Corti, in the immunized animal compared to the control animals (fig. 7B). In reference to the cochlear neurons, half of the spiral ganglion cells were missing and a decrease of cochlear nerve fibers was marked (fig. 8). In reference to the cochlear neurons, half of the spiral ganglion cells were missing and a decrease of cochlear nerve

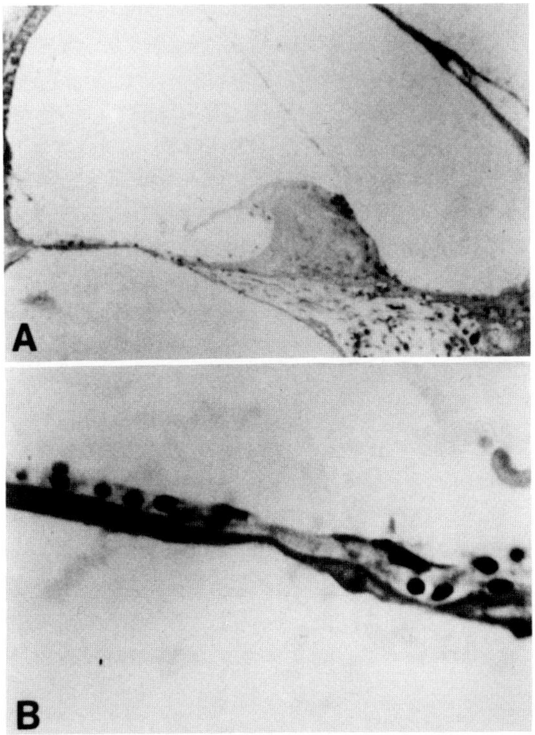

Fig. 7 Cochlear duct and neuron of the CB-11 peptide-immunized mouse (animal No. 12). *A* Low magnification (× 64). The organ of Corti was totally atrophied and neurons were missing. *B* High magnification (× 256). Note the completely shrunken organ of Corti. The precipitates were seen in both the perilymphatic and endolymphatic spaces.

fibers was marked (fig. 8). In addition, the cells' bodies of the residual spiral ganglion cells were swollen and the nuclei were also pyknotic.

No remarkable changes were recognized in the vestibule of any ear tissue from all groups.

Type II collagen whose molecular composition is represented as $[\alpha I(II)]_3$, has been cleaved with CNBr digest into 13 unique peptides which have been characterized with regard to amino acid composition and molecular weight [35]. Although these CNBr peptides are renaturable by stepwise cooling, renatured CB-11 peptides were recently confirmed to be not only the most immunogenic portion on the molecule of type II collagen, but also capable of inducing arthritis [34]. Conse-

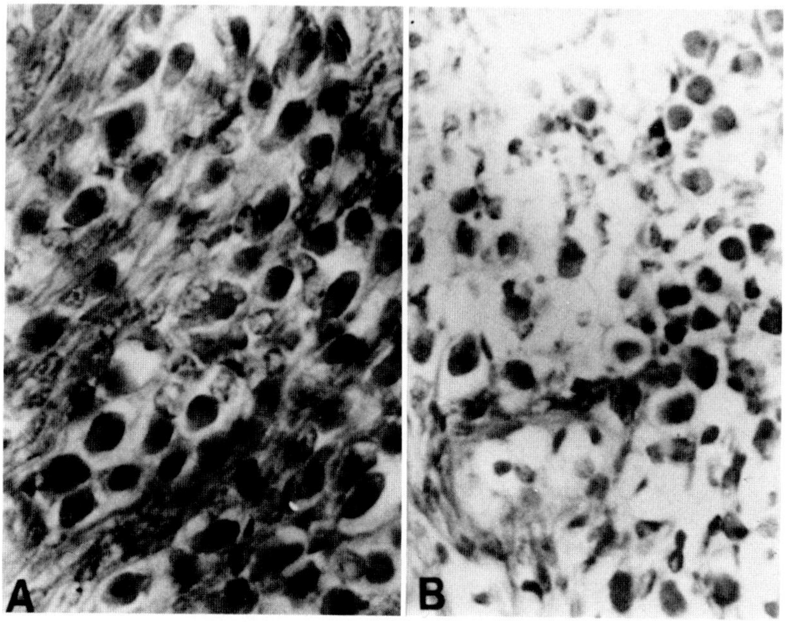

Fig. 8 High magnification of spiral ganglion cells. *A* Control (animal No. 5), × 256. *B* CB-11 peptide-immunized mouse (animal No. 12). Note the marked loss of spiral ganglion cells. The residual cell bodies were also swollen and the nuclei were pyknotic. × 256.

quently, one of the arthritogenic epitopes is suspected to be at least located on CB-11 peptide. In this study, DBA/1J mice immunized with CB-11 peptide developed the same level of sensorineural hearing loss as that induced in CIIn-immunized mice. This hearing loss was one of progessive deafness. A CB-11 peptide immunized mouse at 10 months post-immunization showed deafness. This hearing loss was also associated with severe histologic changes involving loss of both spiral ganglion cells and cochlear nerve and atrophy of the Corti organ. Three out of four CB-11 peptide-immunized mice developed moderate hearing loss 5 months after immunization. These same animals also showed partial loss of the outer hair cells and a mild decrease of cochlear nerve in the basal turn. In addition, dense precipitates, localized in the tunnel of Corti and never seen in the scala tympani, scala vestibuli and scala media, were observed. These precipitates were not detectable in control mice, although simliar precipitates were recognized in the scala media and scala tympani of the CB-11 peptide immunized mouse with the severe hearing loss as well as in the tunnel of Corti. These precipitates may be responsible for the immunologic reactions, such as the deposition of IgG and/or C3. Tested sera showed high antibody titers against native chick type II collagen. No immunohistological sections were performed. Since most of the efferent nerve fibers cross the tunnel of Corti and the afferent nerve fibers toward the outer hair cells run on the base of the tunnel of Corti [37], inflammation in the tunnel of Corti could cause damage that could influence auditory function.

In spite of extensive research, the detailed immune injury mechanism of collagen-induced inner ear lesions still remained obscure. In this study, there was no clear evidence of cochlear vasculitis, an important factor of immunologically mediated lesions. Nevertheless, the present results suggest that the mechanism of inner ear injury was an immunologic reaction in the tunnel of Corti. The immunological assault in the tunnel of Corti led to the loss of hair cells and a decrease of cochlear nerve function followed by retrograde degeneration of spiral ganglion cells.

Further studies are required to ascertain whether or not immunologic reactions are definitely responsible for the precipitates deposited in the tunnel of Corti. However, the data suggest that one of the epitopes on the type II molecule which can induce type II collagen-induced ear disease is CB-11 peptide.

Other Influencing Factors

Collagen-induced autoimmune ear disease occurs in several different animal species. Rats and guinea pigs were the most extensively studied animals, but CIAED can also be induced in monkeys and mice. The lesions of CIAED were mild in chinchillas, rabbits, and cats. Type II collagen immune responses were studied extensively in mice in terms of the induction of arthritis. The immune response gene to type II collagen is linked to $H2^q$ loci. In the rat, it is also linked to AgB loci. Wistar outbred rats and Lewis rats produce these ear lesions. Wistar rats have an immune response to type II collagen, but show only a mild degree of changes in the organ of Corti. In the guinea pig, Hartley and strain 13 types are better responders for the prodution of CIAED. Strain 2 produces less severe lesions. The type of lesion also depends on the degree of immune responsiveness and animal species; e.g. only guinea pigs showed any endolymphatic hydrops. Otospongiosis-like lesions were observed only in rats and, to a lesser degree, in monkeys.

In general, animals immunized with antigens in complete Freund's adjuvant showed relatively more severe lesions than animals immunized with antigens in incomplete Freund's adjuvant. The duration of immunization seems to be a more important factor in producing severe lesions. The strain, and even the source of the animals, are very important factors in autoimmune ear disease, as is the condition of the host animals.

Recently, Cremer et al [38] reported that subclinical or clinical mycoplasma infection in the rat markedly reduced the incidence and serverity of lesions in type II collagen-induced arthritis. Sialoductal adenovirus, widely distributed among laboratory rats, has also been implicated as a nonlesion-producing factor in rats by many researchers. As a result of complications in disease induction associated with certain viral infections, several investigators now use laminar flow rooms to insure induction of pathologic lesions at the maximum level.

We have also recently observed that none of the type II collagen-immunized Lewis rats had developed arthritis or hearing loss in one experiment. These rats are being followed closely at the present time.

The nature of antigens is also important. Chicken type II collagen seems better than bovine for the induction of ear lesions. The native conformation is needed in the rat model, but it does not appear to be an important factor in the guinea pig and mouse models. Other factors that might affect the induction of ear lesions include infection or trauma. Although many factors influence the induction and severity of CIAED, these animal models provide us with an excellent new avenue of inner ear research.

References

1 Cogan, D.G.: Syndrome of nonsyphilitic interstitial keratitis and vestibuloauditory symptoms. Archs Ophthal. *33:* 144 (1945).
2 Lehnhardt, E.: Plötzliche Hörstörungen, auf beiden Seiten gleichzeitig oder nacheinander aufgetreten. Z. Lar. Rhinol. Otol. *37:* 1 (1958).
3 Kikuchi, M.: On the 'sympathetic otitis'. Pract. otol., Kyoto *52:* 600 (1959).
4 Beickert, V.P.: Zur Frage der Empfindungsschwerhörigkeit und der Autoallergie. Lar. Rhinol. Otol. *40:* 837–842 (1961).
5 Sasaki, Y.; Terayama, Y.: Studies on experimental allergic (isoimmune) labyrinthitis in guinea pigs. Acta oto-lar. *58:* 49–64 (1964).

6 Yoo, T.J.: Etiopathogenesis of otosclerosis. A hypothesis. Ann. Otol. Rhinol. Lar. *93:* 28–33 (1984).

7 Yoo, T.J.: Etiopathogenesis of Ménière's disease. A hypothesis. Ann. Otol. Rhinol. Lar. *93:* suppl. 113, pp. 6–12 (1984).

8 Yoo, T.J.; Stuart, J.M.; Kang, A.H.; Tomoda, K.; Townes, A.S.; Dixit, S.: Type II collagen autoimmunity in otosclerosis and Ménière's disease. Science *217:* 1153–1155 (1982).

9 Yoo, T.J.; Tomoda, K.; Stuart, J.M.; Kang, A.H.; Townes, A.S.: Type II collagen induced autoimmune otospongiosis. Ann. Otol. Rhinol. Lar. *92:* 103–108 (1983).

10 Yoo, T.J.; Tomoda, K.; Stuart, J.M.; Cremer, M.A.; Kang. A.H.; Townes, A.S.: Type II collagen induced autoimmune sensorineural hearing loss and vestibular dysfunction in rats. Ann. Otol. Rhinol. Lar. *92:* 267–271 (1983).

11 Yoo, T.J.; Tomoda, K.; Hernandez, A.D.: Type II collagen-induced autoimmune inner ear disease in the guinea pig. Ann. Otol. Rhinol. Lar. *93:* suppl., pp. 3–5 (1984).

12 Yoo, T.J.; Yazawa, Y.; Floyd, R.; Tomoda, K.: Antibody activity in the perilymph from rats with type II collagen-induced autoimmune inner ear disease. Ann. Otol. Rhinol. Lar. *93:* suppl. pp. 1–2 (1984).

13 Yoo, T.J.; Floyd, R.A.; Sudo, N.; Ishibe, T.; Takeda, T.; Tomoda, K.; Yazawa, Y.; Stuart, J.; Choe, I.S.; Ha, S.C.: Influencing factors of collagen induced autoimmune ear disease. Am. J. Otolar. *6:* 209–216 (1985).

14 Pearson, C.M.: Relapsing polychondritis: clinical and immunologic features; in Parker, Clinical immunology, vol. 2, pp. 774–783 (Saunders, Philadelphia 1980).

15 Yoo, T.J.; Shea, J.J.; Shulman, A.; PerLee, J.; Gardner, G.; McCabe, B.: Autoimmune sensorineural hearing loss. Treatment update. J. Otol. Lar., suppl. *19:* pp. 220–227 (1985).

16 Yoo, T.J.; Floyd, R.; Ishibe, T.; Shea, J.J.; Bowman, C.: Immunologic testing of ear disease. Am. J. Otolar. *6:* 96–100 (1985).

17 Yoo, T.J.; Chiang, T.; Dixit, S.; Tomoda, K.; Sudo, N.; Takeda, T.; Seyer, J.; Cremer, M.; Causse, J.B.; Kang, A.H.: Collageneous components of bovine fetal cochlear bone and human stapes bone (submitted, 1986).

18 Yoo, T.J.; Cremer, M.A.; Ishibe, T.; Tomoda, K.: Type II collagen distribution in the ear. Science (to be submitted).

19 Cremer, M.A.; Ishibe, T.; Yoo, T.J.: Type II collagen distribution in the guinea pig fetus (submitted, 1986).

20 Ishibe, T.; Yoo, T.J.; Shea, J.J.; Tomoda, K.: Immunohistochemical studies in Ménière's disease, otosclerosis and tympanosclerosis Abstract. Ass. Res. Otorhinolar. *114:* 92 (1985).

21 Tomoda, K.; Kumazawa, T.; Yoo, T.J.: Immunological basis of Ménière's disease. Br. Otorhinolar. Res. Soc., abstr. No. 17 (1984).

22 Friedman, I.: Pathology of the ear, p. 475 (Blackwell, Oxford 1974).

23 Floyd, R.A.: Ishibe, T.; Kuo, C.Y.; Sudo, N.; Yazawa, Y.; Yoo, T.J.: Type II collagen-induced inner ear diseases in chinchilla. Midwinter Ass. Res. Otolaryngol., abstr. No. 21 (1984).

24 Takeda, T.; Orchik, D.; Yoo, T.J.: Induction of type II collagen autoimmune arthritis and ear disease in monkey (submitted, 1986).

25 Yoo, T.J.; Yazawa, Y.; Tomoda, K.; Floyd, R.: Type II collagen-induced autoimmune endolymphatic hydrops in guinea pig. Science *222:* 65–67 (1983).
26 Lindsay, J.R.: Otosclerosis; in Paparella, Schumrick, Otolaryngology, vol. 2, pp. 1617–1643 (Saunders, Philadelphia 1980).
27 Abramson; Maxwell; Huang; Cheng-Chun; Saporta; Diego: Type II collagen induced bone resorption in the temporal bone of rats. Histological and immunohistochemical studies. Archs Oto-Rhino-Lar. *242:* 183–188 (1985).
28 McCabe, B.F.: Autoimmune sensorineural hearing loss. Ann. Otol. Rhinol. Lar. *88:* 585–589 (1979).
29 Stewart, I.A.; Wilson, R.L.K.: Autoimmune sensorineural deafness. Case report. N. Z. med. J. *697:* 414–415 (1981).
30 Barna, B.P.; Calabrese, L.M.; Hughes, G.B.; Kinney, S.E.: Autoimmune reactivity in Ménière's disease. Preliminary report. Laryngoscope *93:* 410 (1983).
31 Altermatt. H.J.; Arnold, W.; Phfaltz, C.R.: Evidence of serum antibodies against inner ear tissues in the blood of patients with certain sensorineural hearing disorders. Acta otolar. *99:* (1985).
32 Floyd, R.A.; Ishibe, T.; Yazawa, Y.; Yoo, T.J.: Cell transfer of CIAED in guinea pig. Ass. Res. Otolar., abstr. No. 31 (1983).
33 Sudo, N.; Takeda, T.; Yoo, T.J.: Induction of tolerance in CIAED (to be submitted).
34 Terato, K.; Hasty, K.A.: Cremer, M.A.; Stuart, J.M.; Townes, A.S.; Kang, A.H.: Collagen-induced arthritis in mice. Localization of an arthritogenic determinant to a fragment of the type II collagen molecule. J. exp. Med. *162:* 637–46 (1985).
35 Miller, E.J.: Isolation and characterization of the cyanogen bromide peptides from the 1 (II) chain of chick cartilage collagen. Biochemistry *10:* 3030–3035 (1971).
36 Igarashi, S.; Kang, A.H.; Trelstad, R.L.: Physical chemical properties of chick cartilage collagen. Biochim. biophys. Acta *295:* 514–519 (1973).
37 Spoendlin H.: Primary neurons and synapes; in Friedman, Ballantyne, Ultrastructural atlas of the inner ear, pp. 133–164 (Buttersworth, London 1983).
38 Cremer, M.A.: Leary, S.L.; Taurog, J.D.: Infection with mycoplasma pulmonis modulates adjuvant- and collagen-induced arthritis in Lewis rats. Arthritis Rheum. *27:* 943–946 (1984).

T.J. Yoo, MD, Departments of Medicine, Microbiology and Immunology, and Neurosciences Program, University of Tennessee, 956 Court Avenue, H300, Memphis, TN 38163 (USA)

Concepts Immunopathol., vol. 4, pp. 243–260 (Karger, Basel 1987)

Immunoregulatory Defects Associated with Infection with the AIDS Virus, HTLV-III

Richard M. Crapper[a], *Ian H. Frazer*[a], *Ian R. Mackay*[a], *Angelina Iscaro*[a], *David L. Bradford*[b]

[a] Clinical Research Unit of The Walter and Eliza Hall Institute of Medical Research and The Royal Melbourne Hospital, and [b] the Melbourne Communicable Diseases Centre, Melbourne, Australia

Introduction

The acquired immune deficiency syndrome (AIDS) and AIDS-related conditions are known to be due to infection with the retrovirus human T cell lymphotrophic virus, HTLV-III [1], also called lymphadenopathy associated virus, LAV [2], or AIDS-associated retrovirus, ARV [3]. The review will start with a brief description of the evolution of retroviruses including HTLV-III. The retrovirus family is divided into 3 subfamilies – oncoviruses, lenteviruses and spumaviruses: the first two groups have now been clearly implicated as causes of disease in humans. Molecular biological studies have shown that many of these retroviruses including HTLV-I and HTLV-III contain transactivating transcriptional activator (tat) sequences (fig. 1) which greatly enhance transcription of viral and probably cellular genes [4], and this enhanced transcription is considered to be very important in pathogenicity.

Oncoviruses, which are characterized by a capacity to transform cells in vitro and be oncogenic in vivo, include bovine leukemia virus, simian T cell leukemia virus (STLV) and the human T cell leukemia viruses. Lenteviruses, in contrast, cause cytopathic effects on cells in vitro and slowly progressive immunosuppressive disease in vivo. However, there is some overlap between oncoviruses and lenteviruses since HTLV-I and Simian(S)TLV-I viruses can cause immune impairment in vivo, and HTLV-III can be induced to transform some cell lines in vitro. Lenteviruses include the human and simian viruses HTLV–III and STLV-III [5], and the originally described group of ungulate lenteviruses, notably visna

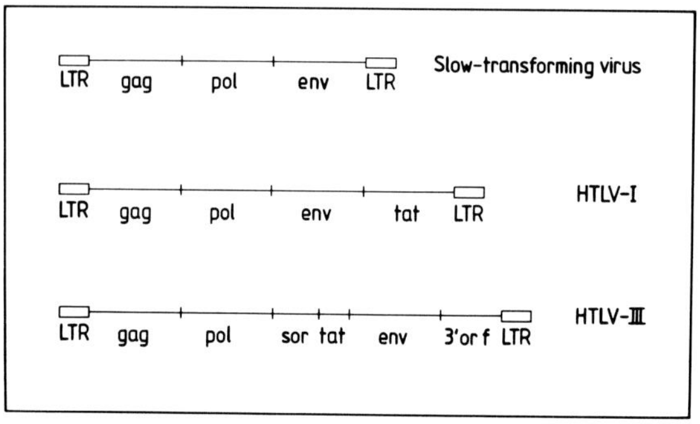

Fig. 1. Molecular structure of the HTLV-III retrovirus, and shown for comparison is the structure of HTLV-I and a slow-transforming or chronic retrovirus (e.g mouse leukemia virus). LTR = Long terminal repeats; gag = gene coding for structural proteins; pol = polymerase gene; env = envelope gene; tat = transactivating transcription element; sor = short open reading frame; orf = open reading frame.

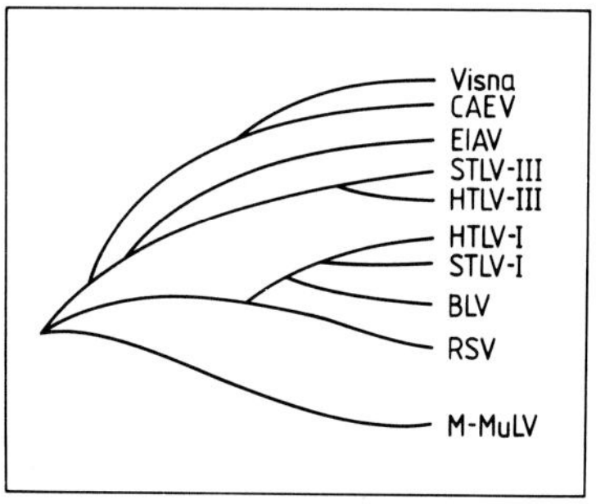

Fig. 2. Evolutionary tree of retroviruses based on percentage homology of pol genes. The length between the branches does not reflect actual divergence times.

virus which is the prototype retrovirus first described in 1949 as an agent causing an indolent inflammatory central nervous system (CNS) disease with wasting in sheep, caprine arthritis-encephalitis virus (CAEV), and equine infectious anemia virus (EIAV) (fig. 2) [6]. HTLV-III is closely related genomically to STLV-III and shares considerable nucleotide sequence homology including the short open reading frame (sor) and 3′ open reading frame (3′ orf) sequences (fig. 1). The AIDS virus HTLV-III most probably evolved from the STLV-III virus which is indigenous to primates in central Africa. STLV-III causes no obvious disease in monkeys in Africa although it does cause an immune deficiency syndrome in captive macaque monkeys from which it was first isolated [7].

The predominant cell type known to be infected by HTLV-III is the helper T lymphocyte (Th). This cell is characterized by the presence of the CD4 surface antigen, recognized by the monoclonal antibodies OKT4 (Ortho) or Leu 3a (Becton-Dickinson). It is most likely that the CD4 antigen actually is, or forms part of the receptor for HTLV-III, since most monoclonal antibodies to CD4 block infection of T helper cells in vitro with HTLV-III [8]. Infection of Th cells in vitro causes cytopathic effects including multinucleate cell formation, vacuolation and cell lysis and may cause in vivo a marked diminution in cell numbers to virtually zero in advanced cases of AIDS. Follicular dendritic (FD) cells of lymph nodes also have been shown in electron microscopic studies to harbor retrovirus-like particles, identified in follicles of hyperplastic lymph nodes of homosexual males with various categories of AIDS [9]; such infection may lead to aberrant antigen presentation with development of exaggerated B cell reactions to various infectious agents and autoantigens, with consequent proliferation of supressor T lymphocytes (Ts) [9]. These processes may be important, either primarily or secondarily, in the loss of Th cells. Another site in which HTLV-III has been identified is the brain, in subjects infected with the virus; the HTLV-III virus is deemed to be directly or indirectly responsible for the progressive dementia or encephalopathy which may occur in infected subjects [10], but the range of cell types which may contain the virus has not been fully established. Thus, studies using in situ nucleic acid hybridization have shown the virus to be present in perivascular aggregates of macrophage-type microglial cells, but whether these cells are infected in the CNS or migrate there after infection [11], and whether central neurones are infected remains to be determined.

Historically, there was in 1980 in the USA an unprecedented occurrence of cases of Kaposi's sarcoma, pneumocystis carinii pneumonia, and other opportunistic infections in homosexual men and to a lesser extent in drug addicts, concentrated in New York City and San Francisco. AIDS was recognised in 1981 as a distinct clinical entity and, by the end of 1981, 216 cases in the USA had been reported to the Centers for Disease Control, Atlanta, Ga. Due to its distinctive epidemiological features, the illness was suspected from the outset to be infectious, and presumably viral, although various co-factors were also incriminated. The first report describing the isolation of the AIDS virus, called lymphadenopathy-associated virus (LAV), was published by Montagnier and colleagues in May 1983 [2] and, in May 1984, Gallo et al. [1] published reports describing the propagation of a similar virus in vitro, thus allowing detailed studies on its characteristics.

AIDS is now definable as an acquired immune deficiency due to infection with the HTLV-III virus together with serious opportunistic infection or certain types of malignancy [12]. The two tumors most typically associated with HTLV-III infection are Kaposi's sarcoma and B cell lymphoma. Since in neither of these can the HTLV-III genome be detected in the malignant cells, another mechanism must be postulated for tumor development or persistence, be this lack of immune surveillance and/or sustained cellular stimulation. The HTLV-III virus is the direct cause of a variety of syndromes or diseases in addition to AIDS, these including lymphadenopathy syndrome (LAS) [13], AIDS-related complex (ARC) in which there is one or more of a variety of systemic disorders including malaise, weight loss, diarrhoea, fevers and sweats in the presence of immune impairment, with or without lymphadenopathy [14], neurological disease including dementia [10], and thrombocytopenia [15].

Assessment of Immune Dysfunction in Relation to AIDS

The comprehensive testing of immune function requires assessment of functions dependent on T and B lymphocytes using both in vivo and in vitro assay procedures. Assays of T lymphocyte function are of most importance. The most commonly used assay of immune function in vivo, and the only one referred to in this article, is recall of delayed-type hypersensitivity to a panel of ubiquitous antigens: this depends on lymphokine-mediated cellular immune function expressed by CD4 lymphocytes, and requires intact afferent and efferent limbs of the immune response. Earlier procedures depending on testing with various panels of antigens have been superceded by a commercially available device (the Multitest, Institut Mérieux, Lyon, France) enabling the simultaneous administration of 7 standardized ubiquitous antigens, tetanus, diphtheria, streptococcus, tuberculin, candida, trichophyton and proteus, to which most normal subjects would have developed previous immunity [16]. The Multitest device overcomes the nonstandardization of previous procedures, the inconvenience of separate injections of antigen and the technical difficulty of ensuring their intradermal rather than subcutaneous injection. A positive response to an antigen is defined as an area of induration present at 48 h of at least 2 mm in diameter: results are expressed as the number of positive responses and the aggregate size for all of the positive reactions. In a study of 110 healthy heterosexual men in Melbourne, anergy (response to none of the 7 antigens) was seen in only 1%, an aggregate score of less than 5 mm was observed in only 5% and the mean aggregate score was 15.3 mm. The correlation in the Melbourne study between reaction scores obtained on two occasions, 3 months apart, was high ($r = 0.88$).

The integrity of cellular immunity in vitro is measured by functional assays, i.e. lymphocyte proliferative response or lymphokine production (interleukin 2, interferon) after mitogen or antigen stimulation, or numerical assays, i.e. determination of numbers of helper (Th) and suppressor/cytotoxic (Ts) T lymphocytes (CD4 and CD8) and the ratio between them (Th/Ts, TCR) [17]. The best characterized cellular defects associated with HTLV-III infection are alterations in absolute numbers and proportions of T cell subsets, and these results will be referred to extensively in this review. In brief, the assay procedure involves separation of blood mononuclear cells by density sedimentation on 'Ficoll-Hypaque', staining with fluoresceinated monoclonal antisera, and then enumeration by flow cytometry. Enumeration of cells microscopically, although slower, is reliable and applicable if flow cytometry is not available or if field studies need to be done. Mean values (±SD) for cell counts ($\times 10^{-6}$/L) obtained from a group of 100 healthy heterosexual men in Melbourne were as follows. Th, 1130 ± 375, Ts, 480 ± 190, and Th/Ts ratio, 2.6 ± 1.1. Taking 2 SD from the mean as the range of normal, the lower limit of normal for men for the absolute Th cell count would be 400 and the upper limit of normal for Ts cells 850.

B lymphocyte function also can be assessed by both in vivo and in vitro techniques. Total serum immunoglobulin G, measured by nephelometry or radial immunodiffusion, is used to determine the degree of polyclonal B cell activation. Specific antibody responses following immunization (and rechallenge) give further information on the integrity of afferent and efferent limbs of the humoral immune response. Finally, the functional capacity of individual B lymphocytes can be determined by measuring immunoglobulin production in vitro following pokeweed mitogen stimulation.

Alterations in T Cell Numbers in Homosexual Men

Early studies from both the USA and England demonstrated that, aside from the profound immune deficiency of men with AIDS, immune functional indices of healthy homosexual men were lower than those of heterosexual men. For example, Kornfeld et al. [18] in 1981 studied 81 homosexual men in New York and found that 50 were asymptomatic and 31 reported weight loss, diarrhea, fever, malaise or lymphadenopathy; in a comparison with a matched group of heterosexual men the asymptomatic homosexual men had decreased Th cells, 644 vs. 813, increased Ts cells, 675 vs. 454 and a lower TCR, 1.1 vs. 1.8, whereas the symptomatic homosexual men showed greater differences, particularly in numbers of Th cells (483) and TCR (0.8). Greater sexual activity was associated with a greater immune impairment, in that subjects reporting 9 or fewer different sexual partners per year had a higher TCR than those reporting more than 9 sexual partners per year. This was the first study to draw attention to the gradation of severity of immune impairment in homosexual men grouped according to their reported degree of sexual activity.

A later study from Detels et al. [19] in Los Angeles reported a comparable degree of immune impairment as assessed by T cell subsets in healthy homosexual men, since 27% of 89 such men had a TCR <0.8; they ascertained that the low TCR was due predominantly to a raised number of Ts cells, seen particularly in men with lymphadenopathy (29% of the study group), whereas in AIDS a low ratio was due more to a decrease in the Th subset. The relationship between homosexual activity and the degree of immune alteration was investigated also by Detels et al. [19] who found that receptive (passive) anal intercourse correlated with increase in Ts cells: 'immune augmentation' was applied to this state. Pinching et al. [20] investigated immune function in 97 asymptomatic homosexual men in London, of whom a high proportion showed immunological abnormalities: decreased TCR (43%), decreased Th counts (15%), monocyte chemotactic defects (10%) and phagocytic defects (27%), anergy to 3 recall antigens (32%), and anergy to PPD (55%). Immune impairment was more severe in those with lymphadenopathy than in those without. The high proportion of abnormalities in this otherwise normal population was remarkable; anergy, for example, was as frequent as in patients with Hodgkin's disease.

A number of other reports appeared during 1983 to 1985 describing alterations in immune function and T cell ratios in homosexual men which confirmed the original studies [21–23] and described a hierarchical series of levels of immune impairment, as follows. Men without lymphadenopathy had a reduced TCR due to increased numbers of Ts cells; men with lymphadenopathy had a further decrease in the TCR due predominantly to increased numbers of Ts cells but with some reduction in Th cells; men with prolonged systemic symptoms had a further reduction in the TCR with a still greater reduction in Th cells; and men with AIDS had a very great reduction in Th cells, usually without a high Ts cell number, so that in the most severely immunocompromised men the TCR stabilized because of the fall in Ts cells. AIDS with opportunistic infections was found to be associated with a more marked immune impairment than AIDS with Kaposi's sarcoma, suggesting that co-factors apart from those causing immune impairment may be important in the induction of this malignancy.

There is a point here needing major emphasis. This is that all of the above-cited data were obtained before identification of HTLV-III as the cause of AIDS and, in particular, before the advent of specific serological tests for detection of carriers of the virus. Hence, it could not be known to what extent the immune abnormalities were due on the one hand to the etiological agent HTLV-III, or on the other hand to various infectious illnesses and life-style factors unique to homosexual men. The fact that the degree of immune dysfunction was greater in the more promiscuous subjects, and those preferentially engaging in receptive anal intercourse, suggests that semen itself may be immunosuppressive, either as a direct effect of seminal plasma [24], or due to an exposure of lymphocytes to foreign HLA antigens present on leukocytes transferred in semen. The issue of the relative contributions to immune dysfunction in homosexual men of HTLV-III infection and other factors is discussed below in the light of experience in Melbourne.

Correlation of Immune Abnormalities with Anti-HTLV-III Status

A detailed prospective immunological study was begun on a group of 100 volunteer homosexual men in Melbourne by us in mid-1983 [25,26]. Results of antibody to HTLV-III and immune function for these men, and for a control group of 100 age-matched healthy heterosexual men, are shown in table I. In remarks below, seropositive will refer to a positive test for antibody to HTLV-III. For the homosexual men, there

Table I. Immune function in relation to seropositivity for anti-HTLV-III in homosexual men

Subjects	Indices of immune function (mean ± 1 SD)					
	IgG g/l	T cells $\times 10^{-6}/l$	Th $\times 10^{-6}/l$	Ts $\times 10^{-6}/l$	TCR	DTH score, mm
Seropositive (n=23)	13.5 ±2.7[b]	1,531 ±546	771 ±249[a]	636 ±289	1.3 ±0.8[b]	12.8 ±8.8
Seronegative (n=77)	11.6 ±2.5	1,581 ±483	894 ±311[a]	529 ±228	1.9 ±1.1[a]	14.5 ±7.5
Controls (n=100)	10.9 ±2.4	1,554 ±469	1,128 ±375	483 ±194	2.6 ±1.1	15.3 ±6.0

This table is based on one from the manuscript: 'Immunological abnormalities in asymptomatic homosexual men: correlation with antibody to HTLV-III and sequential changes over two years' by I. H. Frazer, I. R. Mackay, R. M. Crapper, et al. [39].

[a] $p < 0.01$, [b] $p < 0.001$, compared with controls.

was a significant reduction in both Th cell numbers and the TCR, with a trend for even lower values in seropositive men; there was an increase in Ts cell numbers and a decrease in the DTH score, but with no significant differences between seropositive and seronegative men. The homosexual men had higher levels of immunoglobulin G, with significantly higher levels in the seropositive men. The data for each of these indices of immune function had a Gaussian distribution, but with differing modal values from those of the controls, indicating that there was no subgroup among the homosexual subjects with altered immune function. These Melbourne data are in line with the American and English studies in showing significant degrees of immune abnormality in homosexual men, and the Melbourne data show further that these abnormalities are not wholly explained by infection with HTLV-III.

The mean number of sexual partners in the 2 years preceding the study was also predictive of abnormal cell mediated immunity (CMI), independently of anti-HTLV-III. Thus, the group with abnormal indices of CMI and anti-HTLV reported a mean of 88 partners during this period, and the group without anti-HTLV-III and with abnormal CMI, 46 partners, the group with anti-HTLV and normal CMI, 33 partners, and the group without anti-HTLV-III and with normal CMI, 16 partners. Another infectious agent apart from HTLV-III of importance in predicting abnormal immune function was cytomegalovirus (CMV) since, although the groups with and without abnormal CMI did not differ for the frequency of serum CMV IgG antibody (95 vs. 98%), they did differ in the prevalence of positive semen culture for CMV (9/19 vs. 1/16, $p<0.01$). Of the 9 subjects with abnormal CMI and positive CMV semen culture, 4 had anti-HTLV-III.

Thus, from the above data, it is evident that life-style factors, including the degree of promiscuity, in addition to infection with HTLV-III, are predictors of cellular immunodeficiency in homosexual men. As a comment on the finding that the immunological defects in the seropositive Melbourne men were relatively mild, we could note that when this study was begun, most of the participants would have seroconverted within the previous 1–3 years, and it is known that immune function deteriorates with duration of seropositivity [27]. The possible causes of the immune deficiency in seropositive men are discussed in the final section of the review.

Immunological Indices in Lymphadenopathy Syndrome (LAS) and in Homosexual Men with Constitutional Symptoms

The lymphadenopathy syndrome of homosexual men has been defined as an enlargement of 3 or more extra-inguinal noncontiguous lymph node groups for a period of at least 3 months [13]; the reported incidences in homosexual men from earlier studies have varied from 6 to 29% [18–20]. In our prospective study on 100 homosexual men in Melbourne, lymphadenopathy was observed in 1983 in 4 (4%) of whom 3 were seropositive, and in 1985 in 11 of 80 remaining participants (14%), of whom 9 were seropositive. The lymphadenopathy syndrome has not so far resolved in any of the seropositive men. When lymphadenopathy was observed in persistently seronegative men, this was generally minor in degree and number of nodes involved, was transient and did not fulfil the diagnostic criteria for LAS. However, there are 2 men in our study with LAS who have been persistently negative for anti-HTLV-III; these men may nonetheless be infected but have not yet mounted an antibody response or, alternatively, there may be some other cause for their persistent lymphadenopathy.

Considering only the seropositive men, the frequency of LAS in the Melbourne study increased from 15% in 1983 to 38% in 1985, compara-

Table II. Clinical status and immune function in anti-HTLV-III-positive homosexual men with or without LAS

LAS[a]	Symptoms[b]		TCR[c]		Th cells ($\times 10^{-9}$/l)[d]		Mean T cell number ($\times 10^{-9}$/l)[e]	
	yes	no	< 1.0	≥ 1.0	< 400[f]	≥ 400	Th	Ts
Yes (32)[g]	10	22	25	7	7	25	553 ± 235	695 ± 332
No (40)	4	36	13	27	8	32	676 ± 356	573 ± 265

[a] See text for definitions of LAS and 'symptoms'.
[b] Chi^2 5.12, p = 0.02.
[c] Chi^2 14.8, p < 0.001.
[d] Chi^2 3.79, not significant.
[e] Mean numbers ± 1 SD.
[f] A Th cell count of 400×10^{-9}/l is our lower limit of normal.
[g] Numbers in parentheses or in columns 1–6 represent number of subjects.

ble with the increase in frequency in a large San Francisco cohort study in which in 1984 21% of men had LAS. As 67% of that study group had seroconverted by then, the frequency of lymphadenopathy among the seropositive subjects would be 31% [28]. Further to this, a small prospective study from Finland [29] reported LAS in 3 of 17 seropositive men and, over a follow-up period of approximately 1 year, a further 3 seropositive subjects developed lymphadenopathy, representing 35% of the group.

We began a further study in Melbourne in 1985 to ascertain clinical and immunological features of 72 homosexual men known to be seropositive for anti-HTLV-III; some had symptoms, but most were in employment and seroconversion was judged to have been recent. Generalized lymphadenopathy was detected in 32 (44%) and, compared to those without lymphadenopathy, the LAS subgroup had an increased frequency of symptoms indicative of chronic infection, i.e. night sweats, fever, weight loss, diarrhea, malaise or lethargy for more than 3 months and a lowered TCR (table II). The proportion of men with absolute Th cell numbers below 400×10^9/l did not differ according to the presence or absence of lymphadenopathy, indicating that the reduced TCR in those with lymphadenopathy was due to a relative imbalance of Th and Ts cells. The mean values for numbers of Th and Ts cells in men with and without LAS are shown in table II, and reveal that those with LAS had

Table III. Immune function in anti-HTLV-III-positive homosexual men with or without symptoms

Symptoms[a]	TCR[b]		Th cells[c]		Mean T cell number ($\times 10^{-9}$/l)	
	< 1	⩾ 1	< 400	⩾ 400	Th[d]	Ts[e]
Yes (14)	12	2	10	4	376±271	577±302
No (58)	26	32	5	53	660±275	696±357

[a] See table II for definitions.
[b] Chi^2 7.56, $p < 0.01$.
[c] Chi^2 26, $p < 0.001$.
[d] t 3.4, $p < 0.005$.
[e] t 1.13, not significant.

lower mean numbers of Th cells and higher mean numbers of Ts cells than those without LAS. Constitutional symptoms were present in 14 (19%) of the entire group and of these, very few had a TCR in the normal range (table III); in contrast to patients with LAS, most men with symptoms had a reduced count of Th cells (table III).

These data indicate that among men seropositive for HTLV-III, LAS specifies a group with a different immune response to HTLV-III which is not characterized by a significantly greater immune impairment. Furthermore, in separate studies, we found no difference in DTH score between seropositive men with or without LAS. Those men with symptoms, however, had a marked deficiency in immune function, the majority of these men fitting into the Krause definition of the AIDS-related complex (ARC) [14]. The outcome of LAS remains uncertain since the reported progression to AIDS varies from 2 to 19% [30, 31); in the study reporting progression in 19%, those who did develop AIDS generally had both constitutional symptoms and marked immune impairment beforehand. In the prospective study performed in Melbourne for which there is a follow-up of at least 2 years, none of the 10 participants with LAS has yet developed AIDS. Pending further data, the outcome for a person with LAS remains uncertain, since the syndrome does not resolve spontaneously yet the risk of developing AIDS seems only about 10%. However, for those with constitutional symptoms, whether lymphadenopathy is present or not, there is usually a substantially compromised immunological status and the outlook is worse.

Changes in Immune Function with Time and Relationship to HTLV-III Status and Lifestyle

It is obviously of interest to know which immunological indices may change during prospective follow-up. In the Melbourne cohort study of 100 homosexual men, all immunological indices were measured initially in 1983 and after 1 and 2 years: the data at 1 year, shown in table IV, are expressed as proportional increments of decrements in relation to the value at recruitment, shown in table I. Complete data were available for 84 subjects; data for the 4 who seroconverted during this 1-year period are excluded. The mean serum IgG level did not change significantly but, unexpectedly, the mean TCR increased significantly from 1.7±0.1 to 2.3±0.1 due to an increase in Th cells and a decrease in Ts cells, and the mean DTH score also increased. For a control group of 29 concurrently-studied heterosexual subjects, the T cell counts, TCR, DTH score and IgG level did not differ significantly throughout the study (data not shown). Considering seropositive (20) and seronegative (60) homosexual men separately, the mean serum IgG level increased significantly (table IV) in the former group and fell in the latter; the total T cell count did not change in either group; the TCR ratio increased in both groups due to an increase in Th and a fall in Ts cells, and the DTH score increased in both groups.

The degree of improvement in indices of cell-mediated immunity was assessed according to anti-HTLV-III status. The TCR or the DTH score improved over one year by greater that 100% in 31 of the 84 subjects for whom complete data was available, of whom 9 had anti-HTLV-III, and by 25–100% in 36 subjects, of whom 10 had anti-HTLV-III: both indices improves by 100% or more in 3 seropositive and 13 seronegative subjects and by 25–100% in 4 seropositive and 20 seronegative subjects. On the other hand, there was a deterioration in one or both of these indices over this period by 50% or greater in 8 subjects, of whom 4 were positive for anti-HTLV-III and by 25–50% in 4 subjects of whom 2 were positive for anti-HTLV-III. Thus, improvement in immune function over the first year of the study occurred independently of anti-HTLV-III status, but deterioration was more frequent in those seropositive for anti-HTLV-III. The observed improvement in indices of CMI over 1 year of study could be related to reduction in the number of sexual partners. The average reported number of sexual partners per month for 84 fully-studied subjects decreased from a mean of 11.3 at recruitment to 5.2 after 1

Table IV. Changes in immunological indices in 80 Melbourne homosexual men after 1 year

Group	Change in indices of immune function[a]					
	IgG	T cells	Th	Ts	TCR	DTH score, mm
All subjects (n = 80)	0.98	1.01	1.18	0.84	1.43[b]	1.33[b]
Seropositive (n = 20)	1.26[b]	0.96	1.11	0.87	1.31[b]	1.31[b]
Seronegative (n = 60)	0.87	1.03	1.20	0.82	1.43[b]	1.34[b]

This table is based on one from the manuscript: 'Immunological abnormalities in asymptomatic homosexual men: correlation with antibody to HTLV-III and sequential changes over two years' by I. H. Frazer, I. R. Mackay, R. M. Crapper, et al. [39].

[a] The mean result for each index at 1 year is shown as the ratio of the mean of results at recruitment and after 1 year.

[b] Significantly different from value at recruitment ($p < 0.01$).

year of study; a reduction in the number of sexual partners by more than 50% was reported by 15 of the 60 seronegative subjects and 9 of the 24 seropositive subjects. The mean improvement in the TCR was 56% for the 24 subjects reporting a reduction of >50% in sexual partners and 28% for 60 reporting a lesser or no reduction ($p<0.05$). Similarly, the mean increase in the multitest score was 89% for the 24 subjects reporting a >50% reduction in the total number of sexual partners, and 5% for the 60 subjects reporting a lesser or no reduction ($p<0.01$).

What may be the reasons for this improvement in parameters of immune function? It is now well established that homosexual men have impaired CMI and, as stated before, there are a variety of possible causes for this including the specifically immunosuppressive viruses HTLV-III and CMV, other recurrent infections, drug abuse, especially nitrites, and exposure to the potentially immunosuppressive effects of seminal plasma and foreign HLA antigens. From our studies on the Melbourne cohort, it is obvious that there is a significant degree of immune impairment in men without evidence of infection with HTLV-III (table I), and, as demonstrated by previously cited studies performed prior to a significant spread of HTLV-III [18–20], and also from our studies, the degree of the deficiency is strongly correlated with homosexual lifestyle factors, particularly sexual promiscuity and receptive anal intercourse. Thus, it is encouraging and perhaps to be expected that immune function should improve with a reduction in sexual activity.

That seropositive as well as seronegative men had an improvement in CMI with a reduction in sexual activity is a notable finding. This may be related to 'co-factor effects' given that similar influences are operative in seronegative and seropositive men; or perhaps it may be that with a reduction in sexual activity in seropositive men, there is less immune activation and thus less replication of the HTLV-III virus and hence less destruction of Th cells. As a corollary to this it is now well recognized that, for HTLV-III to be lytic to infected Th cells in culture in vitro, there needs to be activation of these cells, by mitogens in the case of in vitro stimulation [32].

Final Remarks

In this report we have attempted to describe the range and extent of immune impairments observed in homosexual men and their relationship to HTLV-III infection. Indices of cellular immunity assessed by in vivo and in vitro techniques are decreased in a proportion of homosexual men, and the degree and severity of the impairment are more marked in those infected with HTLV-III. The precise cause(s) of the immune defects in seronegative men is uncertain but the degree of immune deficiency correlates with sexual promiscuity, a preference for passive anal intercourse and active CMV infection. Despite the importance of co-factors in determining the degree of immune dysfunction in homosexual men, HTLV-III is clearly adequate in its own right to cause immune impairment and AIDS, as evidenced by the development of these conditions in heterosexual subjects infected by transfusion of contaminated blood or blood products.

The cause of the immune deficiency induced by HTLV-III infection is also not clearly defined. The two principal mechanisms which have been considered to diminish Th cells are direct lysis by HTLV-III, or autoimmune destruction. In favor of the former is the fact that, in in vitro experiments, infection which HTLV-III is sufficient to cause cytopathic and cytolytic changes in cultured T cells, but two reasons argue against this being the only or major explanation. The first is that replication and subsequent damage to the Th cells is seen only in activated T cells in vitro rather than in resting lymphocytes [31], which would be the normal status in vivo, and the second is that studies of peripheral blood lymphocytes from HTLV-III-infected subjects indicate that only a small proportion contain the HTLV-III genome and even a smaller proportion (less than 1 in 10,000) contain replicating virus [33]. Thus, there would seem to be reasonable evidence against direct destruction of Th cells by viral infection as a major lytic mechanism.

The second possibility, that the viral infection triggers an autoimmune response, is well established for a variety of viral agents [34, 35]. Antilymphocyte antibodies are present in the serum of HTLV-III infected subjects [36, 37] and it has been shown by some authors that these antibodies react selectively with Th cells [37]. Several mechanisms might explain this immune reactivity including immunological cross-reactivity between viral and host antigens [34], virus-induced alteration of host cell membranes, or an immune response to HTLV-III envelope proteins bound to the surface of uninfected CD4 positive cells [33]. Th cells with surface-bound antibody would then be eliminated by cellular or complement-mediated cytotoxic mechanisms.

Persistent lymphadenopathy is strongly associated with HTLV-III infection and is reported in some 20–40% of seropositive men. Furthermore, the proportion of subjects with lymphadenopathy increases with duration of HTLV-III infection. Seropositive homosexual men with lymphadenopathy versus those without have a significantly reduced TCR due to both a reduction in Th cells and an increase of Ts cells and men with constitutional symptoms have a further reduction in TCR due also to increased Ts cells and markedly reduced Th counts.

The CD8-positive subset of lymphocytes includes cells mediating both suppression and cytotoxicity (Ts/c or Ts) as it has not been possible to subcategorise these groups. Certainly Ts are elevated in many infectious illnesses and it has been documented that they are increased in acute HTLV-III infection [38]. In the context of response to micro-organisms, particularly viral pathogens, the increase in Ts cells is due mainly to a proliferation of cytotoxic T lymphocytes recognizing viral encoded antigens in combination with class I MHC molecules but this response is usually transient, lasting only some weeks. Our studies revealed a moderate increase in mean numbers of CD8 (?suppressor) cells in seronegative homosexual men and an even greater increase in seropositive subjects. The increase in Ts cells in seronegative subjects may be secondary to an increased frequency of infectious episodes, particularly with CMV for which there is serological evidence of infection in virtually 100% of homosexual men. Men with lymphadenopathy have a greater increase in Ts over those without so-called 'immune augmentation' [22]. It has been postulated [9] that aberrent antigen presentation by HTLV-III-infected dendritic follicular cells in the enlarged nodes may underlie this excessive Ts response. Men who are seropositive and have systemic symptoms have the greatest reduction in numbers of Th cells and these are probably the most immunologically compromised, despite having lower numbers of Ts than seropositive men without symptoms. Hence although Ts cells are raised in seropositive men, the absolute level may not be of major importance in the assessment of immune competence.

Since our prospective studies on well-motivated homosexual males revealed significant improvements in immune function in both seropositive and seronegative men, with the most substantial improvements occurring in those who were able to change their lifestyle the most, we conclude that advice on 'safe sex' practices is relevant to all homosexual men regardless of anti-HTLV-III status.

References

1 Gallo, R.; Salahuddin, S.; Popovic, M.; Shearer, G.; Kaplan, M.; Haynes, B.; Palker, T.; Redfield, R.; Oleske, J.; Safai, B.; White, G.; Foster, P.; Markham, P.: Frequent detection and isolation of cytopathic retroviruses (HTLV-III) from patients with AIDS and at risk for AIDS. Science *224:* 500–503 (1984).

2 Barré-Sinoussi, F.; Chermann, J.; Rey, F.; Negeyre, S.; Chamaret, S.; Gruest, J.; Dauguet C.; Axler-Blin, C.; Vézinet-Brun, F.; Rouzioux, C.; Rozenbaum, W.; Montagnier, L.: Isolation of a T-lymphotropic retrovirus from a patient at risk for acquired immune deficiency syndrome. Science *220:* 868–871 (1983).

3 Levy, J.; Hoffman, A.; Kramer, S.; Landis, J.; Shimabukuro, J.; Oshiro L.: Isolation of lymphocytopathic retroviruses from San Francisco patients with AIDS. Science *225:* 840–842 (1984).

4 Arya, S.; Guo, C.; Josephs, S.; Wong-Staal, F.: Transactivator gene of human T-lymphotropic virus type III (HTLV-III). Science *229:* 69–73 (1985).

5 Kanki, P.; Alroy, J.; Essex, M: Isolation of T-lymphotropic retrovirus related to HTLV-III/LAV from wild-caught African green monkeys. Science *230:* 951–954 (1985).

6 Chiu, I.; Yaniv, A.; Dahlberg, J.; Gazit, A.; Skuntz, S.; Tronik, S.; Aaronson, S.: Nucleotide sequence evidence for relationship of AIDS retrovirus to lenteviruses. Nature, Lond. *317:* 366–368 (1985).

7 Daniel, M.; Letvin, N.; King, N.; Kannagi, M.; Sehgal, P.; Hunt, R.; Kanki, P.; Essex, M.; Desrosiers, R.: Isolation of T-cell tropic HTLV-III-like retroviruses from macaques. Science *228:* 1201–1204 (1985).

8 Dalgleish, A.; Beverley, P.; Clapham, P.; Crawford, D.; Greaves, M.; Weiss, R.:

The CD4 (T4) antigen is an essential component of the receptor for the AIDS retrovirus. Nature, Lond. *312:* 763–767 (1984).

9 Armstrong, J.; Dawkins, R.; Horne, R.: Retroviral infection of accessory cells and the immunological paradox in AIDS. Immunol. Today *6:* 121–122 (1985).

10 Shaw, G.; Harper, M.; Hahn, B.; Epstein, L.; Gajdusek, D.; Price, R.; Navia, B.; Petito, C.; O'Hara, C.; Groopman, J.; Cho, E.; Oleske, J.; Wong-Staal, F.; Gallo, R.: HTLV-III infection in brains of children and adults with AIDS encephalopathy. Science *227:* 177–181 (1985).

11 Gallo, R.: Personal commun.

12 Centers for Disease Control: Revision of the case definition of acquired immunodeficiency syndrome for national reporting–United States. Morb. Mortal. Wkly Rep. *34:* 373–375 (1985).

13 Centers for Disease Control: Persistent, generalized lymphadenopathy in homosexual males. Morb. Mortal. Wkly Rep. *31:* 249–251 (1982).

14 Krause, R.: Koch's postulates and the search for the AIDS agent. Rev. infect. Dis. *6:* 270–279 (1984).

15 Walsh, C.; Krigel, R.; Lennette, E.; Karpatkin, S.: Thrombocytopenia in homosexual patients. Ann. intern. Med. *103:* 542–545 (1985).

16 Frazer, I.; Collins, E.; Fox, J.; Jones, B.; Oliphant, R.; Mackay, I.: Assessment of delayed-type hypersensitivity in man: a comparison of the multitest and conventional intradermal injection of six antigens. Clin. Immunol. Immunopathol. *35:* 182–188 (1985).

17 Frazer, I.; Mackay, I.: A graphical presentation of counts of T lymphocyte subpopulations and Th-Ts ratios. Pathology *17:* 62–63 (1985).

18 Kornfeld, H.; Vande Stouwe, R.; Lange, M.; Reddy, M.; Grieco, M.: T-lymphocytes in subpopulations in homosexual men. New Engl. J. Med. *307:* 729–731 (1982).

19 Detels, R.; Schwartz, K.; Visscher, B.; Fahey, J.; Greene, R.; Gottlieb, M.: Relation between sexual practices and T-cell subsets in homosexually active men. Lancet *i:* 609–611 (1983).

20 Pinching, A.; Jeffries, D.; Donaghy, M.; Munday, P.; McManus, T.; Moshtael, O.; Parkin, J.; Harris, J.: Studies of cellular immunity in male homosexuals in London. Lancet *ii:* 128–130 (1983).

21 Nicholson, J.; McDougal, J.; Spira, T.; Cross, G.; Jones, B.; Reinherz, E.: Immunoregulatory subsets of the T helper and T suppressor cell populations in homosexual men with chronic unexplained lymphadenopathy. J. clin. Invest. *73:* 191–201 (1984).

22 Fahey, J.; Prince, H.; Weaver, M.; Groopman, J.; Visscher, B.; Schwartz, K.; Detels, R.: Quantitative changes in T helper or T suppressor/cytotoxic lymphocyte subsets that distinguish acquired immune deficiency syndrome from other immune subset disorders. Am J. Med. *76:* 95–100 (1984).

23 Mittelman, A.; Wong, G.; Safai, B.; Myskowski, P.; Gold, J.; Koziner, B.: Analysis of T cell subsets in different clinical subgroups of patients with the acquired immune deficiency syndrome. Am J. Med. *78:* 951–956 (1985).

24 James, K.; Hargreave, T.: Immunosuppression by seminal plasma and its possible clinical significance. Immunol. Today *5:* 357–363 (1984).

25 Frazer, I.; Sarngadharan, M.; Mackay, I.; Gallo, R.: Antibody to human T cell

leukaemia virus type III in Australian homosexual men with lymphadenopathy. Med. J. Aust. *141:* 274–276 (1984).

26 Frazer, I.; Mackay, I.; Crapper, R.; Gust, I.; Sarngadharan, M.: Prevalence of antibody to HTLV-III in Melbourne homosexual men. Med. J. Aust. (in press).

27 Jaffe, H.; Feorino, P.; Darrow, W.; O'Malley, P.; Getchell, J.; Warfield, D.; Jones, B.; Echenberg, D.; Francis, D.; Curran, J.: Persistent infection with human T-lymphotropic virus type III/lymphadenopathy-associated virus in apparently healthy homosexual men. Ann. intern. Med. *102:* 627–628 (1985).

28 Jaffe, H.; Darrow, W.; Echenberg, D.; O'Malley, P.; Getchell, J.; Kalyanaraman, V.; Byers, R.; Drennan, D.; Braff, E.; Curran, J.; Francis, D.: The acquired immunodeficiency syndrome in a cohort of homosexual men. Ann. intern. Med. *103:* 210–214 (1985).

29 Valle, S.; Ranki, A.; Suni, J.; Saxinger, C.; Antonen, J.; Lähdevirta, J.; Krohn, K.: Diversity of clinical spectrum of HTLV-III infection. Lancet *i:* 301–304 (1985).

30 Abrams, D.; Lewis, B.; Beckstead, J.; Casavant, C.; Drew, W.: Persistent diffuse lymphadenopathy in homosexual men. Endpoint or prodrome? Ann. intern. Med. *100:* 801–808 (1984).

31 Mathur-Wagh, U.; Spigland, I.; Sachs, H.; Yancovitz, S.; William, D.; Enlow, R.; Winchester, R.; Rorat, E.; Klien, M.; Mildvan, D.: Longitudinal study of persistent generalised lymphadenopathy in homosexual men. Relation to acquired immunodeficiency syndrome. Lancet *i:* 1033–1038 (1984).

32 McDougal, J.; Mawle, A.; Cort, S.; Nicholson, J.; Cross, G.; Scheppler-Campbell, J.; Hicks, D.; Sligh, J.: Cellular tropism of the human retrovirus HTLV-III/LAV. I. Role of T cell activation and expression of the T4 antigen. J. Immun. *135:* 3151–3162 (1985).

33 Klatzmann, D.; Montagnier, L.: Approaches to AIDS therapy. Nature, Lond. *319:* 10–11 (1986).

34 Tardieu, M.; Powers, M.; Hafler, D.; Hauser, S.; Weiner, H.: Autoimmunity following viral infection. Demonstration of monoclonal antibodies against normal tissue following infection of mice with reovirus and demonstration of shared antigenicity between virus and lymphocytes. Eur. J. Immunol. *14:* 561–565 (1984).

35 Boonpucknavig, S.; Udomsangpetch, R.: Autoantibodies in viral infection. J. clin. Lab. Immunol. *10:* 171–172 (1983).

36 Tomar, R.; John, P.; Hennig, A.; Kloster, B.: Cellular targets of antilymphocyte antibodies in AIDS and LAS. Clin. Immunol. Immunopathol. *37:* 37–47 (1985).

37 Dorsett, B.; Cornin, W.; Chuma, V.; Ioachim, H.: Anti-lymphocyte antibodies in patients with the acquired immune deficiency syndrome. Am. J. Med. *78:* 621–626 (1985).

38 Cooper, D.; Maclean, P.; Finlayson, R.; Michelmore, H.; Gold, J.; Donovan, B.; Barnes, T.; Brooke, P.; Penny, R.: Acute AIDS retrovirus infection: definition of clinical illness associated with seroconversion. Lancet *i:* 537–540 (1985).

Dr. I.R. Mackay, The Walter and Eliza Hall Institute of Medical Research, Post Office, Royal Melbourne Hospital, Victoria 3050 (Australia)

Concepts Immunopathol., vol. 4, pp. 261–274 (Karger, Basel 1987)

Reconstitution of Immune Function in AIDS/ARC

A. A. Gottlieb, M. S. Gottlieb, V. E. Scholes

Tulane Medical School and Imreg, Inc., New Orleans, La., USA

The acquired immunodeficiency syndrome (AIDS) is a recently described condition caused by an unusual retrovirus, the human immunodeficiency virus (HIV) [1], which is seen predominantly in male homosexuals, drug addicts, and hemophiliacs [2–4]. The clinical features of the syndrome are associated with a severe deficiency in cell-mediated immunity and include fever, night sweats, lymphadenopathy, weight loss, malaise, opportunistic infections, and malignancies, including an aggressive form of Kaposi's sarcoma. A variety of immunological defects have been described including marked decrease of $T4^+$ (helper) cell numbers and function, decrease in the ability of patients' lymphocytes to produce interleukin-2 (IL-2) and gamma-interferon, variable NK cell activity, and increased nonspecific B-cell function as reflected in hyperglobulinemia coupled with the inability to produce a specific antibody response against foreign antigens such as bacteria, viruses and parasites. The increased susceptibility to infection observed in these patients appears to be principally attributable to the impaired function of the helper T cell ($T4^+$) subset. Reversal of the immune dysfunction does not occur spontaneously, and the disease in its advanced form has a high degree of fatality.

It is essential to recognize that the original definition of AIDS, as promulgated by the Centers for Disease Control [5], is very narrow and reflects only a minor fraction of this very serious public health problem. It is more logical to regard infection with HIV as being able to cause a deficiency of the immune system to variable degrees. That is, some individuals who have been infected with the human immunodeficiency virus (previously referred to as the LAV/HTLV III virus) will have little compromise of immune function, while others will have severe deficiency, and many will fall in between. Those who have severe deficiency are more likely to experience the serious complications of opportunistic infections and malignancies. In a real sense, the basic disease is a destruction of a critical part of the immune system by the HIV from which the clinical sequelae follow as a consequence of the immune defect.

The disease spectrum caused by HIV affects not only homosexuals and others regarded as belonging to high-risk groups, but also heterosexual contacts of those who are infected [6], as well as children whose mothers are infected [7]. In view of these considerations, it is to be expected that the disease will spread into the general population, as has already been observed. The overall spread of the disease may, however, progress at a slower rate than previously, given the availability of a test procedure to detect antibody to HIV, attention to the nation's blood supply, and better public education. Nevertheless, the number of reported cases is increasing and can be expected to increase each year.

As with any disease caused by an infectious agent, two prime objectives are to find a drug that will destroy that agent and a vaccine that will protect uninfected individuals from the disease. A variety of drugs with antiviral activity are being studied, but it is too early to conclude that any one or another of these is safe and effective. Many of these drugs do not cross the blood-brain barrier, and the virus has the ability to integrate into the DNA of the patient thus providing a long-term reservoir of infection which cannot be readily eliminated.

In this context, the development of agents capable of moving a patient's immune system from a state of immune deficiency to one of more normal function would likely have a significant impact on this disease and the patients it affects. Such an agent would not be a cure, since it would not eliminate the virus, but it could control the manifestations and course of the disease. It is also well to point out that if an effective antiviral agent is found, the combination of such an antiviral drug with an immunorestorative agent would be a very logical approach to the treatment of patients with AIDS and AIDS-related complex (ARC).

Various investigators have attempted to restore the immune system of AIDS patients using a number of agents including interferons, interleukin-2, thymic factors and gamma globulin, as well as pharmacologic immunomodulators. However, toxicity to many of these agents remains a problem. Natural and recombinant alpha and gamma interferon have been used, but with minimal success [8–18]. Natural and recombinant

IL-2 (rIL-2) have also been studied by several investigators [19, 20], but sustained restoration of the immune defect in AIDS/ARC has not been seen in vivo with these agents. Fauci and Lane (21) have reported that treatment of AIDS patients with 2×10^6 U/day of IL-2 resulted in increases in total peripheral blood lymphocyte counts, enhanced spontaneous lymphocyte proliferation, minor tumor regressions, and clearing of HIV (HTLV-III) viremia. However, Volberding et al. [22] in reporting their experience in treating AIDS patients with increasing doses of rIL-2, including levels as high as 2×10^6 U/day, concluded that, despite the ability of IL-2 to affect T lymphocyte function in vitro in AIDS, this agent, rIL-2, even at maximal doses, had no in vivo effect in their study and no objective clinical benefit was seen at any dose.

Pharmacologic immunomodulators have been tested in AIDS/ARC patients, and among these, azimexon [8, 25], cimetidine [8, 26] and Imuthiol® (sodium diethyldithiocarbamate, DTC) [27–29] do not appear to have any significant restorative effect. AZT (3′-azido-3′-deoxythymidine) has been shown to have antiviral effects, and in a limited study over a 6-week-period, some beneficial clinical effects were reported, including weight gain, increases in number of T helper cells and return of delayed hypersensitivity to recall antigens in 6/19 patients [52, 61]. It is of interest to note, however, that in this study the return of delayed hypersensitivity was seen in only 6 of the 15 patients who displayed increase in T cell numbers. This raises the question as to whether the increased T cells in all of these patients were indeed functional.

Preliminary data from ARC patients treated with isoprinosine [23, 24, 29–31] suggest marginal clinical and immunological benefits in AIDS/ARC patients. Similar limited results were observed in AIDS patients treated with thymopentin (TP-5) [32, 33]. Ribavirin, an inhibitor of reverse transcriptase activity of HIV, has been reported to enhance mitogen (Con-A) induced proliferative responses but not to affect the response of lymphocytes to antigen [47]. Marginal clinical effects have been noted in patients treated this drug [54]. Methionine-enkephalin has been reported to have immunomodulator properties in that it increases T cell subsets in normal volunteers and cancer patients [55, 56]. Methionine-enkephalin has been tested in six patients with AIDS/ARC and shown to have effects on NK cell activity, mitogen responses, IL-2 production and T4 cell numbers [57]. Since methionine-enkephalin is an opiod peptide, its use as an immunomodulator may not be practical.

As early as 1979, Gottlieb et al. [34–36] had shown that human white blood cells (leukocytes) contained a group of small molecules which were able to affect the expression of delayed-type hypersensitivity in man. These components, when injected intradermally in combination with an antigen to which the recipient had been previously sensitized, produced an accelerated and intensified delayed hypersensitivity response to that antigen. These leukocyte-derived immunoamplifiers did not produce an inflammatory response when injected into the skin by themselves, nor were they able to transfer a new antigenic sensitivity to a non-sensitive recipient. Following the description of the ability of one of these leukocyte-derived immunomodulators, which has now been termed IMREG®-1, to enhance reactions of delayed hypersensitivity to recall antigens, in vitro assay systems were developed to characterize the mechanism of action of this low molecular weight modulator. In particular, the effect of IMREG-1 on the production of antigen-induced leukocyte migration inhibition factor (LIF) and macrophage migration inhibition factor (MIF) were investigated since production of these in vitro lymphokines has been correlated with delayed hypersensitivity response. Addition of IMREG-1 to cultures of peripheral blood lymphocytes accelerated and augmented production of antigen-induced migration inhibitory activity, with the characteristics of this in vitro modulation closely resembling those observed in respect of delayed hypersensitivity reactions in vivo. Furthermore, by selectively enriching peripheral blood mononuclear cells for T cell subsets, it has been demonstrated that the target cell for IMREG-1 amplification of LIF/MIF production is the helper (OKT^+/$Leu3a^+$) T cell subset. This suggests that modulation of helper cell lymphokine (LK) production may at least be partially responsible for the in vivo activity of IMREG-1 [37].

IMREG-1 has been examined for both its effect on production of T cell-derived lymphokines other than LIF/MIF, and for its ability to augment production of specific cytolytic lymphocytes. Inclusion of IMREG-1 in standard culture systems clearly enhances production of IL-2 by normal lymphocytes [38]. This effect is particularly apparent at suboptimal concentrations of the agent used for IL-2 induction, which can be either a mitogen or alloantigen. As was the case for LIF/MIF production, augmentation of IL-2 production by IMREG-1 is a result of IMREG-1 action on the human helper T cell subset [39]. Recent studies indicate that IMREG-1 modulates production of gamma interferon by peripheral blood lymphocytes under conditions where IL-2 production is augmented. This effect appears 24 h later than IL-2 modulation and is linked to the enhancement of IL-2 production [40]. More recently, IMREG-1 has been shown to enhance the expression of the receptor for interleukin-2 on lymphocytes of the $T4^+/Leu3A^+$ phenotype [41]. These results collectively indicate that IMREG-1 exerts a set of important effects on human T helper cells, one of which appears to be the enhancement of IL-2 production by these cells. This in turn leads to augmented production of gamma interferon and the expression of receptors for IL-2. Coordinately, the production of the migration inhibiting lymphokines is enhanced.

The ability of IMREG-1 to augment helper cell function in vitro suggested that this immunomodulator might function as in immunopotentiating agent in individuals with immunodeficiencies characterized by a defect in the T cell subpopulation. In particular, patients suffering from AIDS or ARC display a severe decrease in the number of circulating T helper cells, along with an impairment in T cell dependent immune functions, e.g. IL-2 production. To determine if IMREG-1 might augment immune reactivity in this disease, lymphocytes from patients with AIDS or ARC were examined for their ability to produce IL-2 in response to pythohemagglutinin (PHA) in the presence and absence of IMREG-1. From the data obtained, it was clear that IMREG-1 can enhance the production of IL-2 by peripheral blood lymphocytes from AIDS/ARC patients [43–46]. Similar results were obtained using gamma interferon as the index lymphokine, and it appeared that the augmentation of gamma interferon is attributable to enhanced production of IL-2 [40, 44, 45]. Gamma interferon is important in this context, since patients with ARC whose gamma interferon production is impaired are at higher risk for opportunistic infections.

IMREG-1, when administered in combination with isologous HLA-identical leukocytes to a patient with severly advanced AIDS and Kaposi's sarcoma, resulted in a striking, though transient, improvement of this patient's immune function as reflected in enhanced proliferative responses to mitogens and IL-2 production in response to PHA, and in an increase in $T4^+$ cells to normal levels [38, 40]. Administration of isologous HLA-identical leukocytes alone produced none of these effects [38]. These results strengthened our hypothesis that IMREG-1, acting on a critical population of T helper lymphocytes, can result in improvement of immune function in patients with AIDS.

The ability of peripheral blood lymphocytes to produce IL-2 was measured at 7-day intervals for 21 days following administration of a single dose of IMREG-1 to 22 AIDS/ARC patients. After treatment, more than 75% of the patients displayed enhanced IL-2 production by their peripheral lymphocytes in response to PHA stimulation. The patients who presented with greater than 50 $T4^+$ cells per mm^3 demonstrated enhanced production of IL-2 in response to mitogen in the 7- to 14-day period following the administration of IMREG-1. However, in the group of patients with fewer than 50 $T4^+$ cells per mm^3 on presentation, only some appeared to show enhanced IL-2 production 1 week later [45]. Further supporting evidence that the effects of IMREG-1 are on the $T4^+$ cells is the observation that a relationship exists between the number of $T4^+$ cells in the peripheral blood of AIDS patients and the enhancement of their IL-2 production following IMREG-1 administration under experimental conditions in which $T8^+$ (suppressor) cells do not produce this lymphokine.

On this basis, studies of IMREG-1 were carried out on 29 patients with AIDS and Kaposi's sarcoma to assess: (1) toxicity (if any) to IMREG-1; (2) in vivo immunological response to IMREG-1; (3) in vitro immunological response following in vivo administration of IMREG-1; (4) clinical parameters to be followed in a planned randomized clinical trial. Two groups of patients were followed: (1) patients who where given IMREG-1 once every four weeks for 3 months (n = 15), and (2) patients who were given IMREG-1 once every two weeks for 3 months (n = 14). Upon presentation, all patients failed to respond to a battery of skin test antigens [42, 45, 46].

Patients treated once every 4 weeks manifested a return of delayed hypersensitivity (DTH) to a recall antigen (tetanus toxoid) in 6 out of 16 patients so treated. Delayed hypersensitivity is a fundamental indicator of the ability of the immune system to respond to antigenic challenge, and is perhaps the most important clinical parameter pertaining to immune function that can be followed in such patients. No toxicity to IMREG-1 was observed in any of the patients and no generalized adverse effects were noted among any of the laboratory hematological or biochemical parameters studied. Repeated treatment with IMREG-1 of patients who displayed decreased lymphocyte response to PHA resulted in an increase in responsiveness to PHA stimulation. The proliferative response reached maximum levels 14 days after administration of the IMREG-1 modulator. The first IMREG-1 treatment resulted in the greatest response. Additional, but smaller increases were observed following the second and third doses of IMREG-1. Patients who exhibited high baseline responses to mitogen demonstrated small increases in response following treatment, as compared with those who presented with weaker proliferative responses prior to treatment.

It was observed that the higher the number of $T4^+$ cells prior to treatment, the greater the PHA response following treatment. Ten of fourteen patients (71%) demonstrated an increase in IL-2 production following treatment with IMREG-1. Of those demonstrating an IL-2 response, 50% (5/10) showed a return of DTH and had an average of 20% $T4^+$ cells (299/mm^3) compared with a 25% (1/4) return of DTH and 10% $T4^+$ cells (61/mm^3) in patients who did not respond [46].

Direct comparisons between patients treated biweekly and monthly are difficult, since the patients treated biweekly were more severely ill at the start. However, following biweekly treatment, a greater proportion of patients in this group [69% (9/13)] demonstrated return of DTH. Following biweekly IMREG-1 treatment of patients with more than 50–100 $T4^+$ cells per mm^3 on presentation, the IL-2 response peaked 14 days following the second dose. In patients with fewer than 50–100 $T4^+$ cells per mm^3 on presentation, only a minimal response was noted, but the number of individuals in each group who demonstrated some positive response increased until 60% of the patients showed a small positive response following the 4th biweekly treatment. In the group with more than 50–100 $T4^+$ cells per mm^3 on presentation, all subjects responded following two biweekly doses of IMREG-1; of those six patients who displayed only a small increase in the capacity to produce IL-2, only 2 of 6 were able to recover the ability to manifest DTH to tetanus toxoid.

Viewed collectively, the 29 AIDS patients who were treated with IMREG-1 displayed significant weight gain and clearing of oral candida in those patients who presented with this infection. In this group, there were 11 cases of resistant candida: six of these resolved completely, one additional patient showed significant improvement, and four cases did not progress. No new infections with candida occurred in these patients while on treatment with IMREG-1. It is of interest to note, in this regard, that leukocyte dialysates had previously been reported to be effective in the treatment of refractory candidiasis [58–60]. Additionally, in the group of patients treated biweekly, 11/14 gained weight (an average of three pounds in 3 months), while there was no overall decrease in weight in the patients treated monthly. The weight gain was associated with declines in the level of serum uric acid and creatine phosphokinase. The decrease in these parameters is consistent with a reduction in the relatively rapid rate of cellular and tissue destruction which is characteristic of patients with AIDS/ARC.

An important observation in patients treated with IMREG-1 was a reduction in overall rate of destruction of $T4^+$ cells. Studies of 13 patients with PGL (persistent generalized lymphadenopathy) indicative of ARC showed an overall loss of 13.4 T4 cells per patient month, while those patients who received IMREG-1 monthly, as a group, exhibited a loss of $T4^+$ cells at the rate of 7.2 $T4^+$ cells per patient month, a greater than 40% decrease in the rate of $T4^+$ cell loss. Furthermore, in the group of patients treated biweekly, the overall loss of $T4^+$ cells was reduced to 4.2 $T4^+$ cells per patient month, also, a more than 40 percent decrease in rate of $T4^+$ cell loss. When these groups were matched to include patients with comparable numbers of $T4^+$ cells at the start of treatment, and followed for a comparable time period, the overall rate of destruction of these cells was reduced by more than 80 percent in the group treated monthly compared to the untreated group, and more than 60 percent in a group treated biweekly compared to one treated monthly. These results strongly suggest that IMREG-1 has the ability to reduce the overall rate of destruction of $T4^+$ cells in AIDS/ARC patients, notwithstanding the fact that the HIV virus is still present and continues to infect and destroy the $T4^+$ helper cell population.

These observations are confirmatory of prior laboratory studies which indicate that IMREG-1 does not 'activate' T helper cells for viral infection and expression. It is generally considered that the HIV virus requires an activated T4 cell for replication. Had 'activation' and resultant viral production occurred as a result of treatment with IMREG-1, the rate of destruction of T helper cells in these patients would have increased. In fact, the opposite effect was observed. In laboratory studies, IMREG-1 by itself does *not* induce proliferation or expression of either Ia like antigens or receptors for IL-2 on T helper cells.

Several AIDS/ARC patients have been treated with multiple doses of the IMREG-1 immunomodulators for one year or more. In these treated patients there has been no observed toxicity associated with IMREG-1 treatment. In those with at least a minimum level of residual immunity on presentation, functional immune patterns have returned towards normal, and clinical improvement has occurred.

From these results, it is clear that administration of IMREG-1 leads to reconstitution of immune parameters and documentable clinical benefits in patients with AIDS/ARC. While the results are those of an open study, and a double-blind randomized study is necessary for definitive proof of efficacy, IMREG-1 appears to be an agent that may prove important in treatment of this disease. The attractive feature of this approach is that IMREG-1 is a nontoxic immunomodulator that can promote the natural ability of the $T4^+$ cell to produce important biological regulators such as IL-2 and gamma interferon. In addition to offering the prospect of reconstructing the immune system in patients with AIDS, this approach may be particularly useful in patients with ARC in possibly preventing the progression of that condition to the severe form of AIDS.

It is important to consider the role of both antiviral agents and immunomodulators in treatment of patients with AIDS. The ideal antiviral agent would eliminate the virus completely. In the case of HIV, a retrovirus, this is not likely to occur since the virus integrates into the DNA of the genome which can serve as a persistent reservoir for re-expression in the future. Thus, an antiviral agent that is virosuppressive and non-toxic would have utility for short-term application in patients who manifest virus in body fluids. It is not likely that such an agent would be given prophylactically or on a long-term basis. Rather, such an agent would be used to suppress the virus when it appears. Compounds being tested in this regard include AZT (azidodeoxythymidine), ribavirin and dideoxycytidine [47–54]. It is too early to draw conclusions about the effectiveness or lack of effectiveness of such agents, though isolated reports have suggested encouraging results with AZT and ribavirin [49, 52–54, 61].

Apart from antiviral effects, what effects on the immune system would likely be expected from an antiviral agent? Clearly, if HIV destruction of $T4^+$ cells could be eliminated, one might expect to see an increase in numbers of $T4^+$ cells over the treatment course, and corresponding increases in laboratory parameters of immune function including mitogen responsiveness and IL-2 production. In this respect, the antiviral agent is acting in a fashion similar to the effect of penicillin on pneumococcal pneumonia in which the antibiotic reduces overall bacterial load, allowing the immune system to cope with a lower level of pathogen. A similar effect may occur here, but one must bear in mind that in AIDS/ARC the patient's immune system has been seriously damaged, and requires time for formation of new cellular elements. An immunomodulator having an enhancing effect on $T4^+$ cell function would, therefore, clearly be useful. Thus the combination of an antiviral agent given short-term (to control viral expression) and an immunoenhancer given over the longer term offers a very rational approach to control of the AIDS/ARC problem.

In this context, it is well to ask how one evaluates the efficacy of an immunomodulator in AIDS/ARC. It is important to keep in mind that the key lesion is in the immune system, and the immune deficiency is the disease which results in the serious clinical sequelae such as opportunistic infections and Kaposi's sarcoma. Therefore, it seems reasonable to suggest that correction of the immune deficiency is the end-point which should serve as the primary criterion for efficacy. Given the present state-of-the-art, criteria for restoration of immune function are readily available. The most important of these is restoration of delayed hypersensitivity reactions to antigens to which the patient has been previously sensitized, since this is a direct measure of the ability of the patient's immune system to respond to challenge with a foreign substance. Restoration of immune function can be expected to lead to more classical evidence of clinical improvement that can be demonstrated by clinical indices such as decreased frequency and duration of infections. From a fundamental point of view, immunologic improvement should be considered an end point in its own right.

References

1 Varmus, H., Human Retrovirus Subcommittee, International Committee on the Taxonomy of Viruses (Letter). Human immunodeficiency viruses. Science *232:* 697 (1986).

2 Gottlieb, M. S.; Schroff, R.; Schanker, H. M.; et al.: *Pneumocyotis carinii* pneumonia and mucosal candidiasis in previously healthy homosexual men. Evidence of a new acquired cellular immunodeficiency. New Engl. J. Med. *305:* 1425 (1981).

3 Popovic, M.; Sarngadharan, M. G.; Reed, E.; et al.: Detection, isolation, and continuous production of cytopathic human T lymphotropic retrovirus (HTLV-III) from patients with AIDS and pre-AIDS. Science *224:* 497 (1984).

4 Gallo, R. C.; Salahuddin, S. Z.; Popovic, M.; et al.: Frequent detection and isolation of cytopathic retroviruses (HTLV-III) from patients with AIDS and at risk for AIDS. Science *224:* 500 (1984).

5 Centers for Disease Control: Update on acquired immune deficiency syndrome (AIDS). U. W. MMWR *31:* 507, 513 (1982).

6 Harris, C.; Small, D. B.; Klein, R. S.; et al.: Immunodeficiency in female sexual partners of men with acquired immune deficiency syndrome. New. Engl. J. Med. *308:* 1181 (1983).

7 Oleske, J.; Minnefor, A.; Cooper, R.; et al.: Immune deficiency syndrome in children. J. Am. med. Ass. *249:* 2345 (1983).

8 The Therapy of AIDS and Related Disorders: NIH workshop, Washington 1984 (unpubl. transcript of proc.).
9 Krown, S.E.; Real, F.X.; Cunningham-Rundles, S.; et al.: Preliminary observations on the effect of recombinant leukocyte A interferon in homosexual men with Kaposi's sarcoma. New Engl. J. Med. *308:* 1971 (1983).
10 Real, F.X.; Krown, S.E.; Krim, M.; et al.: Treatment of Kaposi's sarcoma (KS) with recombinant leukocyte A interferon (rIFN-A). Proc. Am. Soc. clin. Oncol. *3:* 55 (1984).
11 Groopman, J.E.; Gottlieb, M.S.; Goodman, J.; et al.: Recombinant alpha-2 interferon therapy for Kaposi's sarcoma associated with the acquired immunodeficiency syndrome. Ann. intern. Med. *100:* 671 (1984).
12 Mitsuyasu, R.; Volberding, P.; Jacobs, A.; et al.: High dose alpha recombinant interferon (IFN) in the therapy of epidemic Kaposi's sarcoma (KS) in acquired immune deficiency (AIDS). Proc. Am. Soc. Oncol. *3:* 51 (1984).
13 Volberding, P., Moran, T.; Abrams, D.; et al.: Recombinant alpha interferon (αIFN) therapy of Kaposi's sarcoma (KS) in the acquired immune deficiency syndrome (AIDS). Blood *62:* suppl. 1, p. 118 A, (1983).
14 Grimm, E.A.; Rosenberg, S.A.: Production and properties of human IL-2; in Fatham, Fitch, Isolation, characterization and utilization of T lymphocyte clones (Academic Press, New York 1982).
15 Nadler, P.I.; the AIDS-Roferon A Study Group: Treatment of the acquired immunodeficiency syndrome (AIDS) with Roferon-A. A randomized double blind, placebo controlled trial. Abstr. Int. Conf. AIDS, Paris 1986.
16 Rozenbaum, W.; Brucker, G.; Duflo, B.; et al.: Treatment of AIDS-related Kaposi's sarcoma by Alpha-2 recombinant interferon. Abstr. Int. Conf. AIDS, Paris 1986.
17 Miles, S.A.; Martinez, O.; Sherwin, S.; et al.: Phase I trial of Recombinant interferon gamma (r IFN-γ) in AIDS related Kaposi's sarcoma (AIDS/KS). Abstr. Int. Conf. AIDS, Paris 1986.
18 Farkin, J.M.; Eales, L.J.; Moshtael, O.; et al.: Results of a trial of recombinant interferon-gamma (Biogen) in patients with the acquired immune deficiency syndrome. Abstr. Int. Conf. AIDS, Paris 1986.
19 Rook, A.H.; Masur, H.; Lane, H.C.; et al.: Interleukin 2 enhances the depressed natural killer and cytomegalovirus-specific cytotoxic activities of lymphocytes from patients with the acquired immune deficiency syndrome. J. clin. Invest. *72:* 398 (1983).
20 Mertelsmann, R.; Einzig, A.; Merluzzi, V.; et al.: Recombinant interleukin-2 and human lymphocyte interleukin-2 are able to restore defective mitogen responses in patients with immunodeficiency states. Blood *62:* suppl. 1, p. 118 a (1983).
21 Fauci, A.S.; Lane, J.C.: Therapeutic approaches to the underlying immune defect in patients with AIDS. Abstr. Int. Conf. AIDS, Paris 1986.
22 Volberding, P.A.; Abrams, D.; Beardslee, D.; et al.: Recombinant Interleukin-2 therapy of acquired immunodeficiency syndrome. Abstr. Int. Conf. AIDS, Paris 1986.
23 Grieco, M.H.; Reddy, M.M.; Manvar, O.; et al.: In vivo immunomodulation by isoprinosine in patients with the acquired immunodeficiency syndrome and related complexes. Ann. intern. Med. *101:* 206 (1984).

24 Tsang, P. H.; Roboz, J. P.; Tangnavarad, K.; et al.: Normalization of T and B lymphocyte function by isoprinosine in homosexual subjects with prodromata of AIDS. Proc. Am. Soc. clin. Oncol. *3:* 59 (1984).

25 Parr, Y. Z.; Mansell, P.; Hersh, E. N.; et al.: Partial immunorestoration in pre AIDS with Azimexon (in preparation).

26 Gottlieb, M. S.; Wolfe, P. R.; Mitsuyasu, R. T.: Immunotherapy of The acquired immune deficiency syndrome; in Gallin, Fauci, Advances in host defense mechanisms, vol. 5 (Raven Press, New York 1984).

27 Brewton, G. W.; Hersh, E.; Reuben, J. M.; et al.: Preliminary observations on Imuthiol Therapy in Symptomatic HTLV-III/LAV infection. Abstr. Int. Conf. AIDS, Paris 1986.

28 Lang, J. M.; Oberling, F.; Aleksijevic, F.; et al.: Immunomodulation with diethyldithiocarbamate (DTC) (Imuthiol®) in patients with LAV/HTVL-III-related illnesses. Abstr. Int. Conf. AIDS, Paris 1986.

29 Pompidou, A.; Telvi, L.; Delsaux, M. C.; et al.: Influence of immunomodulators on T-lymphocytes differentiation and resistance to LAV/HTLV-III infection. Abstr. Int. Conf. AIDS, Paris 1986.

30 Keller, R. H.; Milson, T. J.; Ellingboe, K. M.; Patrick, C. W.: Sequential clinical and immunoregulatory phenotype and functional changes in patients with AIDS and ARC treated with Isoprinosine. Abstr. Int. Conf. AIDS, Paris 1986.

31 Bekesi, J. G.; Tsang, P. H.; Roboz, J. D.: Potentiation of impaired lymphocyte function by Isoprinosine in AIDS patients and prodromal subjects in vitro. Abstr. Int. Conf. AIDS, Paris 1986.

32 Clumerck, N.; Van De Perre, P.; Mascart-Lemone, F.; et al.: Preliminary results on clinical and immunological effects of Thymopentin in AIDS. Inst. J. clin. Pharm. Res. *IV:* 459–463 (1984).

33 Benn, V. J.; Garber, J.; Gottlieb, M. S.; et al.: Thymopentin (TP-5) increases lymphocyte subpopulation levels in persistant generalized lymphadenopathy. Abstr. Int. Conf. AIDS, Paris 1986.

34 Gottlieb, A. A.; Maziarz, G. A.; Tamaki, N.; Sutcliffe, S. B.: The effects of dialyzable products from human leukocyte extracts on cutaneous delayed hypersensitivity response. J. Immun. *124:* 885–892 (1980).

35 Gottlieb, A. A.; Sutcliffe, S. B.: In vivo modification of delayed-type hypersensitivity by small molecular weight components derived from human leukocytes: partial purification of components causing amplification of response. Clin. exp. Immunol. *50:* 434–441 (1982).

36 Gottlieb, A. A.; Sutcliffe, S. B.; Saito, K.; Maziarz, G.; Tamaki, N.; Sakatsuji, K.; Sutherland, C.: Modification of intradermal delayed hypersensitivity by components of leukocyte dialysates. Kahn, Kirkpatrick, Hill, Immune regulators in transfer factor, p. 339 (Academic Press, New York 1979).

37 Gottlieb, A. A.; Farmer, J. L.; Matzura, C. T.; Hester, R. B.; Rosenberg, J. L.: Modulation of Human T cell production of migration inhibitory lymphokines by cytokines derived from human leukocyte dialysates. J. Immun. *132:* 256–260 (1984).

38 Gottlieb, A. A.; Farmer, J. L.; Nishihara, T.: Endogenous immunomodulators from human leukocytes as agents for immunorestoration in patients with AIDS; Szentvanyi, Friedman, Conference Monograph (Tampa, Fla., 1984). Viruses, immunity and immunodeficiency, pp. 287–299 (Plenum Press, New York 1986).

39 Farmer, J. L.; Gottlieb, A. A.: Modulation of human T helper cell production of interleukin-2 by an endogenous leukocyte-derived immunomodulator (submitted).

40 Farmer, J. L.; Benes, E.; Bertucci, D.; Montgomery, A.; Morin, G.; Smith, R.; Alexander, S.; Gottlieb, A. A.: Regulation of gamma-interferon (γ-IFN) production by Interleukin-2 (IL-2) in normals and patients with acquired immune deficiency syndrome. Fed. Proc. *45:* 251 (1986).

41 Farmer, J. L.; Benes, E.; Gottlieb, A. A.: Augmentation of antigen-induced interleukin-2 receptor expression and gamma interferon production by IMREG-1, a leukocyte-derived immunomodulator. 1st IUIS Conf. Clinical Immunology, Toronto 1986.

42 Gill, P. S.; Levine, A. M.; Aguilar, S. L.; DelSignore, C.; Burkes, R. L.; Farmer, J.; Gottlieb, A. A.: Use of leukocyte-derived endogenous immuno-modulator (IMREG-1) in patients with aids. Blood *64:* (1984).

43 Gottlieb, A. A.; Farmer, J. L.; Hester, R. B.; Levine, A.; Gill, P.; Kardinal, C.; Pankey, G.; Flaum, M.: Reconstitution of T cell function in AIDS and ARC patients by use of 504A leukocyte-derived endogenous immunomodulators. Clin. Res. *32* (1984).

44 Gottlieb, A. A.; Farmer, J. L.; Levine, A.; Gill, P.; Flaum, M.; Gottlieb, M. S.: Reconstitution of T cell function in AIDS and ARC patients by the use of the endogenous, leukocyte-derived immunomodulator, IMREG-1. Conf. Int. Soc. Immunopharmacol. on current problems in testing and evaluation of experimental and clinical effects of immunomodulators, Prague 1985.

45 Gottlieb, A. A.; Farmer, J. L.; Levine, A.; Gill, P.; Flaum, M.; Gottlieb, M. S.: Reconstitution of T cell function in AIDS and ARC patients by use of the endogenous, leukocyte-derived immunomodulator, IMREG-1, Abstr. 7th Eur. Immunology Congr. EFIS 1985.

46 Gottlieb, A. A.; Levine, A. M.; Farmer, J.; Kern, C. H., III; Shear, C. L.; DelSignore, C.: Changes in mitogen-induced proliferation and interleukin-2 production in patients with AIDS treated with IMREG-1. Abstr. Int. Conf. AIDS, Paris 1986.

47 Roberts, R. B.; Scavuzzo, D.; Laurence, J.; et al.: Effects of short-term oral ribavirin in high risk patients for AIDS. Abstr. Int. Conf. AIDS, Paris 1986.

48 Matheron, S.; Katlama, C.; Leport, C.; et al.: A ribavirin open trial in AIDS. Abstr. Int. Conf. AIDS, Paris 1986.

49 Laskin, O. L.; Roberts, R. B.; Longstreth, J.; et al.: Pharmacokinetics of ribavirin in patients with AIDS related complex. Abstr. Int. Conf. AIDS, Paris 1986.

50 Balzarini, J.; Mitsuya, H.; Clercq, P. de; Broder, S.: Deoxythymidine potentiates the protective effect of 2^1–3^1 dideoxycytidine against cytopathogenicity of HTLV-III/LAV. Abstr. Int. Conf. AIDS, Paris 1986.

51 Blum, M. R.; Liao, S.; Good, S. S.; et al.: Pharmacokinetics of Azidothymidine (AZT) following intravenous and oral administration. Abstr. Int. Conf. AIDS, Paris 1986.

52 Smith, M. S.; Pagano, J. S.: Effect of azidothymidine (AZT) on LAV/HTLV-III infection of H9 cells in culture. Abstr. Int. Conf. AIDS, Paris 1986.

53 Crumpacker, C.; Bubley, G.; Hussey, S.; et al.: Evaluation of oral ribavirin therapy on immunologic and viral parameters in AIDS and ARC. Abstr. Int. Conf. AIDS, Paris 1986.

54 Lazzarin, A.; Crocchiolo, P.; Chemotti, M.; et al.: Therapeutic trials with IFNα and ribiavirin in LAV/HTLV-III infections. Preliminary results. Abstr. Int. Conf. AIDS, Paris 1986.
55 Plotnikoff, N. P.; Murgo, A. J.; Faith, R. E.; Good, R.: Enkephalins and endorphins. Stress and the immune system (Plenum Press, New York 1986).
56 Plotnikoff, N. P.; Miller, G. C.; Wybran, J.; Nimeh, N. F.: Methionine-enkephalin. T-cell enhancement in Kaposi's sarcoma (AIDS). Abstr. Int. Conf. AIDS, Paris 1986.
57 Wybran, J.; Latinne, D.; Sonnet, J.; et al.: Immuno restorative effect of methionine-enkephaline in ARC and AIDS. Abstr. Int. Conf. AIDS, Paris 1986.
58 Pabst, H. F.; Swanson, R.: Successful treatment of candidiasis with transfer factor. Br. med. J. *11:* 442 (1972).
59 Rocklin, R. C.; Chilgren, R. A.; Hong, R.; David, J. R.: Transfer of cellular hypersensitivity in chronic mucocutaneous candidiasis monitored in vivo and in vitro. Cell. Immunol. *1:* 290–299 (1970).
60 Schulkind, M. L.; Adler, W. H.; Altemeir, W. A.; Ayoub, E. M.: Transfer factor in the treatment of a case of chronic mucocutaneous candidiasis. Cell. Immunol. *3:* 606 (1972).
61 Yarchoan, R.; Weinhold, K. J.; Lyerly, H. K.; et al.: Administration 3′-azido-3′-deoxythymidine. An inhibitor of HTLV-III/LAV replication, to patients with AIDS or AIDS-related complex. Lancet *March 15:* 575 (1986).

Note Added in Proof

Results of a phase III randomized trial of AZT were announced at the International Conference on Antibiotics and Antimicrobial Chemotherapy, New Orleans 1986. The trial included patients with AIDS who had recently recovered from their first episode with Pneumocystis carinii pneumonia and patients with ARC. While 25% of the patients treated with AZT required blood transfusions during the 6-month trial, only 1 of the patients in the treated group died. There were 16 deaths in the untreated group, 5 of whom had ARC. Those patients with AIDS who received AZT had an increase in $T4^+$ cell numbers which fell to baseline levels towards the end of the trial. The increase in $T4^+$ cells continued through the end of the trial in the ARC patients receiving AZT. While these results indicate short-term benefits attributable to AZT, the usefulness of this agent for long-term use and/or broader application to large numbers of HIV-infected patients remains to be established.

A. A. Gottlieb, MD, Tulane Medical School and Imreg, Inc.,
New Orleans, LA 70112 (USA)

Concepts Immunopathol., vol. 4, pp. 275–286 (Karger, Basel 1987)

Immunotherapy of Autoimmune Disease with T Cell Subset Specific Antibodies

S. Sriram, G. E. Ranges

Department of Neurology, Department of Medicine, College of Medicine, University of Vermont, Burlington, Vt., USA

Experimental model systems have contributed enormously to our understanding of autoimmunity and autoimmune disease states over the last three decades. It has become clear that the immune system has a repertoire to recognize and interact with a number of antigens including self, and the development of 'horror autotoxicus', as suggested by Paul Ehrlich, is prevented by a number of immune homeostatic mechanisms. The T cell is a key cellular factor in the biology of self-nonself recognition and hence when these regulatory systems breakdown as in autoimmune disease states, disorder of T cell function is seen [1]. The diversity of autoimmune injury stems from the differences in the autoantigen, the cellular and humoral factors that modify the immune response and the nature of the end organ.

A number of attempts to inhibit T cell function with anti-T cell antibodies have been carried out in experimental disease systems and in humans. Antithymocyte serum has been used extensively to prevent allograft rejection and to suppress the immune response in fulminant autoimmune disease states. However, these therapies were limited by the broad specificities of the antiserum and global suppression of T cell function [2]. Two events changed immunotherapies in the last ten years. Firstly, the introduction of hybridoma technology has spurred the development of monoclonal antibodies with fine specificities that can be generated in large quantities [3, 4]. Several investigators have already used them as antitumor agents, and as agents for immunosuppression to prevent allograft rejection. Therapeutic trials to facilitate human tumor rejection in this manner have already occurred [5–10]. Secondly, with the better delineation of T cell subsets, monoclonal antibodies that identify T cells with different antigen and functional specificities have become available. T cells that express the T4 or Leu 3 antigen in man, or the equivalent L3T4 antigen in mouse, serve the helper/inducer function. The cell surface protein is intimately involved in the recognition of antigen in association with the immune response gene products of the major histocompatibility complex. Monoclonal antibodies directed against the L3T4 antigen prevent all class II MHC antigen restricted T cell function, such as T cell proliferation, antibody response, and T cell killing of class II associated antigen [11–12]. Although the exact function of the L3T4 antigen is not known, it is thought that the L3T4 antigen improves the binding of the Ia antigen complex to the T cell receptor.

Recent studies by us and others have investigated the effects of anti L3T4 antibodies in vivo and the effect of such in vivo therapy on the development of autoimmune disease, both spontaneously occurring and experimentally induced. We discuss here the implications of treatment in vivo with anti L3T4 antibodies, in two experimentally induced autoimmune disease systems, experimental allergic encephalitis (EAE) and collagen induced arthritis (CIA) and the spontaneously occurring lupus-like disease in F_1 (NZB × NZW) mice. These observations lend support to the potential use of such immunotherapy in man when the antibodies become available.

In vivo Therapy of Anti-L3T4 Antibody in EAE

EAE is an autoimmune demyelinating disease that can be induced in a number of experimental laboratory animals by the injection of a homogenate of whole spinal cord in complete Freund's adjuvant. The disease follows autosensitization to myelin basic protein (MBP) [13]. T cells are crucial for the development of EAE [14]; T cells of the Ly-1 phenotype are observed in perivascular cuffs, in the brain and spinal cord [15] and more recently T cell clones that react with the encephalitogenic determinant and express the Ly-1, L3T4 phenotype are sufficient for the induction of the disease [16].

When 100 μg of anti-L3T4 antibodies were administered for 2 days prior to and following immunization with MBP, there was a significant reduction in the incidence of clinical and histological disease when compared with animals that received saline, or Lyt-2 antibody. While 4/15 animals became paralyzed in the anti-L3T4-treated group, 26/30 animals that received normal saline ($p < 0.0001$) and 8/9 animals that received an equal amount of Lyt-2 antibody became paralyzed ($p < 0.001$). Delaying treatment until day 9 (at a time when T cell response to MBP has occurred) was also successful in preventing acute EAE [17].

Prevention of Chronic Relapsing EAE (CR-EAE) with Anti-L3T4 Antibodies

While acute EAE is a monophasic disease either resulting in recovery or death, relapsing EAE is a disease of chronicity characterized by remissions and exacerbations of clinical signs. CR-EAE can be induced by modification of the immunization regimen for acute EAE, but more recently an elegant system of remissions and exacerbations has been observed following passive transfer of MBP-sensitized T cells. CR-EAE is clinically a more relevant model since the disease shows strong similarities to the human demyelinating disease, multiple sclerosis [18–20].

When anti-L3T4 antibodies (100 μg daily for 4 successive days) were administered along with 1×10^7 MBP-sensitized T cell blasts the development of the initial paralytic signs was completely prevented. While 9/10 animals that received 1×10^7 MBP-sensitized T cells and treated with normal saline developed clinical paralysis, none of the 8 animals that were treated with anti L3T4 antibody developed paralytic signs (table I).

To be of clinical benefit any therapy must be successful when therapy is begun after the onset of clinical signs. The benefit of anti L3T4 antibodies in animals in CR-EAE was studied when treatment was begun after the onset of initial paralytic signs. Animals were randomized to either receive anti L3T4 antibody or an equivalent amount of rat Ig after the initial paralytic attack, and observed for the development of clinical relapses. While there was a total of 3 relapses in the L3T4 group, 23 relapses occurred in the rat IgG-treated group (table II). Histological analysis paralleled clinical scores in virtually all animals. Animals that received rat IgG and developed relapses had extensive lymphocytic infiltrations and demyelination in the parenchyma and the periventricular areas of the brain. In the spinal cord, multifocal areas of subpial and parenchymal demyelination was seen at all levels although they were maximal in the lumbar areas. In contrast, animals that received anti-L3T4 antibodies had scanty inflammatory response in all brains examined. In the spinal cord the demyelination was often limited to a single sector such as the posterior or lateral columns [21].

Table I. Incidence of EAE in animals passively transferred with 1×10^7 MBP-sensitized T cell blasts and treated with anti-L3T4 antibodies[1]

	Number of mice	Incidence of disease	Date of onset
Anti-L3T4 antibody treated	8	0/8	–
Saline treated	10	9/10[2]	12 ± 4

[1] SJL/J mice were treated with 100 μg of anti-L3T4 antibody in 0.5 ml of normal saline for 4 consecutive days following passive transfer.
[2] $\chi^2 = p < 0.001$.

Table II. Relapse rate in mice with chronic relapsing EAE following treatment with anti-L3T4 antibodies[1]

	Number of mice	Cumulative relapses	Number of mice that relapsed
Anti-L3T4 treated	11	3	3
Rat IgG treated	14	23[2]	12

[1] SJL/J mice were passively transferred with 1×10^7 MBP-sensitized T cells and at the earliest signs of initial paralysis were randomized to either receive 100 μg of anti-L3T4 antibody in 0.5 ml of saline intraperitoneally, or an equal amount of rat IgG biweekly thereafter.
[2] $p < 0.001$, Wilcoxon-Rank sum test.

Prevention of Type II Collagen-Induced Arthritis with Anti-L3T4 Antibody

Type II collagen-induced arthritis is an inflammatory polyarthritis that displays several characteristics similar to human rheumatoid arthritis. The onset of arthritis is associated with the development of cellular and humoral response to type II collagen, and unlike EAE both are postulated to play a role in the development of disease. Treatment of DBA/1 mice with 100 μg of anti-L3T4 1 day before and 1 day after immunization with type II collagen and twice a week thereafter successfully prevented the development of arthritis. While only 3/25 animals treated in this

Table III. Summary of arthritis and anticollagen titres in DBA/mice immunized with type II collagen in CFA

	IgG titre on day 45	IgG titre on day 70	Incidence of CIA	Mean date of on set
Group A	1,585 ± 333	2,101 ± 755	14/20	39
Group B	412 ± 104	381 ± 172	3/25	62
Group C	863 ± 238	1,748 ± 605	10–22	42

CIA incidence = Number of mice displaying arthritis/number of mice in group. Group A = Control mice immunized with type II collagen and treated with PBS; group B = immunized with type II collagen, injections of 100 μg GK1.5 day –1, +1, 14, 28, 45; group C = immunized with type II collagen; injections of 100 μg GK1.5 days 28, 45.

manner developed disease, 14/20 animals that received saline developed arthritis. When treatment was delayed until day 28, the disease incidence (10/22 animals with arthritis) did not differ significantly from the control group. Treatment with anti-L3T4 prior to immunization substantially lowered the anti collagen response in all animals. When treatment was begun after an established immune response the titre was lower than the nontreated animals at day 45, but by day 70 no significant differences (table III). The failure of the anti-L3T4 treatment to be of therapeutic value when given after the development of a strong immunologic response to collagen may indicate that T cells play a more prominant role during the inductive phase of the disease and thus must be dealt with early in the process. Alternatively, the T cells at the end organ site, i.e. synovium, may not be accessible to the anti-L3T4 antibody [22].

Anti-L3T4 Antibody in the Lupus-Like Syndrome in F1 (NZB × NZW) Mice

Unlike EAE and CIA (NZB × NZW)F_1 mice spontaneously develop a disease that is remarkably similar to systemic lupus erythematosus (SLE) in humans. The disease in characterized by the appearance of antibodies to nuclear antigens by the sixth month of life and the development of a fatal glomerulonephritis. The role of T cells in the pathogenesis has been very uncertain since earlier reports on in vivo therapy with anti

Thy-1 antibodies failed to alter the course of the disease. Wofsy and Seaman have studied the efficacy of anti-L3T4 antibodies in mice (NZB × NZW)F_1 mice with anti L3T4 antibodies when therapy was begun prior to the development of anti-DNA antibodies and alteration of renal function. Such a treatment prevented the development of anti DNA antibodies and prolonged survival. At the end of 10 months while 100% of animals that received biweekly injections of anti L3T4 antibody were alive, none of the animals that received equal amounts of rat IgG and 20% of animals that received saline were alive. These workers have extended the work on the effect of anti-L3T4 antibodies when treatment was begun after the onset of renal disease and development of anti DNA antibodies. Once again they observed that treatment reduced renal disease and prolonged survival [23, 24].

Mechanism of Action of Anti-L3T4

The mechanism by which anti-L3T4 interferes with disease expression in these autoimmune model systems is not fully known. The addition of anti-L3T4 in vitro, blocks all class II, MHC antigen restricted functions. Reports by Marrack et al. [25] indicate that this is accomplished by interfering with the binding of the L3T4 antigen on the T cell with that of the antigen-presenting cell. Under normal circumstances this binding stabilizes the interaction of the T cell receptor and the Ia antigen complex on the antigen-presenting cell surface. However, in vivo, the mechanism of action seems to be more complex.

The monoclonal antibody, anti-L3T4 (GK1.5), developed by Dialynas et al. [12] was the first to define the murine L3T4 antigen and has been used as the antibody source in the three autoimmune models described in this report. In normal healthy mice the injection of anti-L3T4 results within 48 h in the depletion of greater than 90% of the L3T4 population (table IV). The fact that all of the remaining T cells can be accounted for by the Lyt 2+ population indicates that the L3T4+ cells are being eliminated rather than simply reflecting antigen blockage or modulation. Recovery of the T cell population to normal proportions of L3T4 and Lyt 2+ cells occurs in approximately 30 days in the DBA/1 strain. However, strain variation with respect to this parameter might occur as we have noted in the Balb/c strain where recovery is more in the order of 2 months.

Table IV. Depletion of L3T4+ cells by *in vivo* administration of anti-L3T4 antibody (GK1.5)[1]

	Percent positive cells by fluoroscein-activated cell sorter analysis (FACS)			
	Thy-1	Ia	Lyt-2	L3T4
Control				
Spleen	37.0	44.0	16.4	30.5
Lymph node	58.6	23.2	27.5	50.2
Thymus	85.2	7.8	80.3	75.0
GK1.5 treated				
Spleen	21.4	63.0	74.1	6.6
Lymph node	48.7	43.2	41.7	9.6
Thymus	81.3	9.1	78.0	80.7

[1] DBA/1 mice were treated with 100 μg of GK1.5 intraperitoneally, and the lymphocyte population was analyzed by FACS analysis 48 h later.

The isotype of the antibody appears to be critical in its ability to mediate elimination of target cells (GK1.5 bears the IgG2b isotype). Cobbold et al. [26] have reported that of several rat monoclonals with specificity for the Thy 1 antigen only those of the IgG2b isotype were effective in depletion in vivo of T cells and modulating the immune response.

In similar experiments concerned with in vivo treatment of murine tumors with tumor specific antibody, Denkers et al. [27] and, more recently, Kaminski et al. [28] have isolated isotype class switch variants of specific anti-tumor murine monoclonal antibodies and have shown that successful anti-tumor therapy is effective only when using antibody bearing the murine IgG2a isotype.

Cobbold et al. [26] have suggested that the importance of isotype may be reflective of their relative ability to bind complement. However we have performed experiments to test the efficacy of GK1.5 treatment in complement deficient mice. Administration of anti-L3T4 antibody was equally efficient in both C5-deficient and its normal congenic partner in eliminating L3T4-positive cells. While these data do not discount a role for complement as a mechanism for depletion in vivo of L3T4 cells, they do indicate that other mechanisms such as antibody dependant cellular cytoxicity (ADCC) may play an important role.

Administration of anti-L3T4 inhibits both the primary and secondary humoral response to tetanus toxoid while leaving an ongoing response unaffected [Ranges and Sriram, unpubl. observation]. The immunologic basis for these alternations in immune reactivity is currently under investigation. While the primary action of the antibody appears to be that of deletion of L3T4 positive cells, the specific effects of this cell loss are not well understood. The simplest scenario would be that the loss of potentially reactive cells accounts for the decreased immune response. However, other options are just as likely. In the absence of L3T4+ cells, the antigen may induce a state of tolerance, perhaps by eliciting the development of suppressor cells. It is possible that total elimination of L3T4+ cells is not a necessary prerequisite for the observed immunologic alterations. It may be that deletion of some but not all L3T4+ cells will tip the immunologic balance between helper and suppressor activities sufficiently to favor a lowering of the immune response. In our lab we have seen evidence of this in mice which, after long-term treatment with anti-L3T4 in CR-EAE, show an inverted ratio of L3T4+ to Lyt 2+ cells. However, a sizable proportion (roughly 30%) of the L3T4 population remain intact. Nevertheless, these mice remain resistant to recurring relapses. It may well turn out that, as with many other immunologic phenomena, in vivo immunomodulation with anti-L3T4 will be the result of several processes.

Lack of Specificity of Lymphocytes in End Organ: Implication for Antigen-Specific Suppression Therapies

In many experimental and spontaneously developed autoimmune disease states the receptor specificities at the end organ are varied. While the MBP-specific T cell line and clone are sufficient to cause disease, the final mediators of effector function at the end organ are comprised of T cells, B cells, and macrophages with varying specificities. Wekerle et al. [personal commun.] have shown that following injection of ^{14}C-labeled encephalitogenic T cell blasts in vivo the inflammatory exudate is comprised almost completely of non radiolabeled cells. Furthermore, Trotter and Steinman [29] have also shown that specificity of lymphocytic homing is lost once the blood-brain barrier bas been disrupted. These results extend the earlier results of Werdelin and McCluskey [30] who showed that the homing pattern of lymphocytes was an antigen nonspecific process, and T cells of various specificities end up at the inflammatory site.

It is thus becoming increasingly apparent that while many autoimmune diseases may begin as a uni-antigenic disease process, when clinically established, many antigenic epitopes of the initiating antigen, and new antigens released as sequelae of tissue injury augment and sustain the immune process. Analysis of antibody specificities in the cerebrospinal fluid in MS patients and synovial fluid in rheumatoid arthritis has repeatedly shown a broad spectrum of antibody specificities [31]. It may thus not be fruitful to implement antigen-specific therapy in already established disease.

We had earlier suggested that antibody to the cell surface products of immune response gene products (anti-Ia antibody) might be a novel mechanism of immune suppression. Treatment in vivo with anti-I-A antibodies successfully prevented the development of EAE and experimental autoimmune myasthenia gravis, reversed CR-EAE, and also prolonged survival in (NZB × NZW)F_1 mice [32–34]. The uniqueness of this form of therapy was that anti-IA antibodies suppressed the immune response in a haplotype specific manner without producing global immune suppression. Although mice have tolerated anti-IA antibodies in vivo for prolonged duration, their long-term effects in man must be viewed with caution.

Therapy with anti-L3T4 antibody provides an alternate method of immune suppression of established disease but is not without potential side effects. Treatment with anti L3T4 antibodies causes a reduction of helper T cells in lymphoid organs and circulation and a hematological profile not unlike that seen in AIDS. Although mice housed in our animal facility did not succumb to intercurrent infections when treated for prolonged periods of time, such potential complications of long-term therapy remain. It is conceivable that when short-term depletion of specific T cell subsets is required such a therapy might be feasible. This immunotherapy does not cause permanent depletion of thymocytes and there is a return of L3T4+ cells to normal levels when the antibody is discontinued.

While it would be ideal to prevent the development of autoimmune disease states, the possibility of a vaccine does not appear to be feasible. The antigenic specificities of most autoantigens are not known and the individual susceptibility markers are not well characterized. Hence, it will be impossible to tolerize individuals to all the potential disease-causing autoantigens. While we await answers to these questions, therapy with anti-L3T4 antibodies will add an additional drug to our armamentarium of immunosuppressive regimens in the treatment of established autoimmune disease.

References

1 Smith, H. E.; Steinberg, A. D.: Autoimmunity: a perspective. A. Rev. Immunol. *21* (1984).

2 Meischer, P. A.; Beris, P.: Immunosuppressive therapy in the treatment of autoimmune disease. Springer Semin. Immunopathol. *7:* 69–90 (1984).

3 Kohler, G.; Milstein, C.: Continuous culture of fused cells secreting antibody of predefined specificity. Nature, Lond. *256:* 495 (1975).

4 Goding, J. W.: Antibody production by hybridomas. J. Immunol. Methods *39:* 285 (1980).

5 Miller, R. A.; Mahoney, D. G.; McKillop, J.; Levy, R.: In vivo effects of murine hybridoma monoclonal antibody in a patient with T-cell leukemia. Blood *58:* 78 (1981).

6 Riz, J.; Pesando, J. M.; Sallan, S. E.; Clavell, L. A.; Notis-McConarty, J.; Rosenthal, P.; Schlossman, S. F.: Serotherapy of acute lymphoblastic leukemia with monoclonal antibody. Blood *58:* 141 (1981).

7 Dillman, R. D.; Shawler, D. L.; Sobol, R. E.; Collins, H. A.; Beauregard, J. C.; Wormsley, S. B.; Rayston, I.: Murine monoclonal antibody therapy in two patients with chronic lymphocytic leukemia. Blood *59:* 1036 (1982).

8 Cosimi, A. B.; Colvin, R. B.; Burton, R. C.; Rubin, R. H.; Goldstein, G.; Kung, P. C.; Hansen, W. P.; Delmonico, F. L.; Russell, P. S.: Use of monoclonal antibodies to T-cell subsets for immunologic monitoring and treatment in recipients of renal allografts. New Engl. J. Med. *305:* 208 (1981).

9 Cosimi, A. B.; Burton, R. C.; Kung, P. C.; Colvin, R.; Goldstein, G.; Lifter, J.; Rhodes, W.; Russell, P. S.: Evaluation in primate renal allograft recipients of monoclonal antibody to human T-cell subclasses. Transplant. Proc. *13:* 499 (1981).

10 Prentice, H. G.; Janossy, G.; Skeggs, D.; Blacklock, H. A.; Bradstock, K. F.; Goldstein, G.; Hoffbrand, A. V.: Use of anti-T-cell monoclonal antibody OKT3 to prevent acute graft-vs-host disease in allogeneic bone-marrow transplantation for acute leukaemia. Lancet *i:* 700 (1982).

11 Wilde, D. B.; Marrack, P.; Koppler, J.; Dialynas, D. P.; Fitch, F. W.: Evidence implicating L3T4 in class II MHC antigen reactivity monoclonal antibody GK 1-5 (anti L3T4a) blocks class II MN4HC antigen specific proliferation, release of lymphokines and binding by cloned murine helper T lymphocyte lines. J. Immun. *131:* 2178–2186 (1983).

12 Dialynas, D. P.; Wilde, D. B.; Marrack, P.; Pierres, A.; Wall, K. A.: Characterization of the murine T-cell surface molecule designated L3T4 recognized by monoclonal antibody GK 1-5. Expression of L3T4a by functional T-cell clones, appear to correlate primarily with class II MHC antigen reactivity. Immunol. Rev. *74:*30 (1983).

13 Ortiz-Ortiz, L.; Weigle, W.O.: Cellular events in the induction of experimental allergic encephalomyelitis in rats. J. exp. Med. *144:* 604–620 (1976).

14 Pettinelle, C.B.; McFarlin, D.E.: Adoptive transfer of EAE in SJL mice after in vitro activation of lymph node cells by myelin basic protein. J. Immun. *127:* 420–1425 (1981).

15 Sriram, S.; Solomon, D.; Rouse, R.V.; Steinman, L.: Identification of T-cell subsets and B, lymphocytes in mouse EAE brains. J. Immun. *129:* 1649 (1982).

16 Trotter, J.; Sriram, S.; Rassenti, L.; Jen chow, C.H.; Fritz, R.; Steinman, L.: Characterization of T-cell lines and clones from SJL/J and (Balb/c×SJL/J)f, mice specific for myelin basic protein. J. Immun. *134:* 2322–2328 (1985).

17 Waldor, M.K.; Sriram, S.; Hardy, R.; Herzenberg, L.A.; Lanier, L.; Lim, M.; Steinman, L.: Reversal of experimental allergic encephalomyelitis with monoclonal antibody to a T-cell subset marker. Science *227:* 415 (1985).

18 Lassman, H.; Wisnieski, H.M.: Chronic relapsing EAE. Cliniopathological comparison with multiple sclerosis. Archs Neurol. *36:* 490 (1979).

19 Lublin, F.D.; Maurer, P.H.; Berry, R.G.; Tippett, D.: Delayed relapsing experimental allergic encephalomyelitis in mice. J. Immun. *126:* 819 (1981).

20 Mokhtarian, F.; McFarlin, D.E.; Raine, C.S.: Adoptive transfer of myelin basic protein sensitized T-cells produce chronic relapsing demyelinating disease in mice. Nature, Lond. *309:* 356 (1984).

21 Sriram, S.; Roberts, C.A.: Treatment of established CR-EAE with anti L3T4 antibodies. J. Immun. (in press).

22 Ranges, G.E.; Sriram, S.; Cooper, S.: Prevention of type II collagen induces arthritis by in vivo treatment with anti L3T4. J. exp. Med. *162:* 1150 (1985).

23 Wofsy, D.; Seaman, W.E.: Successful treatment of autoimmunity in $(NZB \times NZW)F_1$ mice with monoclonal antibody to L3T4. J. exp. Med. *161:* 378 (1985).

24 Wofsy, D.; Seaman, W.E.: Antibody to the helper T-cell antigen L3T4 retards advanced lupus in NZB/NZW mice. Clin. Res. *34:* 100a (1986).

25 Marrack, P.; Endres, R.; Shimonkivetz, R.; Zlotnic, A.; Dialynas, D.; Fitch, F.; Kapplar, J.: The major histocompatibility complex restricted antigen receptor or T-cells. Role of the L3T4 product. J. exp. Med. *158:* 1077 (1983).

26 Cobbold, S.P.; Jayasuriya, A.; Nash, A.; Prospero, T.D.; Waldman, H.: Therapy with monoclonal antibodies by elimination of T-cell subsets in vivo. Nature, Lond. *312:* 548 (1984).

27 Denkers, E.E.; Badger, C.C.; Ledbetter, J.A.; Bernstein, I.W.: Influence of antibody isotype on passive serotherapy of lymphoma. J. Immun. *135:* 2183 (1985).

28 Kaminski, M.S.; Kitamura, K.; Maloney, D.G.; Cambell, M.J.; Levy, R.: Importance of antibody isotype in monoclonal antiidiotype therapy of a murine B cell lymphoma. A study of hybridoma class switch variants. J. Immun. *136:* 1123 (1986).

29 Trotter, J.; Steinman, L.: Homing of lymphoid cells in EAE. J. Immun. *131:* 1286 (1983).

30 Werdelin, O.; McCluskey, R.T.: The nature and specificity of mononuclear cells in experimental autoimmune inflammations and the mechanisms leading to their accumulation. J. exp. Med. *133:* 1242 (1971).

31 Mattson, D.H.; Roos, R.P.; Arnason, B.G.W.: Isoelectric focusing of IgG eluted

from multiple sclerosis and subacute sclerosing panencephalitis brains. Nature, Lond. *187:* 335–337 (1980).

32 Steinman, L.; Rosenbaum, J.T.; Sriram, S.; McDevitt, H.O.: In vivo effects of antibodies to immune response gene products of experimental allergic encephalitis. Proc. natn. Acad. Sci. USA *78:* 7111 (1981).

33 Waldor, M.K.; Sriram, S.; McDevitt, H.O.; Steinman, L.: In vivo therapy with monoclonal anti-I-A antibody suppresses immune responses to aceylocholine receptor. Proc. natn. Acad. Sci. USA *80:* 2713 (1983).

34 Adelman, N.E.; Watling, D.L.; McDevitt, H.O.: Treatment of $(NZB \times NZW)F_1$ disease with anti-I-A monoclonal antibodies. J. exp. Med. *158:* 1350.

35 Rosenbaum, J.T.; Adelman, N.E.; McDevitt, H.O.: In vivo effects of antibodies to immune response gene products. I. Haplotype-specific suppression of humoral immune responses with a monoclonal anti-I-A. J. exp. Med. *154:* 1694.

S. Sriram, MD, Department of Neurology, College of Medicine, University of Vermont, Burlington, VT 05401 (USA)

Subject Index

A2 11, 148
A2 line 148
A2 T cell line 148
A2b 149, 150, 159
  arthritogenic clone 153
  clone 149, 151–153
  T cell clone 153
A2 cell line 12, 150, 158, 159
A2c 159
A2c clone 159
AA 156, 157, 160, 163
  CFA-induced 152
Abnormalities, cytokine 189
Accessory cells 178
  antigen-presenting 178
Acetylcholine receptors 12, 156
  autoantibodies 43
Acquired immune deficiency 246
Acquired tolerance 26
Actin 4, 49, 51
  antibody 50
Activated killer (AK) 5, 78
Activators, polyclonal 144
Activity
  colony-stimulating 186
  leukocyte mobilizing factor 123
Acute phase reactants 173
Adenomas 92
Adjuvant arthritis (AA) 10–12, 147, 148
AgB loci 239
AIDS (acquired immune deficiency syndrome) 20, 243, 245, 246, 248, 249, 253, 261–263, 265, 283
  immune function 261
  virus 19, 243, 244
AIDS/ARC 20, 268, 269
  immune defect 263
  patients 20, 262, 265, 266, 268
AIDS-associated retrovirus (ARV) 243
AIDS-related complex (ARC) 20, 246, 253, 262, 265, 269
AIDS-related conditions 243
AISNHL 218, 219
Albumin 4
  autoantibodies 59
Alleles, HLA class II 161
Alloantigen 264
Alloantisera 201
Allogenotopes 205
Allograft rejection 275
Alternative pathways 104
AMLR 205
Analogues, synthetic peptide 123
Analysis, limiting dilution 28
Anaphylatoxin inactivator 8, 104, 110, 112
Anergy 248
  specific cellular 161
  to PPD 248
Angiogenesis 187
  tumor 187
Angiogenin, recombinant 188

Animals
collagen-immunized 233
NC-deficient 89
Ankylosing spondylitis (AS) 12
Antibodies
acetylcholine receptor 156
antiactin 49
antialbumin 49
anticollagen 49, 171
anticytochrome C 49
anticytoskeleton 50
anti-DNA 11, 22, 57, 62, 130, 139, 154, 156, 280
anti-idiotype (id) 52, 60
anti-idiotypic 156
antifetuin 49
anti-immunoglobulin 171
anti-L3T4 22, 276, 277, 284
antilaminin 86
antilymphocyte 257
antimyoglobin 49
antireceptor 12
anti-T cell 22, 275
anti-Thy-1 280
antithyroglobulin 49
antitransferrin 49
autoreactive 35
class II monoclonal 4, 63, 81, 92, 123, 153, 154, 156, 157, 181, 245
monoclonal anti-DNA 56, 156
monoclonal anti-HLA class II 205
monoclonal DNA 154
natural 42, 49, 59
natural antitubulin 48
natural monoclonal 60
neutralizing 183
polyspecific 63
T cell 275
thyroid-stimulating 157
Antibody 104
anti-C3 113
anticochlear 215
anti-ds DNA 57
anti-Ia 283
anti-L3T4 279, 281
cochlear 216
isotope 281
monoclonal 117, 178
monoclonal anti-HLA-B27 146
natural 60
Antibody dependent cellular cytotoxicity (ADCC) 281
Antibody responses, antigen-specific 110
Anti-DNA antibody (F227), NZB/NZW F1 56
Anti-DNA antibody, monoclonal 57
Anti-DNA autoantibodies, monoclonal 55
Anti-ds DNA 55
Antigen 179, 275
antibody complexes 104
bacterial 148, 149
CD4 245
cell surface 81
class I MHC 14, 182
class II 14, 182, 184, 201, 206, 210, 211
collagen-type II 223
common 162
complex 160
cross-reacting 4, 58
HLA class I 206
Ia-like 268
intracellular 54
labyrinthine 217
Leu-3 276
mammalian 154
microbial 154, 163
mycobacterial 162
murine L3T4 280
murine leukemia virus 135
mycobacterial common 162
NK-associated 92
nuclear 54
nucleic acid 154
presentation 181
presenting cell 23
Qa-5 81, 82
recall 248, 263, 266
self 35, 163
serologically defined 202
streptococcal 145, 157
T4 276
T-dependent 7, 108
Thy-1 81, 281

ubiquitous 246
Antigen expression, HLA class II 205
Antigen MT 159
Antigenic determinants 158
Antigenic mimicry 10, 12, 154, 157
Anti-L3T4 antibody in EAE, therapy of 276
Anti-L3T4 antibody, therapy with 283
Antisera, anti-TNF 87
Antiserum
anti-fraction 1 116, 117
anti-I-J 27
Anti-TAC 178
Antithymocyte serum 275
Antitumor activity 85
NC 88
Antitumor agents 275
Antiviral agent 269
ARC 253
immune function 261
patients 263
Arthritis 145, 147, 157, 158, 160, 163, 231, 279
adjuvant 144, 146, 150
autoimmune 150
bystander 149
collagen-induced 231
collagen type II-induced 150
induction 239
reactive 145, 146
rheumatoid 283
seronegative reactive 145
streptococcal-induced 145
type II collagen-induced 240, 278
Arthritis in man, type II collagen-induced 22
Arthritogenic
A2b 149
A2b clone 159
Asialo-GM1 markers 81
Assays, NC 86
Auditory dysfunction 215
Auricular chondritis 217
Autoantibodies 3, 5, 42, 43, 52, 59, 62, 65, 132
anti-BrMRBC 45, 46, 61, 64, 65
anti-DNA 4, 52, 54, 58, 61, 65, 130
antierythrocyte 131, 135, 138
anti-gp70 130
anti-HB 44, 48
anti-HOL 48
anti-I 48
antitubulin 49
anti-X 44, 47, 48
human anti-DNA monoclonal 57
lupus 53, 55, 62, 63
lupus monoclonal 56
lupus monoclonal anti-DNA 57, 61
monoclonal 54, 67
monoclonal anti-DNA 55–57, 63, 64
multispecific 5
natural 42, 43, 48, 49, 52, 53, 59, 61, 64
natural monoclonal 51, 52
normal 67
pathogenic 3, 44
polyspecific natural 61
Autoantibody 48, 132
Autoantibody idiotype, anti-DNA monoclonal 56
Autoantibody precursor cell, anti-BrMRBC 60
Autoantigen 16, 45, 48, 50, 59, 64, 184, 201, 245, 275
cryptic membrane 44
normal hidden 44
Auto-antiidiotype 66
Autoimmune
arthritis 11
destruction 256
disease 1, 5, 9, 10, 12, 25, 37, 43, 129, 130, 138, 148, 275, 276, 282, 283
hemolytic anemia 9, 129
hydrops 221
injury 19, 275
model 280
phenomenon 217
process 200
reaction 215
reactivity 161
response 217, 257
Autoimmune disease
human 147, 163
immunotherapy 21, 275
spontaneous 235

Autoimmune disorders 144, 161
Autoimmune ear disease 232
collagen-induced 239
Autoimmune sensorineural hearing loss (AISNHL) 215, 217, 219
Autoimmune states 200
Autoimmunoregulation 5
Autoregulation 36
Autoregulatory 36
Autoimmunity 11, 12, 15, 17, 42–44, 156, 158, 161, 201, 215, 275
human 154
natural 43
sensorineural hearing loss 17
type II collagen 217, 218
Autoreactive B cell 59
Autoreactive clones, natural 64
Azimexon 20
AZT (3′-azido-3′-deoxythymidine) 20, 263

B cell
activation 51, 118, 120, 139
autoreactive 42, 44, 51, 59
CR-negative 108
polyclonal 138, 247
X-autoantigen binding 47
B cell clones, autoreactive 60
B cell subsets, NZB 138
B cells 3, 5, 9, 46, 47, 58, 63, 67, 77, 82, 95, 118, 130, 183, 245, 261
$Lyb5^+$ 53
$Lyb5^-$ 53
lymphoma 246
memory 113
murine 179
NZB 130
B clones, autoreactive 61
B lymphocyte 8, 9, 20, 52, 59, 135, 201, 246, 247
B27 allele 145
B-27 lymphocytes 12
Bacterial antigens 50
Bacterial epitopes, cross-reactive 157
Barrier, blood-brain 262, 282
Basement membrane, glomerular 154
Basophils 104
BCG 147, 157
Bence-Jones, proteins 50
B-LCL, autologous 34
Borrelia burgdorferi 146
Bovine leukemia virus 243
Brain antigens 49
BrMRBC, autoantibodies against 61
Bromelin 44

C3 7, 103, 104, 108–110, 113, 118, 122
activation 104
breakdown 120
convertase 104
CoVF-convertase treated 121
deficiency 8, 109, 122
degradation 118
degradation products 123
fragments 7, 8, 104, 109, 112, 121
immunoregulatory role 107
native 104, 111
receptors 7, 8, 108
structure 104
C3 fragments 7, 8, 104, 109, 112, 121
suppressive 109
C3a 7, 105, 109, 115, 122
human 111
receptors 8
synthetic peptide 110
C3a-des-arg 8, 110, 112
inactive 122
C3b 105, 106, 112, 121
degradation products 122
fragments 9, 105, 112
C3c 112
C3d 112
C3dg 113
C3d-K 113, 121, 123
C3-FP 121
C3g 118
C4 109
deficiency 109
Campylobacters 145
Candida 267
Caprine arthritis-encephalitis virus (CAEV) 244
Carboxypeptidase 112

Carcinomas
- breast 92
- colon 92

Cardiolipin 55, 63, 154
- autoantibodies to 55

Carriers
- detection 249
- tolerance to 134

Cartilage 150, 153
- cell-mediated immunity to 157

Catabolin 172
Cathepsin G 107
CB-11 peptide 18, 231, 239
CBA/N mice 52, 53
CD4 247
- helper cells 178
- lymphocytes 246
- positive cells 257
- surface antigen 245

CD8 247
- positive 257

cDNA probes 206
Cell
- natural cytotoxic 77
- surface proteins 55

Cell degeneration, spiral ganglion 221
Cell line
- BP specific 149, 159
- tumor-specific 179
- WEHI-164 80

Cell-mediated immunity (CMI) 250
- deficiency 261

Cells
- allocytotoxic 31
- antigen-presenting 173, 181, 280
- asialo GM-1^+ 89
- autoaggressive 24, 28, 36
- autocytotoxic 2, 24, 28, 32, 35
- autoreactive 201
- autoregulatory 2, 28, 35
- autosuppressor 24, 35
- B 135
- blood mononuclear 247
- CD8 257
- cultured synovial lining 201
- dendritic 26, 183, 206
- DR7 203
- effector 171
- endothelial 185, 221
- enlarged Lyt-2^+ T 132
- follicular dendritic (FD) 245
- ganglion 228
- helper T 283
- hemopoietic progenitor 184–186
- IL-2 receptor-bearing 178
- immunocompetent 27
- infected 181
- L3T4 132, 281, 282
- Langerhans 173
- lectin-stimulating 179
- lymphoid 5
- Lyt-1^+ suppressor T inducer 111
- Lyt-2^+ suppressor 111
- mast 104
- microglial 245
- mononuclear 175, 219
- murine 111
- natural killer (NK) 78, 86, 110, 113
- NC 77, 78, 86, 88
- non-adherent synovial 205, 208
- null 136
- osteoclast precursor 188
- peripheral blood mononuclear (PBM) 175, 183, 184
- plasma 131, 136
- regulatory 24, 32, 35, 36
- rheumatoid synovial dendritic 175
- self-reactive 1
- sensitized 228
- spiral ganglion 227, 229
- suppressor 2, 27, 36, 113, 282
- synovial 175, 181, 183, 206
- synovial dendritic 173
- T 111
- T helper 111, 138, 245, 247
- T suppressor 111, 132, 158, 247
- target 110
- thymic-derived 26
- thymic epithelial 26
- veto 3, 36

Cellular
- anergy 161
- immunity 247
  - indices 256

Cellular (cont.)
  immunodeficiency 251
Chain, invariant 209
Chemotactic defect 248
Chlamydiae 145
Chondrocytes 211
Chondroitin sulfate 152
Chronic relapsing EAE (CR-EAE) 277
CIAED 18, 229, 231, 239, 240
  cell transfer 227
  immunopathology 227
  serum transfer 228
Cimetidine 20, 263
Class II
  antigens 16, 17
  expression 204, 211
  genes 204
  MHC products 178
  molecules 201, 204
  subsets 205
Class II molecules, hybrid 204
Classical pathway 104
Clonal deletion 1, 2, 24, 27, 36
  theory 27, 42, 59
Clonal elimination 27
Clones
  autoimmune 160
  forbidden 42
  self recognizing 158
CMI
  abnormal 251
  impaired 255
CMV 19, 255
  IgG antibody 251
CNBr peptides 237
Cobra venom factor (CoVF) 7, 8, 107, 108
  treatment 103
Cochlea 216, 228
Cochlear
  nerve 221
  vasculitis 219
Cogan's syndrome 215
Collagen 4, 15, 177, 187, 219
  antibodies 49
  arthritis 148
  autoimmunity 226
  bovine type II 221
  chicken type II 231, 239, 240
  disease 215
  immunity 217
  native bovine type II 228, 229
  type II 11, 150, 231
    immunity 150
  type II epitope 231
Collagen-induced arthritis (CIA) 22, 276
Collagen-induced autoimmune ear disease (CIAED) 18, 227
Collagenase 176
Colonies, clonal growth 186
Colony-stimulating factor (CSF) 13, 172, 184, 188
Combining site, antibody 63
Complement 7, 8, 103, 108, 109
Complement
  activators 107, 109
  deficiency 109
  depletion 107, 109
  hemolytic 103
  molecules 123
  proeins 104, 123
  surface receptors 108
  regulation 122
Core protein 11, 150, 152
Corynebacterium parvum 89
CP hybridomas 45
CP idiotype 47
C-reactive protein 176
CR-EAE 277, 283
Crista ampullaris 217
  degeneration 225
Cross-reactivities
  idiotypic 61
  immunological 257
CSF-1 185
CSFs 15, 185, 186
CTL
  activity 86
  clones 87
  lines 87
  mediated target lysis 86
CTLL assay, murine 180
CTLL IL-2 assay 180
Cyclosporin A 25, 150, 176

Cytokines 13–15, 171, 177, 183
non-immunological effects 187
rheumatological 171
Cytomegalovirus (CMV) 6, 251
Cytopathic effect, viral 183
Cytoskeleton proteins 51, 59, 60
autoantibodies 48, 53
Cytotoxic T lymphocytes 257
Cytotoxicity
antibody-dependent 182
natural cell-mediated 77

Defect, Xid 53
Defects, immunological 261
Deficiency, immune 262
Degeneration, cochlear nerve 219
Degradation products, C3b and C3b 112
Delayed type hypersensitivity (DTH) 152, 246, 263, 264, 270
Dementia, progressive 245
Demyelination 277
Dendritic cells 1, 14, 26
rheumatoid synovial 13
Dendritic follicular cells, HTLV-III infected 258
Determinants
antigenic 158
cross-reactive 152
Diabetes 147
Diabetes mellitus 12, 157, 204
Dideoxycytidine 269
Disease
autoimmune 42, 129, 130, 133, 139, 152
autoimmune demyelanting 276
immune complex 123
immunopathic 181
infectious 161
Reiter's 146
rheumatological 176
Diseases, acute viral 146
DNA 4, 54, 59
antigenicity 58
autoantibodies 53
double-stranded 156
normal autoantibodies 48
DNA autoantibodies, polyspecificity 54
Dot immunobinding assays 206
DP 201, 205, 206
DQ 201, 205, 206
B chains 203
molecules 204
DR 201, 205, 206
molecules 16
DR1 202
DR3 162, 204
DR4 202, 204
haplotype 204
Drug addicts 245, 261
Drugs, antiviral 262
dsDNA 4, 60
antibody 50
DTH 152, 254, 267
DW4 202–204
DW10 202, 204
DW13 202
DW14 202
DW15 202, 203

EAE 160, 276, 278, 283
acute 277
relapsing 277
Ear, autoimmunity 215
Ear disease 18
autoimmune 231, 240
collagen-induced 219
human autoimmune 227
immunologic criteria 229
Ear immune injury 228
Ear-swelling 152
Effector cell, human NC 93
Effectors
NC 88
NK 88
Elastase 107
Elastin, antibodies 49
ELISA assays 229, 231
Encephalitogenic determinant 276
Encephalopathy 245
Endolymph 219
Endolymphatic
duct 219
hydrops 17, 217, 219, 221, 227, 240
Endothelial cells 14

Eosinophil
CSF 185
differentiation factor 185
Epitopes 231, 239
antigenic 283
arthritogenic 239
cross-reactive 146, 157, 158, 160
mimicking 158
normal tissue 157
RA specific 205
self cross-reactive 163
self-mimicking 160
suppression-inducing 162
Equine infectious anemia virus (EIAV) 244
Erythrocyte antigens, autoantibodies 47
Erythrocytes
bromelin-treated 45
isologous 59
Experimental allergic encephalomyelitis (EAE) 22, 43, 276
Experimental autoimmune thyroiditis (EAT) 147

Factor
angiogenesis 188
bone resorbing 176
epidermal cell activating 172
fibrogenic 172
H 108, 112
lymphocyte-activating 172
macrophage angiogenesis 188
mononuclear cell 172
osteoclast-activating 176
proteolysis-inducing 172
vascularization 172
Fc fragment of IgG, autoantibodies 59
Fetuin 4
Fibroblasts 14, 15, 181, 183, 185, 187
activation 175
dermal 175
synovial 14, 182
Fibrosis 15, 187
Flow cytometry 131, 247
Forbidden clones 3, 12, 158, 163
Fraction 1 115, 116, 119
Fraction 2 113, 115, 119, 121
Fragments
complement 108, 109
complement activation 7
peptidoglycan-polysaccharide 10
Functions, class II, MHC antigen-restricted 280

Ganglion cells 228
Ganglion degeneration 219
Gammaglobulin 262
antibodies 49
Gamma-interferon 84, 93, 261, 264
Gammapathies, malignant monoclonal 62
Gastric parietal cells 4
G-CSF 186
Gene
dominant suppressing 138
immune response 139, 239
MHC-linked 161, 163
NZW immune response 130
recessive enhancing 138
Genetic gates 138
GM-CSF 14
Globulin 51
Glomerular basement membrane 67
Glomerulonephritis 139, 279
immune complex 58, 131, 139
poststreptococcal 11, 154
Graft-vs-host (GVH) disease 25
Granulocyte 171
CSF (G-CSF) 185
Graves' disease 12, 157
Guinea pig fetus, collagen distribution 230
Guinea pigs
strain 2, 227
strain 13, 227

H 106
$H2^q$ loci 239
Haplotype, HLA class II 201
Haptens 50
HB auto-AG 44
Hearing loss 17
Helper cell function 265
Helper cell lymphokine (LK) 264

Helper T cell 23, 113, 264
human 264
Helper T lymphocyte 133, 245
Hemagglutinins, natural 42
Hemolysis 106
Hemolytic anemia 9, 10, 47, 48, 131, 136, 138
autoimmune 43, 138
Coombs-positive 47
murine 3
Hemophiliacs 261
Heparan sulfate 4
proteoglycans 11
Hepatitis 6, 146
Herpes 6
Heterosexual men 247
Histocompatibility antigens, class II 15
Histones 54
HIV 262, 263, 268, 269
antibody 262
infection 20, 261
HLA
antigens 249
association 161
class II antigens 201
class II probes 205
HLA-B27 antigen 10, 156
HLA-D
products 208
region 200, 201
region antigens 201
region products 202, 206
subregions 15
HLA-DR 184, 201
HLA-DR4 162
HNK1 93
Hodgkin's disease 248
Homosexual 255, 262
males 245, 248, 249, 251, 254, 256, 261
Homosexual men
seronegative 257
seropositive 257
Horror autotoxicus 35, 275
HTLV-I 243
HTLV-III 19, 243, 244, 249, 251, 253, 255
antibody 249
genome 257
immune response 253
infections 19, 247, 249, 256, 257
virus 246, 256
Human
cartilage 153
granulocyte-macrophage CSF (GM-CSF) 185
immunodeficiency virus (HIV) 20, 261
NK 93
SLE 54
tumor rejection 275
urinary CSF 185
Hybrid determinants 204
Hybridoma 51, 52, 56, 61
anti-BrMRBC 60
monoclonal antibody, collagen-specific 230
technology 275
Hybrids (NZB×NFS) F1 131
Hyperactivity, B cell 130
Hyperglobulinemia 261

I 106
Ia antigen 15, 200, 201, 206, 208, 209, 276, 280
aberrant expression 200, 205
hyperexpression 200, 205
Ia protein 206
Idiotype
anti-CP 60
CP 45, 61
cross-reactive 52, 60
D23 61
E7 61
Idiotype-anti-idiotype interactions 36
Idiotypic structures 57
IFN 6, 84, 181, 183, 184
IFN-α 182, 183
IFN-β 182
IFN-γ 13, 14, 16, 182–184
IFN-γ gene 182
IgD, surface 130
IgG, antibodies 49
rheumatoid factor 177
IL chain 210
IL-1 13, 173, 175, 177–179, 182, 187, 188
suppression 177

IL-2 6, 8, 13, 20, 84, 85, 92, 93, 121, 176, 263, 264
  gene, human 178
  human 178
  receptor 9, 21, 85, 132, 133, 138, 178
  recombinant 178
  synthesis 113
IL-3 6, 84, 176
Immune
  abnormalities 249
  augmentation 248
  complexes 173, 177, 218
  defect 262
  deficiency 245, 248, 251, 270
  dysfunction 246, 249
  function 262
  impairment 248, 253, 256
  regulation 103, 161
  response 12, 109, 114, 122, 123
  surveillance 246
Immune complexes
  circulating 147
  disease 9
  glomerulonephritis 130
Immune function, T cell-dependent 265
Immune response
  cellular 179
  complement regulation 107, 109
  genetic control 160
  intrasynovial 171
  type II collagen 239
Immune response gene, RA-specific 202
Immune suppression, global 283
Immunity
  antimicrobial 161
  antitumor 77
  cell-mediated 161, 225
  residual 268
Immunization, type II collagen 229
Immunoamplifiers, leukocyte-derived 264
Immunocytes 227
Immunodeficiency, X-linked 131
Immunofluorescence 226, 228
Immunofluorescent staining 218, 221
Immunoglobulins, monoclonal 4
Immunologic
  abnormalities 248
  indices 251
  regulation 42
  response 181
  tolerance 24, 130
Immunomodulators 269
  leukocyte-derived 264
  pharmacologic 262, 263
Immunoperoxidase 217
Immunopotentiating agent 265
Immunoregulation 103
  complement 7, 122, 123
Immunoregulatory
  defects 243
  fragments 8
Immunorestorative agent 262
Immunosuppression 8, 120, 275
Immunotherapy 275, 276
  cancer 157
Immuthiol 20, 263
IMREG-1 modulator 21, 264–266, 268
Infection
  intercurrent 145
  Klebsiella 156
  microbial 145
  opportunistic 249, 262, 265
  rheumatic disease 145
  streptococcal 145
Infectious
  diseases 144
  tolerance 2, 27
Infective agents 145
Inflammation 171
  rheumatic 145
  rheumatoid 171
  synovial 13, 171, 183
Inflammatory disease, rheumatological 146, 188
Influenza 146
INFs 20
Inner ear lesions, collagen-induced 239
Interferon 92, 247, 262
  alpha 181, 262
  beta 181
  gamma 172, 176, 178, 181, 187, 208, 262

Interleukin-1 (IL-1) 172, 177
Interleukin-2 (IL-2) 29, 172, 177, 247, 261, 262, 265, 269
  receptor 265, 268
Interstitial keratitis 215
Invariant chain (Ii) 206, 210
Ir genes, MHC-linked 160
Isoprinosine 20, 263

Joint diseases, inflammatory 185
Joint, rheumatoid 181
Juvenile rheumatoid arthritis (JRA), seropositive 204

Kallikrein 107
Kaposi's sarcoma 245, 246, 249, 265, 270
Keratinocytes 173
Klebsiella 12, 146, 156
  antigens 55, 146
Klebsiella bacteria, ankylosing spondylitis (AS) 156

L3T4
  antibodies 276
  antigen 22, 276
  murine 280
$L3T4^{+}$ cells 23, 280, 283
Labyrinthitis, experimental allergic 216
Laminin 86
LAS 253
LAV/HTLV-III virus 261
LCM virus 82
Lentiviruses 243
  ungulate 243
Leprosy 161
  lepromatous 147, 161, 162
  tuberculoid 161, 162
Leu-3a 245
Leukocyte mobilizing factor (LMF) 107, 119, 264
Leukocytes, HLA-identical 265
Leukophoresis 180
LIF/MIF 264
Limiting dilution analysis 29, 35
Link protein 150
LMF 121
LPS 118
Lupus
  anti-DNA autoantibodies, polyspecificity 54
  autoantibodies, polyspecific 54
  immunogen 54, 57
Lupus erythematosus 9, 129
Lupus-like syndrome 276, 279
Lupus mouse strains, autoimmune 54
Ly1
  B cells 47, 52, 59, 65
  L3T4 phenotype 276
  Lyb-6 surface marker 52
Lyme arthritis 146
Lymphadenopathy 248, 252, 257
  associated virus (LAL) 243, 246
  syndrome (LAS) 246, 251
Lymphoblastoid cell lines (B-LCL) 31
Lymphocyte activating factor 177
Lymphocytes 2, 7, 13, 103, 157, 181, 211, 228, 249
  antibodies 49
  activated T, B 172
  autocytotoxic 1, 24
  autoreactive 42, 158
  autoregulatory 1, 24
  B27-positive 156
  CD8-positive 19
  cytolytic 264
  cytotoxic 27
  effector 27
  homing 282
  human T 110, 111
  murine splenic 110, 112
  peripheral blood 129, 157, 187
  proliferative responsive 247
  regulatory 27
  self-reactive 66
  sensitized 229
  synovial 179
    fluid 157
    membrane 13
  T helper 19, 265
  thymic 25
Lymphokines 7, 29, 85, 104, 188, 204, 208, 247, 264, 265
  T cell-derived 264
Lymphotoxin 188

Lysis
NC 80, 88
NCMC 84
NK 80
target cell 86
Lyt-2 antibody 276
Lyt-2+ T cells 135

M proteins, streptococcal 11, 154
Macrophage
activating factor (MAF) 182
CSF 185
migration inhibition factor (MIF) 264
Macrophages 5, 7, 8, 14, 77, 95, 103, 104, 111, 112, 171, 172, 206, 226, 282
Malaria 6
Malignancies 262
Mast cells 15, 187
MBP 276
MC1 16, 202
epitope 202
M-CSF 185, 186
Mediator, leukocyte endogenous 172
Melanomas 92
Membrane
receptors 211
synovial 181, 205
Ménière's disease 17, 215, 219, 223
Men
seronegative 256
seropositive 256
Meromyosin 51
Meth-A 79
Meth-113 79
Methionine-enkephalin 263
MHC 161
alleles 161
class II glycoproteins 201
class II molecules 202
Mice
arthritis 231
autoimmune 133, 138
BALB/c 132
complement-deficient 281
EAT 152
New Zealand 129, 130, 133, 138, 140
NFS 134
NZB 9, 131–133, 135
NZW 134
(NZB×NFS) F_1 130, 131, 134, 135
Migration inhibiting lymphokines 265
Migration inhibitory activity, antigen-induced 264
Mimicry 11, 154
antigenic 144, 158
structural 150, 157, 162, 163
Mitogen 118, 179, 265
Mixed lymphocyte response (MLR) 113, 201, 205
Mixed lymphocyte typing 202
Moloney leukemia virus 77
Monkeys, macaque 245
Monoclonal antibodies 11, 157, 218, 245, 275, 276, 280, 281
anti-RNA 57
anti-T cell 22
Monoclonal antibody (HNC-1) 93
Monoclonal Ig, human 49
Monocytes 173, 185, 211, 248
Monocytes/macrophages, peritoneal 186
Mouse
bg/bg mutant 89
CB-11 peptide-immunized 235
Mouse erythrocytes
autoantibodies 44
bromelin-treated 44, 65
NZB 3
YAC-1 110
Mouse red blood cells, bromelin-treated 53
MRL lpr/lpr mouse 56
MT 152, 159, 160, 162
Multi-CSF 185
Multi-lineage CSF 185
Multiple myeloma 50
Multiple sclerosis 12, 147, 157, 277
Mumps 146
Murine
multi-CSF 185
NC 92
Murine NC, human equivalent 79
Mutant mice, NK-deficient 92
Mutant mouse, NK-deficient 91

Myasthenia gravis 12, 43, 147, 156, 157
experimental autoimmune 283
Mycobacteria 10, 144, 153, 157, 160, 162
atypical 159
Mycobacterium leprae 161
Mycobacterium tuberculosis 10, ,11, 148
Mycoplasma infection 240
Myelin basic protein (MBP) 10, 22, 147, 149, 276
Myeloma proteins 58
Myelomas, nonsecreting 51
Myoglobin, antibody 50
Myosin 51, 60
antibody 50

Native C3 114
Natural autoantibodies 44
anti-DNA 62
antierythrocyte 62
antithyroglobulin 62
antitubulin 62
monoclonal anti-DNA 63
Natural cytotoxic (NC), cells 5, 77
Natural killer (NK) cells 5
Natural killer cytotoxicity 110
NC
activity 80, 83, 84, 86, 87, 90, 93
cell 6, 8, 79, 80
effector cell 6
lysis 79, 86, 87
target recognition 87
NCMC
effector cell, human 92
system 77, 80, 81
Neonatal tolerance 1
Neovascularization 188
Nerves, peripheral 161
Network theory 66
Neutrophils 173, 186
New Zealand mice, tolerance defects 133
New Zealand white (NZW) 9
NK
cell activity 83, 85–87, 90, 110, 178
cells 5, 20, 77, 79–81, 90, 93, 261, 263
target 87
target lysis 87
Nonlymphoid tumors, NCMC-sensitive 93
Non-self 156
Nuclear antigen, antibody 279
Nucleic acid hybridization, in situ 245
Null cells 6, 81, 95, 131, 135
proliferation 131
NZB mice 44, 48, 53, 129–131, 133, 135, 136, 138
old 132, 133

OAF 15, 188
OKT4 245
Oligosaccharides 152
Oncoviruses 243
Osteoarthritis 152, 188
Osteoblasts 176, 188, 226
Osteoclast-activating factor (OFA) 13, 172, 188
Osteoclastic cells 226
Osteoclasts 176, 188
Osteocytes 226
Oral candida 267
Organ of Corti 215, 216, 219, 221, 228, 229
Otosclerosis 17, 215, 218, 225
Otospongiosis-like lesions 217, 225, 240

Pannus formation 148
Parietal cells, antibodies 49
Pathways
alternative 103
classical 103
PBL 33, 209
Pemphigus vulgaris 43
Peptide CB-11, immunoregulatory 123
Peptides, cyanogen bromide 231
Peptidoglycan-polysaccharide 145
Peptidoglycans, bacterial 154
Perineural vasculitis 219
PFC, anti-BrMRBC 45
PGL 268
Phagocytic defects 248
Phagocytosis 106
Phenotype, autoantibody 65
Phospholipid cardiolipin 11
Phospholipids 55

Plaque forming cell (PVC) assay 44
Plasma cells 136
Plasmin 107
Platelets 55
Pleuripoietin 185
Pneumococcal polysaccharide (SSS-III), tpye III 132
Pneumocystis carinii pneumonia 245
Polyarthritis 146
  inflammatory 278
Polychondritis, relapsing 217
Poly-IC 89
Polynucleotides 55
Populations, NCMC 88
Proliferation
  anti-Ig-induced 118
  B cell 118
  LPS-induced 118
  T cell 118
Prostaglandin E_2 176
Prostaglandins 111
Protective clone 159
Proteins
  acute phase 176
  complement 109
  cytoskeleton 62
  fraction 2, 116
  sarcolemmal membrane 154
Proteoglycan 10, 12, 16, 17, 150, 152, 153, 210
  cartilage 153, 156
  fragments 152
Proteus 156
Purified protein derivate (PPD) 149
Pyrogen, endogenous 172

Quick-blot 206

RA 13, 152, 162, 177, 179, 180, 183, 189, 201, 202, 205
  ASLC 206
  disease-susceptibility gene 202
  patients 180
  susceptibility genes 205
  synovial effusions 13
  synovial membrane 208
Rabbit erythrocyte 104
Radial immunodiffusion 247
Radioimmunoassay (RIA) 183
Radioimmunometric assay 179
Rats
  collagen-immunized 226
  EAE 152
  Lewis 160
Reactions, graft-versus-host 144
Reactivity
  autoimmune 161
  DTH 152
Reagent, anti-idiotypic 57
Receptors 181
  antigen 150
  C3a 111
  CR2 121
  cell surface 178
  IL-2 131, 178, 182, 265
  polyspecific 63
  preparations 123
  surface IgM 130
  thyrotropin 157
Recombinant inbred lines, NZB 135
Regulatory
  cells 28
  proteins 106
Reissner's membrane 221
Rejection allograft 36
Response
  acute phase 177
  allocytotoxic 32
  autocytotoxic 32
  cellular immune 180
  lymphocyte 122
Restriction, MHC 77, 78
Retrovirus human T cell lymphotrophic virus (HTLV-III) 243
Retroviruses 243, 261, 269
RFLP patterns, RA-specific 205
Rheumatic diseases 13, 175, 210
  inflammatory 145
Rheumatic fever 10, 11, 145
  acute 145, 154
Rheumatoid arthritis 10, 11, 145, 154, 171, 178, 188, 200, 283
  autoimmunity 200
  factors 11, 55, 154

joint 177
synovium 185, 187
Rheumatological
diseases, IL-1 175
disorders 179, 183, 186, 189
Ribavarin 21, 263, 269
RI lines, NZB×NFS 139
RNA, quick-blot 206
RNP 54
Rubella virus 146

Salmonella 145
Saccular
degeneration 221
macula 228
Saccule 227
Sarcolemmal membrane proteins, myocardial 11
Scala tympani 216
Scleroderma 15, 175, 187
SEA-X 47
Secreting cells, anti-BrMRBC 46
Secretion, lymphokine 112
Self 156
antigens 34, 144, 148, 158
epitope 162
reactivity 163
tolerance 1, 5, 12, 24–27, 32, 42, 60, 66, 133, 158–160
Self-nonself recognition 275
Seminal plasma 249
immunosuppressive effects 255
Sensory hearing loss 216
Seroconversion 252
Serum
anti-C3-deficient 117
C3-deficient 116
sickness 58
Shigella 6, 145, 156
Sialoductal adenovirus 240
Simian (S)STLV-I viruses 243
Simian T cell leukemia virus (STLV) 243
Sjögren's syndrome 180
Sm 54
Soluble C3d 120
Spectrin 51, 60
Spiral ganglia 216, 221, 228
degeneration 217, 219, 221
Splenomegaly 131
Spondylitis, ankylosing 146
Spongiosis, collagen-immunized 226
Spumaviruses 243
STLV-III 243, 244
Strain 2 239
Strain 13 239
Streptococcal M protein, MAb 231
Streptococcus
group A 11, 145, 154
group B 145
Streptococcus agalactiae 145
Stria vascularis 216, 221
Sudden hearing loss, bilateral 215
Suppression
immune 283
T cell-mediated 133
Suppression therapy, antigen-specific 282
Suppressor
cells 3, 27, 36
factors 180
function 132
Suppressor T cells, non-antigen-specific 111
Surveillance, NK 89
Sympathetic otitis 215
Synovial
cells 13, 14, 16
membrane 179, 181, 183
inflammatory reaction 148
pannus 205
rheumatoid 15, 171
Synovial fluid 181, 186, 200
IL-2 179
Synovitis 175
Synovium 187, 205, 208, 279
Syphilis
biologically false-positive test 154
false-positive test 11
Systemic lupus erythematosus (SLE) 11, 43, 50, 52, 67, 129, 156, 175, 177, 180, 184, 189, 279
human 53
mouse 53

Systemic sclerosis 180
Systems
NCMC 88, 89
NK 89

T amplifier activity 9, 133
T cell
amplifier 133
blasts, encephalitogenic 282
clone 159, 276
defect 265
enlargement, Lyt-2+ 136
function 275
proliferation 276
ratios 249
receptor 276, 280
regulatory 132
signals, regulatory 138
subsets 247, 264, 275
suppressor 133
T cell function, class II MHC antigen-restricted 276
T cell growth factor (TCGF) 177
T cell killing 276
T cell line 148, 149, 152
MBP-specific 282
MT-specific 148
T cells 2, 5, 6, 12–14, 21, 23, 35, 77, 91, 95, 111, 121, 139, 147, 158, 177, 179, 183, 185, 279, 282
activated 178
antigen-reactive 157
autoaggressive 25
autoproliferative 35
autoreactive 1, 2
cytotoxic 3, 113
effector 163
Lyt-2+ 131, 136
MBP-sensitized 277
regulatory 9, 144, 158
suppressor 161
suppressor-inducer 159
T helper cells 8, 9, 19, 21, 118, 245, 248, 250, 252, 254, 256
T lymphocytes 1, 2, 9, 16, 26, 130, 149, 180, 182, 246
autoreactive 3
cytotoxic 5, 36
effector 149
helper 182, 184
suppressor 161, 245
T suppressor (Ts) cells 8, 10, 12, 19, 248, 250, 253
T suppressor function 138
T4 cell 261, 263, 265, 267–269
T8+ (suppressor) cells 266
TAC 85
Target cell
NC-susceptible 93
NK-resistant 95
NK-sensitive 90, 93, 94
Target lysis, NC 95
Target recognition 86
NC 85
Targets
Meth-113 92
Meth-A 92
WEHI-164 6, 80, 81, 87, 91, 94
TCR 248, 250, 252, 254, 257
Technique, immunoblotting 62
Tetanus toxoid 267
Therapy, anti-Ia 211
Thymic epithelial cells 2
Thymic factors 20, 262
Thymocyte, mouse 175
Thymocytes 26, 49, 283
Thymopentin 20, 263
Thymus 25, 27
grafts 26
Thyroglobulin 4
antibody 50
TNF 6, 8, 87, 91, 95
recombinant murine 87
TNP 51
Tolerance 25, 42, 136, 150, 181, 229, 282
acquired 3, 35
B cell 9
breaking 177
defect 138
induction 229
lymphocytes 26
neonatal 27
partial 157
resistance 131, 138

self 36
T cells 2, 27
T helper cell 135
Tolerogen 27
TP-5 21
Transblot technique 218
Transcriptional activation sequence 243
Transferin 4, 81
antibody 50
autoantibodies 59
Transplantation, bone marrow 1
Trypanosomes 6
Trypsin 107
Tuberculoid leprosy 162
Tuberculosis 147, 157
Tubulin 51
antibody 48, 50
Tubulointerstitial nephritis, autoimmune 148
Tumor angiogenesis factor 15
Tumor cell lines
NC 89
NK-susceptible 89, 90
Tumor line, murine B cell 110
Tumor necrosis factor (TNF) 6, 87, 188
Tumor system
Meth-A 83
WEHI-164 83
Tumors
human nonlymphoid 92
NC-susceptible 89
NK resistant 89
spontaneous 88
surveillance 78
Tunnel of Corti, immunological reaction 239
Twins, dizygotic 24

Type I collagen 226
Type II collagen 17, 216, 218, 221, 225, 227–229
antibodies 219, 231
autoimmunity 17, 218
epitope 18
immune response 239

Urokinase 107
Utricles, vacuolar degeneration 217

Vestibular dysfunction 216, 225
Vestibuloauditory disorder 215
Veto cell 3, 36
Vimentin 55
Viral infection 181, 257, 268
HTLV-III 19
Viremia, HIV (HTLV-III) 263
Viruses
human T cell leukemia 243
immunosuppressive 255
Visna virus 243

Waldenström's macroglobulinemia 50
WEHI-3 cells 84
WEHI-164 6, 79, 81, 87, 91, 94
Western-blot 206

X antigen 47
Xid gene 135
Xid mice 53, 66

YAC-1 87, 94
Yersinia 146, 156
Yersinia entero-colitica 12, 157

Zymosan 108